Body Fluids in Surgery

Body Fluids in Surgery

A. W. WILKINSON
Ch.M. F.R.C.S.E., F.R.C.S., F.A.A.P. (Hon.)

Nuffield Professor of Paediatric Surgery, The Institute of Child Health of the University of London; Surgeon, The Hospital for Sick Children, Great Ormond Street, London

Fourth Edition

CHURCHILL LIVINGSTONE
EDINBURGH AND LONDON 1973

CHURCHILL LIVINGSTONE
Medical Division of Longman Group Limited

Represented in the United States of America by Longman Inc., New York, and by associated companies, branches and representatives throughout the world.

First Edition 1955
Second Edition 1960
Third Edition 1969
Fourth Edition 1973

ISBN 0 443 01021 8

Printed in Great Britain

Preface to Fourth Edition

The objects of this book remain those of the first edition, first to provide enough information for a basic understanding of the behaviour of the body fluids in health and disease and secondly an account of the management of the disturbances of body fluids which occur in surgical patients. Moreover it is still written primarily for those who are responsible for the care of surgical patients; even more now than 18 years ago the surgeon must be responsible for the detailed management of the disturbances in fluid balance in his patients, whether his patient is an infant or a decrepit elderly adult.

In the four years since the last edition of this book there have been some interesting changes in emphasis in the pre- and post-operative treatment of surgical patients of all ages. The use of gastric and intestinal aspiration, especially with long tubes, combined with intensive efforts to replace the loss of gastrointestinal secretions before emergency operative relief of the primary lesion has tended to decline in most clinics. In a few centres however the rapid injection of large volumes of various combinations of replacement solutions has persisted with variable benefit to the patient. The increased use of combinations of powerful antibiotics and the prolonged use of intravenous infusions have been followed by the inevitable rise in the incidence of serious infections with Gram-negative organisms and fungi and of 'septic shock'.

Magnesium depletion has now achieved the clinical distinction and importance which was occupied by potassium 25 years ago in patients of all ages. This long-delayed interest in the clinical importance of disturbances of this mineral seemed to justify a separate chapter on magnesium as part of the extensive revision and rearrangement of this new edition. The small increase in the total number of pages is due more to complete resetting of the type than to any large increase in the number of words in the text. The section on intravenous feeding has been largely rewritten in conformance with recent changes in practice, improvements in the solutions of amino acids and the wide availability of reliable fat emulsions based on soya bean oil.

In response to the helpful and constructive comments of a number of reviewers of the previous edition short sections have been introduced on such subjects as diabetes insipidus and mellitus, and the space given to the influence of the adrenal cortical hormones has been increased. No excuse is made for a small increase in the sections on disturbances in the newly born. Paediatric surgery, especially when it is concerned with the neonate, is one of the few branches of surgery in which real improvements in results have been achieved in the last 15 or 20 years, due mainly to the better pre- and post-operative care of very small babies with major congenital anomalies as the result of the application of new knowledge of neonatal physiology and the wider recognition of the importance of modification of environmental conditions to the benefit of the baby. If the work of Caldwell, Cuthbertson and others on the influence of environmental temperature and humidity on the metabolic response to injury could be applied to the treatment of surgical patients of all ages after major operations the daily destruction of thousands of tons of human muscle and the expenditure of countless millions of calories derived from human tissue could be spared in the population of temperate climates. The implications of this work for those who live in tropical climates are unknown and await direct observations on the indigenous people of those areas. Some further information has been added about the effects of certain tropical climates on body composition and the way in which these effects can be modified or treated in surgical patients, but much more study of the normal behaviour of the indigenous population of tropical areas is still needed.

Like their other authors, I am once again greatly indebted to Messrs Churchill Livingstone for the expeditious way in which they have produced this book.

LONDON, 1973 A. W. W.

Preface to First Edition

There are few short cuts or routine answers for the surgeon who has to solve the problems set by the patient who has suffered large losses of body fluids. His therapeutic decisions must be based on a knowledge of normal body composition, an accurate and detailed history of the illness and fluid loss of the individual patient and an understanding of the effects these disturbances will have on structure and function. Although previous experience will modify his interpretation of the clinical features and the treatment he adopts, the deeper his understanding of the physiology of the body fluids the closer will such treatment approach the ideal. There seems to be a need not only for advice in the management of the common disturbances of equilibrium in the composition and distribution of the body fluids, but also for a set of simple rules on which to base a routine of treatment in all sorts, sizes and conditions of patients. Such a set of rules does not exist; to make allowances for individual variations within the so-called limits of normal of sex, age, stature and nutritional state, is difficult if not impossible in a universal scheme of diagnosis and treatment. Moreover, the speed and chemical delicacy of the complicated interrelated compensatory reactions which follow the loss of body fluids of any kind are perhaps too little appreciated by most clinicians in their search for therapeutic simplicity.

In this book an attempt has been made to provide in a convenient form, first, sufficient information for a basic understanding of the behaviour of the body fluids in health and disease, and secondly an account of the management of the disturbances of the body fluids which occur in surgical patients. It has been written primarily for those responsible for the care of surgical patients in the belief that the detailed management of disturbances of fluid balance in his patients rightly remains the responsibility of the surgeon.

Until about 1939 our knowledge of the physiology of the body fluids was almost confined to measurements by chemical methods of concentration of substances dissolved in plasma and extracellular fluid, and of the volume of plasma and of extracellular fluid. During the last 15 years developments of the dilution technique especially with the aid of radioactive and stable isotopes have led to the evolution of new methods for the estimation of the volume of red cells, plasma, total body water, intracellular water, total exchangeable sodium, potassium and chloride and many other constituents of the body fluids and tissues. From the narrow view given by studies of concentrations of constituents we have progressed to a wider understanding of the total watery environment of the cells and of the total quantities of substances in solution and combination inside as well as outside the cells.

However, it remains important to recognise that even these newer methods of measurement do not provide a complete picture of what happens in the body and that the values obtained are subject to errors and variations, especially in disease and after injury; the greatest value of these measurements is to be derived from the comparison of the results of repeated observations in the same subject. Many of the methods require complicated apparatus and personal skill and are still suitable only for research purposes or occasional use. Their wider adoption will depend to some extent on further simplification and improvement. The basic knowledge which has been obtained, however, has already been incorporated in our understanding of the behaviour of the body in several circumstances. The value of the application of this new knowledge to the treatment of surgical patients is another reason for attempting to express in simple terms some of the advances in this field, and as far as seems possible or justifiable to relate them to the common clinical disturbances which are liable to complicate modern surgical procedures.

Until a few years ago it was generally believed that the transfer of substances across capillary membranes was due to such relatively simple processes as filtration and diffusion, while transfer through the cell wall depended on the selective permeability of the cell wall to different substances. It now appears that transport across the cell wall may depend rather on active secretory processes requiring the expenditure of considerable energy and demanding complex metabolic processes for its accomplishment. The convenient arbitrary division of body fluids into intracellular and extracellular portions is now clearly of limited value and although helpful to an understanding of some problems of fluid and ionic distribution, does not give any idea of the dynamic existence of minerals and water in the body.

In this book emphasis has been placed on the clinical as opposed to the laboratory approach to the patient. Even the most complete laboratory data at present obtainable will give only a limited understanding of the state of the patient at a particular moment. Repeated visits to the bedside at regular intervals do not cost the patient any blood or discomfort and are commonly more rewarding than the perusal of reports of biochemical estimation of the composition of his body fluids. The hardest thinking must be done before any blood is withdrawn for chemical examination, and the examination of this blood should be planned to show if possible whether the clinical diagnosis is right or wrong. This is not to say that biochemical estimations are not of value in clinical surgical practice. Only by the continued application of the scientific method of measurement to the study of surgical problems can any improvement in our present state of ignorance be expected. As a spur to assiduous study at the bedside and in the laboratory a proper sense of humility is required against the background of lack of knowledge and imperfect understanding of the behaviour of the body in normal and diseased conditions.

To keep this book reasonably short much material and many references have been excluded which would have had places in a comprehensive review of this subject. Nevertheless sufficient references are given to provide an ample introduction to the original work. Most writers are more or less deeply impregnated with and indebted to the work of those who have preceded them; in this field the debt to Gamble, Coller, Moyer, Darrow, Cuthbertson, Marriott and McCance, to mention only a few of the pioneers, is heavy and will endure. To my chiefs, the late Sir John Fraser, Sir James Learmonth and Professor W. C. Wilson my debt is a more personal one. To them I owe the stimulation of my interest in the study of shock and other disturbances of the body fluids in surgical patients, and the encouragement and opportunities for investigation on which that interest was nourished and grew. The late K. W. Lane first aroused a biochemical interest which has been maintained and its practical application made possible by Dr C. P. Stewart, to whom and to his colleagues I am indebted for much assistance during the last 18 years. To the members of the staffs of hospitals in Edinburgh and Aberdeen, and especially to Mr T. McW. Millar and Mr W. A. D. Adamson, I am greatly indebted for allowing me to study and to treat patients under their care and for giving me the advantages of their watchful interest and experienced advice in the interpretation of the confusing problems I encountered. From the many resulting discussions at the bedside and elsewhere are derived in no small part the opinions expressed in this book.

I am indebted to Messrs Butterworth & Co. Ltd. for allowing me to incorporate material from a chapter in *Surgical Progress* 1953 for the sections on shock, anuria, loss of intestinal secretions and plasma substitutes and for allowing me to reproduce part of Table II, Table V and, in a modified form, Table IV. Tables XII–XV are modified from similar diagrams by Gilman and Brazeau by kind permission of Dr A. Gilman.

Messrs E. & S. Livingstone Ltd. have produced this book with their usual high skill and craftsmanship, and I am very grateful to them for all their help.

October, 1955 A. W. W.

Contents

CHAPTER ONE

The Content and Distribution of Water, Sodium and Potassium in the Body

It is not usually difficult to collect and measure the total volume and even the concentrations of some of the constituents of fluid which is lost by vomiting, discharge from a fistula or in the stools. To make the fullest use of these measurements there must be some knowledge of the composition of an individual body at the outset of an illness as well as at particular stages during treatment; with such information the effects of the fluid losses in producing the clinical disturbance may be judged, as well as the margin of tolerance which remains and the rate, type and quantity of replacements which are needed. Unfortunately no two human bodies are exactly alike and the range of variation about the mean for age, sex, weight or height is large. There is no close relationship between weight, height, fatness, muscle mass or bone weight, and therefore estimates of the body content of water, sodium, potassium or any other constituent which are not based on direct measurements in the individual but are calculated from so-called standard tables must be subject to large errors. In spite of this, such estimates are often of great value in judging the effects of disease and in designing suitable treatment.

RELATIONSHIP BETWEEN BODY FAT AND WATER

The quantity of water in the human body has usually been assumed to be a fixed proportion, about 70 per cent, of the total body weight; the observed body weight has also been used for the calculation of plasma and extracellular fluid volume in attempts to control fluid replacement therapy with greater accuracy. It is now evident that when such estimates ignore the presence of storage fat in the body they may be very inaccurate and misleading. Hardy and Drabkin (1950) found that blood volume might vary from 70 ml per kg body weight in a very obese subject to 105 ml per kg in a very thin one; yet Gibson and Evans (1937) had shown that in subjects of about average nutrition blood volume was closely related to height. Allen *et al.* (1956) analysed a large number of their own and published determinations of blood volume, and concluded that the fat content of the body is the most important variable factor and that in general blood volume is related more closely to a combination of body weight and the cube of the height than to height or surface area, to a cubic rather than a square function.

The acute changes in volume and distribution of water and electrolyte which are associated with surgical operations and inflammation of all kinds do not involve body fat. During many kinds of disease and after injury the catabolism of storage fat to provide energy may cause a large loss of weight which is another source of error in the calculation of fluid volumes from whole body weight.

Fat floats on water, and fat people are more buoyant than lean ones. When the fat content of a body increases, the density of that body in water diminishes and its specific gravity becomes less. By weighing a body in air and when submerged in water its specific gravity can be directly measured, and from this figure the fat content of the body can be calculated. Behnke (1942) found that fat content had an important bearing on the functional efficiency of the body and that excessively fat men had a poor tolerance for high-altitude flying or deep diving. It is well known that, in general, unduly fat people are not good subjects for surgical procedures, and this has been commonly ascribed to their poor mechanical efficiency. Obese patients are more difficult to move in bed, cough with more difficulty and have to exert themselves more because of their larger bulk; some are so fat that they cannot sit up without help and a few become breathless and cyanosed if laid flat in bed.

From an analysis of the body composition of a large number of men, Behnke postulated a basic body structure of relatively constant composition which he called the 'lean tissue mass'. This consists of 70 per cent water, 20 per cent solids and an irreducible minimum of 10 per cent of structural fat. This type of composition is not peculiar to the human species. It was found in six species of small animals, including the guinea-pig and monkey, that although the fat content varied widely the lean tissue mass was fairly constant, and when excess fat was excluded the lean tissue mass contained about 73 per cent water (Pace and Rathbun, 1945; Rathbun and Pace, 1945).

When storage fat is superimposed on this basic structure, the body weight increases, and although the weight and composition of the lean tissue mass do not alter, the percentage of water in the whole body decreases. The fat content of the body may vary from 10 per cent to nearly 50 per cent of the total body weight, and in excessively obese subjects the body water may be less than 40 per cent of the total body weight.

TABLE I

The effect of increasing the fat content of the body

	Total body weight (kg)	*Fat*			*Solids (kg)*	*Water*	
		Basic (kg)	*Storage or Excess*			*% body weight*	*litres*
			kg	*% body weight*			
Basic structure	60	6	—	—	12	70·0	42
Average man	70	6	10	14·2	12	60·0	42
Fat man	80	6	20	25·0	12	54·0	42
	90	6	30	33·0	12	44·5	42
Very fat man	100	6	40	40·0	12	42·0	42
	110	6	50	45·5	12	38·0	42

The effect of increasing the body content of fat is shown in Table I and Fig. 1. For the sake of clarity, the basic quantities of water, solids and structural fat have been shown unchanged throughout, although small changes do occur. The basic structure is that of an unusually thin person without any storage fat. The normal individual is represented by the second block diagram (Fig. 1), and he contains water equivalent to 60 per cent of his body weight and storage fat equal to 14·2 per cent of body weight; this is the composition of an average healthy male subject. In the remaining four block diagrams, as the proportion of fat increases the proportion of body water falls, and this relationship is also shown in Fig. 2, in which the declining percentage of body water and the increasing percentage of fat are plotted against body weight. The fat content of healthy adults normally increases with age (Brožek and Keys, 1952) from 10 per cent at the age of 20

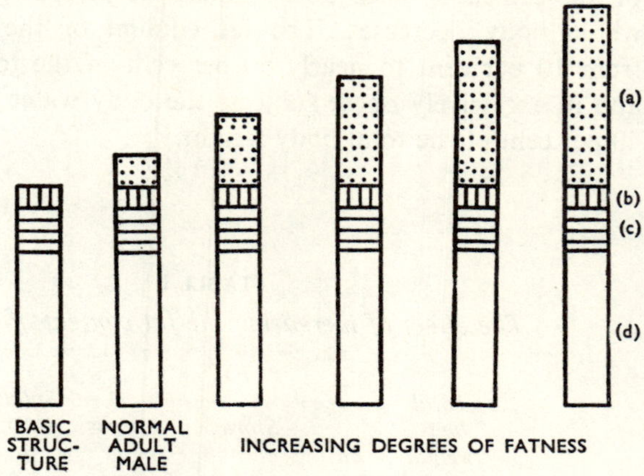

TOTAL BODY WEIGHT						
Stones	9st 6lb	11st	12st 8lb	13st 8lb	15st 10lb	17st 4lb
Lb	132	154	176	190	220	242
Kg	60	70	80	90	100	110
STORAGE FAT						
Kg	0	10	20	30	40	50
% Body Weight	0	14	25	33	40	45
TOTAL BODY WATER						
Litres	42	42	42	42	42	42
% Body Weight	70	60	54	45	42	38

Key.—(*a*) Excess or 'Storage' fat; (*b*) Essential or structural fat; (*c*) Lean tissue solids; (*d*) Water

FIGURE 1. The effect of increasing the fat content of the body.

years to 25 per cent at the age of 55 years, and females are usually fatter than males. (For the fat content of babies and children see p. 265)

Because of the practical difficulties associated with direct measurement in surgical patients of total body water and its subdivisions such as extracellular fluid and plasma volumes, it is often useful to be able to calculate the total body water of a patient from body weight. The inverse ratio between fat content and body water renders such calculations from total body weight misleading unless allowance is made for excess of storage fat. McCance and Widdowson (1951) suggested that calculations of this kind should be based not on the actual measured weight of the patient but on the 'ideal weight' of the individual, and this is probably the best method to employ in clinical practice. 'Ideal weight' is a function of sex, height and age, and can be obtained from standard tables such as those of the Metropolitan Life Insurance Company.

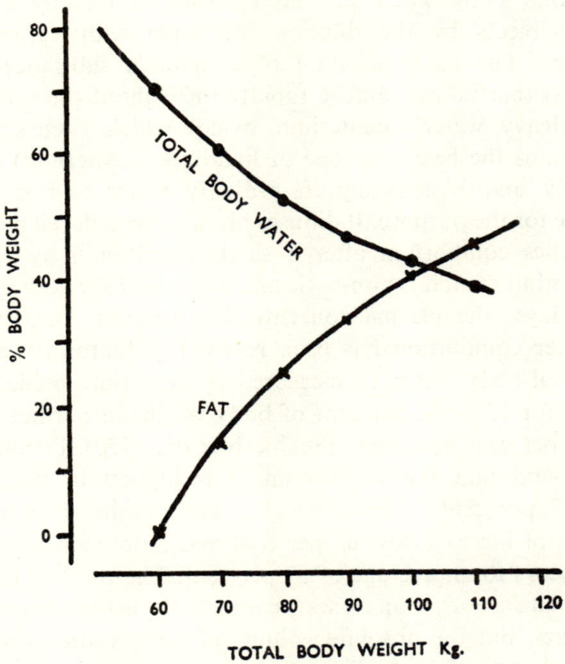

FIGURE 2. Relationship between rising fat content and declining water content.

Allen *et al.* (1956) collected data from which they have derived formulas with which both the blood volume and the fat content of any individual can be calculated. They believe that their method of calculation is accurate in spite of variations in race, age, sex, obesity, malnutrition or the periodic effect of sex hormones. By means of these formulas the actual fat content of an individual can be calculated from his observed weight and can be compared with the previous state in health if the earlier healthy weight is known.

For fat content the formulas are:

Males: $A = 0{\cdot}685$ T.B.M. $- 5{\cdot}86\, H^3 + 0{\cdot}42$ kg

Females: $A = 0{\cdot}737$ T.B.M. $- 5{\cdot}15\, H^3 + 0{\cdot}37$ kg

(A=fat content in kg. *T.B.M.*=body weight in kg. H=height in metres.)

BODY CONTENT OF WATER

The total body water has been measured directly in normal human subjects by the dilution technique with various tracer substances. The main essential of a suitable substance for this purpose is that it shall diffuse rapidly throughout the water of the body. 'Heavy water' (deuterium oxide) which occurs naturally and contains the heavy isotope of hydrogen (deuterium) is similar chemically and biologically to ordinary water and is an ideal substance for the purpose. It diffuses rapidly through cell membranes and reaches equilibrium after a single injection in two to three hours in adult men, it is non-toxic and about half the dose is excreted in nine days; the plasma concentration remains constant for 19 hours after equilibrium has been reached (Elkinton *et al.*, 1944).

The total body water, as measured by deuterium oxide dilution, accounts for 55 to 62 per cent of body weight in normal men and 50 to 52 per cent in women (Schloerb *et al.*, 1950). Edelman *et al.* (1952) found that the water content is highest in the newborn infant, 77 per cent of body weight, falls rapidly during the first 6 months of life to below 65 per cent and more slowly during the next 10 years to an average of 59 per cent. The ratio of total body water to surface area increases progressively up to about the age of 12 years, but the absolute volume of body water is highest in males aged 16 to 40 years. From puberty onwards the water content of males is about 7 per cent higher than that of females, but falls slightly in both sexes after the age of 50 years. They concluded that the average water content of healthy adults is 61 per cent of body weight in males and 54 per cent in females, the difference being due to the higher fat content of females after puberty.

DISTRIBUTION OF BODY WATER

It has been customary to consider that in the living organism water does not exist free and unattached, but that as water of hydration it forms part of the complex ionic equilibria which make up cell substance and the body fluids; much of the water probably exists in apparently loose combination as a gel. The total quantity of water in the body is related to the total quantity of cations, particularly of sodium and potassium, which in their turn govern the total content of anions and their associated water.

TOTAL CONTENT OF SODIUM AND POTASSIUM

Sodium and potassium appear to be the most important of the cations in the control of water, for although they account for only a small proportion of the total mineral content of the body they are its most active components (Table II). The total quantities

TABLE II

Total cation content of the 70 kg male body

	g	*mEq*
Magnesium (Mg^{++})	23	2000
Potassium (K^{+})	130	3400
Sodium (Na^{+})	90	3900

Note: The values of sodium and potassium are derived from published dilutional studies with ^{24}Na and ^{42}K quoted in the text and for magnesium are from Widdowson *et al.* (1951).

Normal composition of plasma

Cations (mEq/litre)		*Anions (mEq/litre)*	
Na^{+}	140	Cl^{-}	103
K^{+}	5	HCO_3^{-}	25
Ca^{++}	5	HPO_4^{--}	2
Mg^{++}	2	SO_4^{--}	1
		Organic acids	5
		Protein	16
	152		152

of sodium and potassium in the body can be estimated directly only by the chemical analysis of the whole body. Apart from the difficulty of obtaining bodies for this purpose, the disease which kills the patient may cause much alteration in the composition of the body. Widdowson *et al.* (1951) analysed four bodies and found wide differences in composition related to age and pre-existing disease.

The dilution principle employing the radioactive isotopes of sodium and potassium is widely used in research but is of limited value for routine clinical purposes. This method measures the quantities of sodium and potassium in the body with which the injected radioactive material equilibrates or exchanges, or the 'exchangeable sodium (Na^e) or potassium (K^e)'. Suitable doses of ^{24}Na and ^{42}K are injected intravenously and urine is collected for 22 hours and at the end of 23 and 24 hours. From the specific activity of the last two specimens the dilution of the injected radioactive materials can be calculated, corrections being applied for decay and the measured quantities excreted in the urine during the 22 hours of equilibration. Both sodium and potassium have a quick primary phase of equilibration lasting about 30 minutes which may be much modified by variations in the activity and blood flow of organs such as the kidneys and liver, and a slow phase which is complete after 18 to 20 hours. The cumulative error of the method may amount to ± 5 per cent and significance cannot be given to changes in total body content of less than 250 mEq. With improvements in methods it is now possible to determine simultaneously total body water, total exchangeable sodium, potassium and chloride, red cell mass and plasma volume (Boling, 1963).

The whole body content of potassium can also be measured by counting in a suitably modified liquid scintillator the emissions of the naturally occurring isotope ^{40}K from the whole body (Garrow, 1965).

Moore *et al.* (1954) combined their own large volume of data with that of Forbes and Perley (1951) and concluded that in healthy male adults the total exchangeable sodium (Na^e) amounts to 42·1 mEq per kg body weight and the total exchangeable potassium (K^e) to 46·3 mEq per kg body weight. For a typical 70 kg male adult this implies exchangeable contents of 2947 mEq sodium and 3241 mEq potassium (Table III). They had previously estimated that 95 per cent of the total potassium in the body was exchangeable with isotopic potassium so that the total body content of potassium is probably in the region of 3410 mEq (130·0 g) for the theoretically typical male adult weighing 70 kg. They have also estimated that in the case of sodium about a quarter of the total body content

TABLE III

Total quantities of sodium and potassium in the body

Exchangeable K $= 46{\cdot}3$ mEq per kg body weight
$= 3241$ mEq in man weighing 70 kg.

Exchangeable K $= 95\%$ total content of K.

Total content of K $= \dfrac{3241 \times 100}{95}$ in man weighing 70 kg
$= 3411$ mEq.

Exchangeable Na $= 42{\cdot}1$ mEq per kg body weight
$= 2947$ mEq in man weighing 70 kg.

Of the Na in bone, 55% is not exchangeable and this quantity is equivalent to about 25% of total body Na.

∴ Exchangeable Na = about 75% total body Na.

∴ Total content of Na $= \dfrac{\text{Exchangeable Na} \times 100}{75}$
$= \dfrac{2947 \times 100}{75}$
$= 3929$ mEq.

situated in the bones is not exchangeable, and from this estimate and their figure for exchangeable sodium it can be calculated that the total body content of sodium is about 3920 mEq (90·0 g).

The manner in which the total exchangeable sodium and potassium are theoretically distributed in the body depends on the concentrations ascribed to sodium and potassium in the intracellular fluid. This in turn depends on the methods which are used to measure the volumes of total body water and extracellular fluid from which the intracellular fluid volume is deduced. For example, Corsa *et al.* (1950) concluded that the intracellular concentration of potassium was 125 mEq per litre, a value which was also obtained by Ikkos *et al.* (1954) when they measured total body water with antipyrine and extracellular fluid with inulin or thiosulphate; when Ikkos *et al.* used heavy water to measure total body water, their value for intracellular potassium concentration was 112 mEq per litre, as was found also by Deane and Smith (1952).

About 98 per cent of the total potassium is in the intracellular fluid, mostly in skeletal muscle, at a concentration of about 112 mEq per litre, and only about 2 per cent is in the extracellular fluid at a concentration of about 5·0 mEq per litre. It was formerly assumed that there was comparatively little sodium in the intracellular fluid, nearly all of it being extracellular. It is now possible to assign to sodium a different distribution, which is shown in detail in Table IV. In the 12 litres of extracellular fluid there are 1680 mEq of sodium at a concentration of approximately 140 mEq per litre. From histochemical analyses Hastings (1941) estimated that the intracellular sodium concentration was 16·9 mEq per litre, but Deane and Smith (1952), who used isotopic sodium,

TABLE IV

*Partition of body fluids, sodium and potassium**

70 kg man (11 st or 154 lb)

Total body water=60 per cent body weight=42 litres

	Extracellular fluid			*Intracellular fluid*	
	Plasma	*Interstitial fluid*	*Transcellular fluid*	*Soft tissues*	*Bone*
%Total body water	7	17	6	60	10
Volume (litres)	3	7	2	26	4
Sodium	44% of total 39·6 g or 1723 mEq Av. 140 mEq/litre			9% of total 8·1 g or 352 mEq Av. 15 mEq/litre	47% of total 42·3 g or 1840 mEq Av. 460 mEq/litre
Potassium	2% of total 2·6 g or 67 mEq Av. 5 mEq/litre			98% of total 127·4 g or 3312 mEq Av. 112 mEq/litre	

*This scheme of distribution is arbitrary and is based on standard assumed volumes for plasma, interstitial fluid and intracellular fluid. The distribution of sodium has been calculated from these volumes and from the concentration shown in the table for extracellular fluid and soft tissues, non-exchangeable bone sodium being taken as 25 per cent of the total body sodium and 55 per cent of bone sodium (Table III).

put the figure as high as 37 mEq per litre. Edelman *et al.* (1954) estimated that bone sodium was equal to about 23 mEq per kg body weight or a total of 1610 mEq in a 70 kg male adult. If Deane and Smith's figure for total intracellular sodium is corrected for bone sodium, a figure of 15 mEq for the soft tissue is obtained, which agrees well with Hastings' estimate. On this basis the body sodium can be distributed as is shown in Table IV. Although there is almost as much sodium in bone as in the rest of the body, 80 per cent of the sodium which is not in the bones is situated in the extracellular fluid.

SUBDIVISIONS OF BODY WATER

INTRACELLULAR WATER

The largest subdivision of the water of the body is that of intracellular fluid (70 per cent of total body water) (Table V).

TABLE V

Partition of body water

	% *Total body water*	% *Ideal body weight*	*Volume (litres) in 70 kg adult*
Total body water	—	60	42
Intracellular fluid	70	42	30
Extracellular fluid	30	18	12·6
Interstitial fluid	17	10·5	7·35
Transcellular fluid	6	3·5	2·45
Plasma	7	4·0	2·8

This has a complex distribution in many small compartments separated from each other by two cell membranes and a layer of interstitial fluid. The intracellular water forms part of the protoplasm of the cells and is associated with potassium, the most important intracellular cation, and with phosphate, the main intracellular anion. The sodium content of intracellular fluid is low except in the skeleton, but nearly half of the sodium of bone is 'exchangeable' with sodium elsewhere in the body. All exchanges of intracellular fluid take place through the extracellular fluid and depend on the maintenance of an adequate volume of extracellular fluid as an environment for the cells. The volume of the intracellular fluid can be measured only indirectly, as the difference between the volume of total body water and extracellular fluid. Any attempt to follow closely the day-to-day changes in intracellular fluid volume and composition is therefore limited by the difficulties and errors associated with repeated measurement of total body water and extracellular fluid volumes.

EXTRACELLULAR WATER. The extracellular water of the body

amounts to about 30 per cent of the total body water and forms the environment of the cells. It is subdivided into intravascular, interstitial and transcellular portions. The intravascular fluid (7 per cent of body water or 4 per cent of 'ideal' body weight) is situated within the blood vessels, whereas the interstitial part of the extravascular extracellular fluid lies outside the blood vessels and amongst the cells of the tissues of which it forms the immediate environment. Transcellular fluid includes fluid which is extracellular but not interstitial, such as the cerebrospinal and synovial fluids, urine in the collecting tubules and urinary tract, fluid in the ducts of glands and in the alimentary tract as well as in the eyes and ears. It accounts for 6 per cent of the total body water or about 3·5 per cent of the ideal body weight.

The most important cation in extracellular water is sodium, and the content of potassium is very small; chloride and bicarbonate are the predominant anions of this fluid. Apart from the large protein content of intravascular fluid there are only small differences in chemical composition between intravascular and interstitial fluid. The volume of the extracellular fluid can be measured by the dilution of a substance which passes freely through the walls of the blood capillaries but does not enter freely into the cells of the body. Many substances have been used, but most (like thiocyanate) enter the cells to some extent or (like inulin) reach equilibrium in plasma and interstitial fluid rather slowly, so that some of the injected material is excreted before equilibrium is achieved. Others, like sucrose, may be partially metabolised before they reach equilibrium; with thiosulphate, inulin and mannitol the values obtained are low (16 per cent of body weight), whereas with thiocyanate or radioactive chlorine, bromine or sodium the values are high (26 per cent of body weight). Measurement of extracellular fluid volume is easy but inaccurate.

Plasma volume may be measured by the dilution principle using albumin labelled with radioactive iodine (^{131}I) or the blue dye T1824 (Evans' blue) which is adsorbed on to plasma albumin.

Blood volume can be measured directly by the dilution principle using red cells labelled with radioactive chromium (^{51}Cr) for red cell volume and ^{131}I or T1824 for plasma volume. It may also be calculated from either measured plasma volume or red cell volume using the ratio 0·910 (s.e. $\pm$0·026) for total body haematocrit to venous haematocrit (Chaplain *et al.*, 1953). In the past the blood volume of adults has often been estimated from body weight (75 ml per kg) or surface area (2·68 litres per m^2 surface area) but both methods may give very misleading figures. Allen *et al.* (1956) found that their formulas gave accurate results in spite of wide variations in sex, age, nutrition and race; there was no variation between the sexes before puberty and although blood volume in non-pregnant women was 600 ml less than males of the same height and weight, in pregnancy it was a litre more. Blood volume varied with the phase of the menstrual cycle and in both sexes declined with age.

For blood volume their formulas are:

Men and boys: $B.V. = 0{\cdot}417H^3 + 0{\cdot}045\ T.B.M. - 0{\cdot}03L$

Adult women: $B.V. = 0{\cdot}414H^3 + 0{\cdot}0328\ T.B.M. - 0{\cdot}03L$

Nadler *et al.* found that these formulas can be improved by correction factors and their revised formulas are:

Men: $B.V. = 0{\cdot}3669H^3 + 0{\cdot}03219\ T.B.M. + 0{\cdot}6041L$
Women: $B.V. = 0{\cdot}3561H^3 + 0{\cdot}03308\ T.B.M. + 0{\cdot}1833L$

(B.V.=blood volume in litres. H=height in metres.
T.B.M.=body weight in kg. L=litres.)

The intravascular fluid, although small in total volume, circulates rapidly within the blood vessels and exchanges across the capillary walls with the interstitial fluid. The latter flows amongst the cells and exchanges occur between it and the intracellular fluid. The normal volume relationship of about 1:3 between plasma and interstitial fluid is maintained in spite of very large daily exchanges of fluid. It has been estimated that there is a daily transfer of 1100 litres of fluid between plasma and interstitial fluid, and each day up to 8 litres of fluid are secreted into and reabsorbed from the intestine. The great permeability of capillary and cell walls to water is illustrated by the rapid equilibration of heavy water in the living body, a 'steady state' being reached in both cells and extracellular fluid within about two hours of injection.

Water and other constituents of cells are constantly in movement and exchanging between cells and their environment. Such arbitrary subdivisions of body water as have just been described are helpful in the visualisation and interpretation of changes in body composition only if it is remembered that they are descriptive of momentary endpoints in a continuously changing process of equilibration.

CELLULAR MEMBRANE PERMEABILITY AND FLUID EXCHANGES

Electron microscopy has shown (Robertson, 1964) that every cell has not only a boundary where it ends but a membrane at that boundary and in some cases within the cell as well. This 'unit membrane' as Robertson has called it is formed of two layers and varies in thickness from 5 to 10 nm and its two sides have different properties. There is a negative charge on the inside surface and a positive charge on the outside surface and the membrane acts as a most efficient insulator. Robertson has suggested that the unit membrane is composed of rod-like molecules, one pole of which is hydrophilic and the other is hydrophobic, and that on the surfaces of the membrane there is a layer of macromolecules. The rods have their hydrophilic ends directed outwards and the hydrophobic poles turned inwards towards each other.

Substances may cross a membrane in several ways. In solution or in association with water molecules a solute may simply flow through pores which are holes in the membrane. A solute may dissolve in the membrane and diffuse through it in solution or it may combine with a 'carrier' molecule, which is part of the membrane, and then diffuse through the cell to be released at the opposite free surface. Active transport is a form of carrier transport which depends on the expenditure of energy. A state of equilibrium implies that the flow in both directions is equal rather than that flow has ceased. Any membrane may be a mosaic of areas of different degrees of porosity and permeability and there may be some with specific permeabilities for particular substances.

The rate of transfer through a membrane depends firstly on the number of molecules bombarding its surface, that is on the concentration of the solution, and also on the ratio of the concentrations of a substance on the two sides of the membrane. It also depends on the number, type and shape of the so-called 'pores' in the membrane and the relation between the shape and size of the molecules to be transported and the pores of the membrane, and on the solubilities of the solute and solvent in the cells of the membrane.

The cell membrane does not completely segregate sodium and potassium since it is permeable to both, and in some cells, such as those of the nervous system, specialised function appears to depend largely on the electrical effects of variations of this kind on chemical transfer. The different rates at which sodium and potassium cross cell boundaries probably depend primarily on certain inherent properties of the ions, but the difference is not completely understood. Potassium is known to penetrate a cell boundary more rapidly than sodium; the diameter of the potassium ion is only 0·3 nm while that of sodium is 0·45 nm, and this property may be enhanced by the electrical charges on the cell membrane and by transient local changes in pH (Baldwin, 1949). Although all ions carry a positive or negative electrical charge and equality exists between the total sum of the cations and anions and their respective electrical charges, local potential differences across cell walls and in nerves not only exist but are perhaps the basis of much selective function.

Sodium is the most important cation in the extracellular fluid, the total volume of which is related closely to the total body content of sodium. Sodium passes freely across the capillary wall and cannot play any decisive part in the allocation of extracellular fluid between plasma and interstitial fluid. The control of the passage of fluid across the capillary wall in both directions is believed to depend on two pairs of factors. First, the hydrostatic pressure of the plasma within the vessels and the colloid osmotic pressure of the interstitial fluid move fluid from the plasma into the interstitial fluid. Secondly, the hydrostatic pressure of the interstitial fluid outside the vessels and the osmotic pressure of the plasma proteins inside the vessels, which have both been increased by the outflow of fluid from the capillaries, move water back into the vessels from the interstitial space. This general hypothesis depends on the supposition that the capillary membrane is permeable to water and sodium, potassium, chloride and bicarbonate but not to plasma albumin and globulin. Although broadly true for the normal peripheral capillaries, this hypothesis does not apply in all circumstances. Since the classic work of Lister there have been many observations of the variable behaviour of the capillary circulation.

In some circumstances there may be an outflow of fluid at the arteriolar end of a capillary and inflow at its venous end, and under other conditions outflow throughout the length of a capillary, the fluid returning into the same or another vessel or through the lymphatic channels (Chambers, 1948). The hydrostatic pressure in the portal venous capillaries is so low that fluid exchange would be impossible if these vessels were not unusually permeable to albumin and thus allowed fluid to cross their walls. The increased peripheral capillary permeability to albumin which is a prominent feature of the inflammatory reaction is associated with a very large local increase in the volume of interstitial fluid and in the rate of its formation, and in the volume of lymph leaving the part.

The lymph vessels open out of the so-called interstitial space and offer another channel of drainage from this space. This is particularly useful for the removal of protein from this space, especially during inflammation, but also allows of the easy return to the blood of the small quantities of plasma proteins which are lost from even normal capillaries. When the intravascular colloid osmotic pressure is lowered by reduction of the concentration of plasma protein or when the outflow of fluid containing protein from the capillaries is increased by an elevation of venous pressure, for example in cardiac disease, the lymph flow also increases.

The movement of water between extracellular and intracellular fluids has been supposed to be controlled by osmosis in such a way that the osmotic pressures of the two fluids remain equal on the two sides of any membrane no matter how the composition of the fluids varies. This view depends on the assumption that all cell membranes are freely permeable to water and that osmotic equilibrium is not disturbed by the active transport across cell membranes of water alone, unaccompanied by other materials.

It was originally thought that the high concentration of sodium outside and the low concentration of sodium inside cells arose in some unknown fashion during the original development of the cell, and was thereafter maintained throughout its lifetime by the cell wall becoming impermeable to all cations. Observations on excised muscle and red blood corpuscles have shown that both sodium and potassium may enter and leave cells, according to the nature of the medium, its content of sodium or potassium and its pH. Dean (1941) suggested that these active exchanges of cations might be explained by the existence of a 'pump' system. When potassium was forced or pumped into cells, there might be a complementary output of sodium, and inward movement of sodium was accompanied by a complementary output of potassium. Maizels (1949) has pointed out that the presence of a large amount of relatively static protein and organic phosphate within the cells would permit the active uptake of potassium but would oppose the output of sodium. The permeability of the cell wall to cations, diffusable anions and water would lead to progressive diffusion into the cell until it burst. The chief cation of the environment of the body cells is sodium, and the cells require some means of extruding sodium if they are to keep their cation content steady and if they are to survive. Maizels has shown that this occurs in non-nucleated red cells. He has also suggested that the active extrusion of sodium does not necessarily imply the active uptake of potassium, and that the passage of potassium into cells is passive and secondary to the extrusion of sodium.

The concentration of cation is higher inside the cells than in their surrounding medium, and this intracellular hypertonicity has been explained in various ways. Robinson (1950, 1953) showed that tissue slices remain normal only so long as their oxygen uptake is normal, and when this is depressed by cyanide they swell up because of absorption of water from the medium. He suggested that the hypertonic state of the intracellular fluid can be maintained only by the expulsion of water as fast as it enters. This expulsion of water requires the 'active transport' or 'secretion' of water out of the cells, a process which involves the expenditure of energy. Active transport is dependent on an adequate supply of oxygen and its utilisation by cellular enzyme systems. When oxygen is lacking or its utilisation is interfered with, the cells swell because water accumulates within them. It has been shown also that when adequate oxygen is made available to such swollen cells they shrink if they have not been anoxic for too long a period of time. Although little is yet known about the active transport of water, it is not surprising that such a process exists for the control of water content by cells of which water is so large a component, and which live in an even more watery medium. Such control may increase the stability of the individual cell and give it some independence of its medium, even although that medium so largely conditions the behaviour and ultimately determines the survival of the cell.

Ussing (1952) has explained in a similar way the low sodium content of cells in a medium with a high sodium content, the sodium which diffuses into the cell being as rapidly expelled by an active process of extrusion. The maintenance of a high potassium content by cells in a saline medium was shown by Terner *et al.* (1950) to be dependent on the presence of oxygen, glucose and L-glutamate in the medium; the absence of any one of these caused a loss of potassium from the cells, but restoration of the missing substance to the substrate was followed by restoration of the potassium content of the cells.

Even if it is possible for free water to traverse cell boundaries, it seems likely that on the whole there is a close association of water with cation and anion shifts which are normally accompanied by the movement of water.

WATER BALANCE

The maintenance of the water content of the body depends on the preservation of a state of balance between daily intake and output or loss of water, both of which may normally vary within wide limits. For the present purpose the requirements of water intake are best considered in the light of what is known of water loss from the body.

WATER LOSS

Water loss may be divided into two parts: first, the extrarenal loss in the form of insensible water loss as vapour in the expired air or through the skin, or as liquid in the faeces and sweat; and secondly, the renal water loss as the urine.

Extrarenal Water Loss

INSENSIBLE WATER LOSS. This is made up of two components. The first is the water vapour which saturates the expired air and which varies in quantity with the rate and depth of respiration. The second component consists of the water vapour which diffuses through the skin into the surrounding air. This kind of loss depends on the difference in water content of the body and its environment, and its rate varies with body temperature and thus with metabolic rate, with the temperature and humidity of the environment, and with the clothing or bedding covering the body. Insensible water loss by vaporisation plays an important part in the dissipation of the heat generated by metabolism, and hence in the regulation of body temperature, and is essential for survival. It should be regarded as inevitable and as the primary water requirement of the body which continues and must be satisfied so long as the body is alive, regardless of the water requirements for urine formation and abnormal losses of body fluids. It is distinct from the loss of water by sweating, which depends on the secretion of sweat by the sweat glands. Sweating is an accessory means of promoting heat loss by the evaporation of water when the body temperature tends to rise because of an increase in heat production, reduced heat loss due to excessive clothing, or elevation of the temperature or humidity of the environment.

The environment can supply the heat for evaporation of water from the skin even when the temperature of the skin and the environment are the same, but only if there is a sufficient gradient in humidity between them.

The average insensible loss of water through the skin and in the expired air was estimated by DuBois (1936) to be 0·5 g of water per kg body weight per hour in adults (840 g of water per day in a 70 kg man); a similar estimate was made by Gamble (1947) as the result of repeated weighing of normal adults under varying circumstances, and he showed also that this basic rate of loss was increased by clothing and by changes in environmental conditions. Newburgh *et al.* (1937) found that loss of water vapour from the skin of normal men varied with the air temperature when they were naked, but when they were lightly clothed the loss varied little over a wide range of temperature. They concluded that when a man is comfortable in his environment about one-quarter of the heat produced in the body is dissipated by insensible water loss, even when the calories consumed vary from 2200 to 3600 per day, or when 6 per cent of body weight has been lost by dehydration. Estimation of insensible water loss from metabolic rate gives a higher figure than the other methods, but being based on energy expenditure and thus related directly to heat production, approaches the true figure more closely; for example, a subject metabolising 2500 calories per day and dissipating one-quarter of this heat by insensible water loss will evaporate $(2500/4)\times(1/0{\cdot}58)$ ml of water per day $=1077$ ml water regardless of his body weight.

It is usually assumed that metabolism rises by 7 per cent for each 1° F rise in body temperature (13 per cent per 1° C), so that an increase in insensible water loss results from pyrexia. Metabolic rate is increased after accidental or surgical injury.

When a nude adult is exposed to a temperature of less than 80° F (26·6° C) body temperature falls, but when it drops 1·5° C shivering is stimulated which tends to raise the body temperature. Between 80° and 84° F (26·6 and 28·8° C) body temperature at rest will remain steady. The closer the environmental temperature approaches that of the body the more does maintenance of heat loss and body temperature depend on the evaporation of water secreted as sweat. The rate of evaporation of water from the surface of the body depends on the humidity of the ambient air as well as its temperature and rate of flow over the body.

Sweat

The evaporation of sweat provides an additional means of dissipating body heat especially when at low relative humidity the environmental temperature exceeds 84° F (29° C) or heat production is very large; when the humidity is higher, sweating begins at lower temperatures. Whether sweating is noticeable depends on how rapidly it evaporates, which in turn is related to the humidity as well as to the temperature of the environment. The volume of sweat varies widely between individuals in the same circumstances, and up to 3 litres may be produced in an hour or 10 litres in a day; such very high rates of sweating are not maintained for long and the rate falls off as exposure to heat is prolonged even if all the lost water is replaced. Ladell (1945) suggested that this was due to fatigue of the sweat glands, which also were less able to regulate the mineral content of the sweat.

Sudden exposure to a high environmental temperature may cause acute disturbances of body fluid equilibrium. This is more likely and important in the small proportion of people who appear to have a poor capacity to make the necessary homeostatic adjustments in the composition and volume of the sweat and urine. Prolonged exposure may reduce the capacity of a patient to deal with the effects of even an uncomplicated surgical operation. This incapacity is now of new importance, for whereas formerly such a patient might have had some time to recover during a sea voyage of three or four weeks from the tropics to Europe he is now more likely to return in one day by air. It is now common for people to arrive in the tropics by air without any acclimatisation.

The confusion which has long been associated with the group of disorders which are caused by exposure to heat has partly arisen from the terminology which has been used. By far the most serious and important disturbances are *heat exhaustion*, a disturbance of the content and distribution of water and electrolytes in the body, and *heat stroke* and *hyperpyrexia*, disturbances due to failure or impairment of the processes involved in body temperature regulation. There is no essential difference between heat stroke and hyperpyrexia except that heat stroke is conventionally used for the more severe and fatal forms of this disturbance of temperature regulation.

Heat exhaustion (formerly type I heat exhaustion) affects the apparently well-acclimatised man who has been working daily in the heat; it is characterised by a pale sweating skin and slight elevation of the body temperature and pulse rate; the patient appears 'dehydrated' and to have lost weight, there is haemoconcentration and he passes small quantities of dark concentrated urine containing little sodium or chloride. Muscle cramps may begin before or during treatment (Ladell, 1957). This condition appears to be the result of a chronic depletion of water, sodium and potassium, and affects both intracellular and extracellular fluid. This is primarily due to repeated incomplete replacement of the daily sweat losses incurred during working hours and is indicated by a low urinary volume. Ladell (1947) found that up to two litres of water must be lost from the body before the volume of the saliva decreases or a basal urinary volume is achieved. During acute exposure to heat, if water is drunk freely but the salt intake is low, the continued small loss of sodium in the urine leads to reduction in extracellular fluid volume although there is no intracellular dehydration. If instead, however, too little water is drunk but supplementary salt is taken, the total body sodium content is well maintained but extracellular fluid volume must be maintained by the withdrawal of water from the cells leading to an intracellular dehydration (Ladell, 1955). In both types of this disturbance the circulatory collapse is the result of reduction in extracellular fluid volume, but in the first this may be associated with a low serum sodium concentration while in the second type serum sodium concentration may be raised. After long exposure to heat, when there is depletion of both intracellular and extracellular fluid, the consumption of a lot of water may cause dilution of the extracellular fluid and muscle cramps but is not likely to cause circulatory collapse. If on the other hand more salt than water is given, especially as hypertonic saline, after an initial improvement there is usually a circulatory collapse. Thus heat exhaustion may be due to drinking too little water in great heat, or to severe exertion combined with the inadequate consumption of water or salt.

Hyperpyrexia is sudden in onset, affecting a man who works normally in the morning, may fall mildly ill at midday, collapses suddenly during the afternoon and if not treated promptly is dead by sunset. This is due to failure to dissipate the heat of metabolism and may be related to the production of too little sweat, as well as to high environmental temperature and humidity. Extra exertion in a very hot environment may increase the production of heat beyond the capacity of the body to lose it. This may be due to unsuitable clothing, poor air movement due to bad ventilation, inadequate sweating because of prickly heat or other skin disorders, or because of an inherent low limit of tolerance of the individual to climatic extremes. It is more likely in those who are not used to climatic extremes or who have been recently ill, for example with enteritis. Shibolet *et al.* (1967) found that patients with heatstroke could be divided into three groups. Those who were unconscious for more than ten hours died within three days, most of those who were comatose for less than ten hours and all those who were in coma for less than six hours recovered. Those who died showed severe disturbance of blood clotting, most of those in the second group had severe disturbance of renal and liver function which improved after five days, but this sort of functional disturbance was mild or absent in the last group. After collapse the unconscious patient has a burning hot skin and may be sweating, a rectal temperature of 105° to 107° F and stertorous breathing. Without treatment all these patients will die. The body must be cooled at once by being wrapped in a wet sheet and laid in the draught from a fan until the rectal temperature falls to 102° F. Ice bags should not be used as they induce local vasoconstriction which interferes with heat loss. Individuals who normally sweat less than their companions may have a poorer tolerance to extreme heat and therefore should probably be protected from it. Shibolet *et al.* (1967) have emphasised the importance of the prevention of heatstroke which most commonly affects the active young adult during, for example, military training, work or sport in unfavourable climatic conditions. The risk of heatstroke is increased by even minor illness, excessive fatigue, too prolonged exertion and lack of water, and can be reduced by common sense.

It is believed that prolonged *prickly heat* may upset sweating function sufficiently to cause *tropical anhydrotic asthenia* (formerly called type II heat exhaustion). This disturbance of heat regulation characteristically comes on gradually towards the end of the tropical summer after prolonged exposure to heat and is associated with an inability to sweat properly, moderate pyrexia (up to 101° F), loss of energy and the passage of copious quantities of dilute urine containing little chloride or sodium. Such individuals recover slowly over a period of about six weeks in a cool environment on a full diet, and according to Ladell (1957) cannot be more rapidly cured by the administration of saline. The exact cause and the mechanism of this disturbance remain obscure.

FAECAL WATER LOSS. The rate of water loss in the faeces varies with the rate of passage of material through the intestine, especially the colon, and on the degree of dryness of the stools when passed. During fasting, the stools are small and contain little water, but on a normal diet it is usual to allow for the loss of up to 200 ml water per day in the faeces. This quantity is approximately equal to the water of oxidation of the food consumed. When large quantities of mucus are lost, for example in some forms of malignant disease of the colon and rectum, or when many loose stools are passed as in ulcerative colitis, up to a litre or more of water, as well as large quantities of minerals, may be lost from the bowel each day.

Renal Water Loss

The renal glomeruli filter about 180 litres of fluid from the 1100 litres of plasma which flow through the kidneys each day. About 85 per cent of this filtrate is absorbed isosmotically in the proximal convoluted tubules. With the exception of rather less than one per cent of the original volume which forms the urine, the remainder of the water is absorbed in the distal tubules. The minimum volume of water required by the kidneys for urine formation varies with the total quantity and with the nature of the solutes which are to be excreted, or the 'osmotic load', and on the ability of the kidneys to excrete a concentrated urine. The solute or osmotic load varies with the food intake and with the metabolic state of the patient; it is raised by tissue catabolism after injury and in many diseases, and by the production of keto acids when fat metabolism is incomplete. Normal urine is hypertonic in comparison with plasma, and by producing concentrated urine the kidneys play an important part in conserving body water. Gamble (1954) has shown how closely the water requirements for urine formation are related to the concentrating capacity of the kidneys, the minimum urine volume for a given solute load varying from about 500 ml at a urine specific gravity of 1032 (1250 mosmol per litre) to 750 ml at a specific gravity of 1020 (800 mosmol per litre), and 1300 ml at a specific gravity of 1016 (600 mosmol per litre). When the intake of water is restricted, the requirements for insensible loss as vapour through the skin and in the expired air must first be satisfied; if the available water then remaining for urine formation is insufficient to dissolve the solute load, either additional water must be obtained from the body fluids or some of the solute load must be retained in the body. When water is consumed in excess of the requirements for insensible loss and the minimum urine volume, the excess is excreted by the kidneys as additional urine water. A healthy adult with normal kidneys can excrete the daily solute load in 500 to 800 ml of urine.

THE TOTAL MINIMUM DAILY EXPENDITURE OF WATER. In a temperate climate for an adult weighing 70 kg insensible water loss amounts to about 1000 ml, 200 ml or more may be lost in the faeces and 500 ml as urine, in all about 1700 ml. In the past too little attention has been paid to the effects on the water turnover of hospital patients of the large variations in environmental humidity which are inevitable in the continental type of climate. On the other hand there has been too much emphasis on forcing up the volume of urine by large intravenous infusions to an arbitrary level often much above the minimum requirements. Ladell (1947) has shown that in a temperate climate a resting adult eating an ordinary diet needs to consume only 800 to 900 ml water per day to remain in water balance.

WATER INTAKE

On an ordinary diet about 12 g water are produced from each 100 calories metabolised, equal to a total of 300 g or more water per day; and the water content of the solid food which varies from 60 to 95 per cent provides about 300 g or more in addition. The daily consumption of water by drinking varies widely; some normal people drink as little as a pint (560 ml) per day, but the average consumption by patients in hospital is about 800 to 1000 ml per day. In certain occupations which involve heavy water losses by sweating, a gallon or more (4 litres) may be regularly consumed daily. These wide individual variations in water intake and turnover deserve greater recognition and respect when the daily water requirement of the individual surgical patient is being considered. It may be a greater hardship and more harmful for some patients, especially if they are elderly, to drink 5 or 6 pints each day than for others to do without water entirely.

Regulation of Water Content of the Body

Of the organs concerned with water exchange, the skin, pulmonary alveoli and air passages are rather passive agents of exchange and only the kidneys have any regulatory effect on water expenditure. The insensible loss of water is dependent on environmental temperature and humidity and on the rate of production of heat or energy consumption of the body. The water content of the body is the important factor which initiates change of rate in turnover in the kidneys. The absorption of water by the distal renal tubules is controlled by the antidiuretic hormone secreted by the posterior lobe of the pituitary gland under the influence of nervous impulses originating in the supraoptic nucleus; this centre responds to impulses received from osmoreceptors sensitive to changes in the water content of the blood (Verney, 1947, 1954). The antidiuretic hormone mechanism responds to changes in blood composition which are the result of excessive loss or ingestion of water, and produces either oliguria (antidiuresis) or increased water output by the kidneys. The osmoreceptors appear to be particularly sensitive to acute changes in the composition of the blood and do not invariably respond so sensitively to chronic or gradual alteration of a degree which if produced acutely would invoke a sharp response.

Control of water output by antidiuretic hormone is generally independent of the output of cations such as sodium and potassium and the rate of excretion of these ions may remain steady in spite of a large diuresis induced by the copious drinking of water. Following the ingestion of a large quantity of water there is a lag period before diuresis begins while the normal circulating antidiuretic hormone is destroyed; the diuresis can be inhibited by injection of antidiuretic hormone. That this control of the volume of the urine is by an antidiuretic hormone emphasises the importance of close limitation of the loss of water by a body of which 70 per cent is water and which must exist in a drier environment.

Thirst

The sensation of thirst is not well understood. Cannon (1918) believed that thirst had a local origin in a dry mouth. He supposed that the salivary glands, which are normally responsible for keeping the mucous membrane moist, suffered from the general lack of water in the body and did not secrete enough saliva to prevent the local discomfort and unpleasantness which constitute the feeling of thirst. Claude Bernard (1856) showed by experiment on a horse with an oesophageal fistula and a dog with a gastric fistula, that when these animals were thirsty they drank almost continuously, pausing only for short periods of rest, and he concluded that thirst was not a local sensation but a response to some general demand to raise the water content of the body to a normal quantity. His results have been confirmed by Adolph (1947), who found that in thirsty men, and in dogs with oesophageal fistulas, the water deficits were closely related to the quantity of water consumed in slaking thirst or to the urge to drink. It seems evident that water is roughly measured in the pharynx as it is drunk. The urge to drink to satisfy a lack of water can be abolished temporarily by sham drinking, by contact of water in the throat, or alternatively and more lastingly by placing water in the stomach through a tube.

The intravenous injection of a hypertonic solution of sodium chloride (Leschke, 1918) or sodium bicarbonate (Arden, 1934) causes intense thirst, but after the injection of the same quantity of an equally hypertonic solution of potassium chloride thirst is not experienced. Gilman (1937) found that the intake of water was much larger when the osmotic pressure of the plasma was increased by the injection of a hypertonic solution of sodium chloride than when urea was used. Wolf (1950) raised the plasma osmotic pressure gradually by injecting hypertonic saline and found that thirst began when the osmotic pressure had risen by 1 to 2 per cent, a figure which resembles Verney's estimate for the threshold of release of antidiuretic hormone in the dog. Andersson and McCann (1955) have produced evidence for the existence of a 'drinking centre' in the hypothalamus.

The way in which the water content of the body is restored after depletion depends on the type of water loss which has occurred. When water has been lost in association with sodium in extracellular fluid depletion, sodium and water must be replaced in order to maintain tonicity as the volume of extracellular fluid is restored; if sufficient sodium is not introduced, the excess water will be excreted. One of the remarkable features of extracellular fluid depletion is the absence of thirst, until it is remembered that thirst, being a stimulus to drink water, would lead to the dilution of the remaining extracellular fluid; it is interesting too that McCance (1936) found that sodium depleted normal subjects lost all sense of taste and smell, but that this returned soon after the consumption of 15 g of sodium chloride.

Neither thirst nor antidiuretic activity is aroused by changes in the volume of body fluids provided there is no accompanying change in the concentration of sodium or in total osmolarity. A loss of water alone stimulates both thirst and the output of antidiuretic hormone and this is a more effective process than the response to an increased body water content, the absence of thirst and a diuresis; an excess of water is fortunately uncommon except following the too lavish intravenous infusion of glucose solution or after bowel washouts with water.

Intense thirst is experienced by severely injured patients suffering from shock and usually subsides as blood volume is restored by transfusion; this kind of thirst seems to be closely related to the acute reduction in blood volume consequent on blood or plasma loss, and may well be due to the transfer of interstitial and intracellular fluid as part of a compensatory reaction to the acute lowering of blood volume, with the production of intracellular dehydration and hypertonicity. Severe thirst is also common after major surgical operations, even when there has not been a large loss of blood; beginning about 6 to 12 hours after operation, it lasts for 36 hours or more, and may persist for up to 6 or 7 days in patients who receive prolonged intravenous infusions,

During the first 24 or 36 hours after operation, thirst can be relieved only for short periods of time, 15 to 20 minutes, by the consumption of water, tea or other fluids, and is not relieved by the intravenous infusion of isotonic saline or glucose solution. The period of most intense thirst after operation corresponds in time to the rapid loss of potassium from the cells and to a marked loss of weight. It seems possible that during this period thirst is due chiefly to intracellular dehydration and is a normal effect of injury; transient relief follows wetting of the mouth and pharynx even when the fluid is not swallowed, and practically none of it is absorbed. The best relief is obtained by washing out the mouth with ice-cold water, and in practice this is more effective than drinking. When after operation the intake of water is stopped for 48 hours, the intense thirst which is experienced from about 12 to 30 hours after operation often diminishes or disappears entirely before any water is drunk (Wilkinson, 1956b). If large quantities of fluids are drunk, the stomach appears to be incapable of absorbing or transmitting them and they are usually vomited. When following operations on the alimentary tract the patient is allowed to drink unlimited quantities of fluid, but distension of the stomach is prevented by aspiration, thirst often increases. As the quantity of fluid drunk increases, there is an even greater increase in the volume of fluid aspirated, and very large quantities of sodium and chloride, as well as of water, may be lost in the fluid sucked out of the stomach. Presumably the increasing thirst is due to an increased transfer of water from the cells, leading to 'intracellular dehydration'.

CHAPTER TWO

Sodium

NORMAL CONTENT AND DISTRIBUTION

In a normal subject nearly 44 per cent of the total body sodium is in the extracellular fluid and only 9 per cent is in intracellular fluid, the remaining 47 per cent being in bone. About 45 per cent of the sodium in bone is exchangeable and may take an active part in the continuous rapid interchange of sodium in the body; thus in all about 74 per cent (66 g) out of the total of about 90 g in the body is freely available for so-called metabolic purposes and the compensation of abnormal loss from the body (Table VI).

TABLE VI

Distribution of sodium in the body

Total content 90 g =3915 mEq/70 kg (11 stones)

	% of Total	*g*	*mEq*	*Exchangeable*	*Available*
Extracellular fluid	44	39·6	1723	all	74% total
Intracellular fluid	9	8·1	352	all	66 g
Bone	47	42·3	1840	45%=19·0 g 827 mEq	2900 mEq

The quantities of sodium and chloride excreted in the urine vary with the intake and with losses by vomiting, diarrhoea or by excessive sweating due to climatic or occupational factors.

SODIUM EXCHANGES

SWEAT

Sweat is produced chiefly by the cholinergic eccrine glands, which are distributed all over the body. Unlike the insensible water loss through the skin, sweat contains all the plasma ions, the most important being sodium and chloride, but is always hypotonic compared with plasma or extracellular fluid. Sweating is caused by a rise in skin and rectal temperature. The rate of sweating is probably not much affected by moderate water deficiency but may stop when dehydration is very severe; it is certainly reduced by the drinking of 0·5 per cent saline and by the administration of drugs of the atropine group. About 50 per cent of the sweat is secreted on the trunk, 25 per cent on the legs and the rest on the arms, head and neck.

The sweat glands are partly under the influence of adrenal cortical hormones and the composition of sweat varies greatly. When a normal subject is made to work hard for a short time in a hot room he secretes larger volumes of sweat containing much higher concentrations of sodium and chloride than he would do if he had become acclimatised over a period of days to an equally hot climate (Ladell, 1945). The mineral content of sweat varies so widely that average figures cannot be given. Schwartz and Thaysen (1956), who stimulated sweating with acetyl-β-methyl-choline, found that the sodium concentration varied from 6 to 85 mEq per litre but was always lower than the plasma concentration, whereas the potassium concentration varied from 5 to 21 mEq per litre and was always higher than that of the plasma. The concentrations of sodium and chloride in sweat are related also to the intake of these ions and usually decline when their total body contents fall; when the salt intake exceeds that necessary to maintain sodium and chloride balance, the concentrations of sodium and chloride in the sweat rise.

It is well known among men working in hot humid environments and by dwellers in hot climates that the taste of the sweat on their skin affords a good indication of the salt content of the body; after heavy sweating a salt 'frost' may be seen on the cheeks and upper lip and the disappearance of the normal salty taste from the sweat is commonly taken as an indication for the consumption of extra salt. Dill *et al.* (1933) stated that part of the process of acclimatisation to a hot climate was expressed in a reduction in the sodium content of the sweat. This has been confirmed by the work of Conn (1949, 1956) and others on adrenal cortical hormones, particularly aldosterone; failure to reduce the chloride and sodium content of the sweat during acclimatisation is an indication of adrenal inadequacy or failure. Conn found that in healthy men adrenal influence was so marked that they could be maintained in sodium balance on an intake of only 5 g sodium chloride (85 mEq sodium) per day in spite of copious sweating caused by heavy work in a hot environment. Compared with plasma, sweat contains more water than sodium, but the repeated replacement of sweat loss by water alone leads to sodium depletion. When the body is depleted of water, replacement is stimulated by thirst, but there is no comparable stimulus to the replacement of sodium, and the natural processes of regulation of water and sodium content are different. Sodium content is regulated by conservation, or stabilisation of the body content, by processes which reduce sodium loss by lowering its concentration in secretions such as sweat and urine, probably under the immediate influence of adrenal cortical hormones. With increasing use and speed of air travel there is more chance than ever before that unacclimatised passengers may occasionally have to undergo emergency surgical operation in the tropics; if they can be nursed in air-conditioned accommodation, severe disturbance of body fluid equilibrium by excessive sweating and mineral loss can be largely avoided. There is still too little information on which to base estimates of water and sodium requirements in hot and humid environments during the first week after a major operation or severe injury, and judgement is even more difficult in unacclimatised patients and during sudden 'heat waves' in otherwise temperate climates.

Renal Regulation of Sodium

Except during the first six days or so after injury, or during inflammation due to other casues, when sodium intake exceeds the extrarenal losses the excess is excreted in the urine. In adults the glomerular filtration rate varies from 90 to 150 ml per minute with an average rate of 120 ml per minute, or 70 ml per m^2 of body surface area per minute, and is not much affected by the state of hydration as long as the individual continues to eat; only about 0·5 to 2 ml of urine are formed per minute, which if maintained results in the excretion of 720 to 3000 ml urine in 24 hours. At a plasma sodium concentration of 140 mEq per litre, 16·8 mEq sodium will be filtered each minute, or if the rate is steady about 24,000 mEq in 24 hours (equivalent to 15 times the total extracellular sodium), yet only about 100 mEq may be excreted in the urine. At a steady glomerular filtration rate of 120 ml per minute, 173 litres of filtrate (4 times the total body content of water) would be formed in 24 hours, but less than 1 litre might be excreted as urine. Such high rates of filtration are not maintained for long periods, and there are variations in sodium and potassium excretion between night and day. Even so, very large volumes of glomerular filtrate are formed and a high proportion of this filtrate is reabsorbed in the proximal tubules with little or no modification in its content of sodium, potassium, chloride or bicarbonate (isosmotic reabsorption). Other substances, in particular urea, are not reabsorbed, and so their concentration in the remaining fluid in the renal tubules increases.

In the distal tubules the remainder of the glomerular filtrate is further modified by selective reabsorption and secretion by the tubular cells. This treatment of the filtrate by the distal tubular cells removes most of the remaining water and sodium and reduces the concentration of sodium in glomerular filtrate, which is the same as that of the plasma, to the varying concentrations of sodium found in the urine in the different states of sodium content of the body. Since the renal tubular cells are themselves probably subject to changes in chemical composition similar to those which occur in other cells of the body in states of deficiency or excess, the tubular cellular function is liable to alteration when the body content of the biologically important ions is disturbed. It is for this reason that in advanced stages of deficiency or excess of certain constituents renal tubular function may be upset and can be restored only by specific correction of the disturbance. The small alteration in composition of large volumes of fluid which occurs in the proximal tubules by the isosmotic absorption of water, sodium, potassium, chloride and bicarbonate without urea is an example of a convenient and primitive biological process which avoids secretion with its high energy requirements. Similar processes are found in the daily large turnover of secretions, containing up to 100 mEq sodium in the alimentary tract, and in the peripheral capillary circulation.

Glomerular filtration rate depends on the renal blood flow, and both may fall when blood and especially plasma volume are reduced. The administration or consumption of water, by increasing extracellular fluid volume and so plasma volume, increases glomerular filtration but not always the sodium content of the filtrate; although the urinary sodium output may rise during water diuresis, this is not an invariable consequence, and the control of sodium excretion is not well understood. Desoxycorticosterone acetate causes sodium retention by the tubules regardless of the sodium concentration in plasma. The most powerful conservation of sodium is effected by aldosterone, which is about 30 times as effective as desoxycorticosterone acetate.

There is normally a reciprocal relationship between the dietary intake of sodium and the output of aldosterone which falls when sodium intake rises and rises when it falls. Although aldosterone probably acts mainly on the distal tubules it may also have effects on the proximal tubule as well. It now seems likely that other factors apart from aldosterone and glomerular filtration rate are concerned in the output of sodium in the urine such as the osmotic pressure in the peritubular space and the variation in absorptive capacity of different nephrons, and at present it is impossible to predict the relative importance of these factors in particular circumstances.

Sodium in Bone

The importance of the skeleton as a reservoir of the mineral constituents of the body is now recognised. Harrison *et al.* (1936) found that half of the sodium in bone was osmotically inactive and soluble in acid but not in water or strong alkali, and they thought that it was part of an apatite complex. The vast surface of the crystals in bone provides an enormous area for the adsorption of sodium, magnesium and potassium in ideal circumstances for a dynamic equilibrium with the extracellular fluid (Robinson, 1951). Bergstrom and Wallace (1954) suggested that sodium might be withdrawn from such a site in bone when the extracellular fluid equilibrium was disturbed by the loss of sodium from the body. Much of the exchangeable sodium can be removed from the bones of experimental animals in a few hours after the artificial induction of severe acidosis and the decalcification of bone in chronic renal acidosis, or in lactation implies that at least part of the sodium content of human bones is labile; there is, however, no evidence that bones can store minerals in excess of their of their normal content.

It is recognised that in some circumstances the results of careful metabolic balances cannot be reconciled with calculations of the total sodium content of extracellular fluid or of the whole body; Moore (1954) suggested that in such circumstances sodium might have been mobilised from bone. Loss of sodium from bone has been shown in animals in acute sodium depletion or with adrenal hypofunction; similar shifts of sodium might occur in patients especially after losses by diarrhoea or sweating, in diabetic acidosis, or prolonged restriction of sodium intake or use of mercurial diuretics.

Normal Intake and Output

It is difficult to decide how much sodium constitutes a normal daily intake because of the compensatory mechanisms which guard against its depletion. As Ladell (1957) has pointed out, phylogenetically man is a tropical animal and the sweating state is a normal one for the species, but he doubts whether it is natural for the human species to have the high salt intake which is so common in the so-called Western civilisation. He has suggested that the addition of salt to food is a luxury and an addiction and has resulted in habituation to a lower daily plane of aldosterone production, but this attitude perhaps ignores the ancient purpose of preventing the putrefaction of meat in a hot climate by bleeding the animal during slaughtering and thereafter applying salt as a preservative. It is clear that a wide range of sodium intake can be tolerated by people with satisfactory renal and adrenal function.

In a temperate climate the average daily intake is probably in the region of 80 to 100 mEq per day (5 to 6 g as sodium chloride). About 70 to 90 mEq (4·5 to 5·5 g as sodium chloride). may be lost in the urine and less than 10 mEq in formed faeces, with varying but usually negligible quantities in sweat (Table VII). Some people habitually consume more and others less than 5 or 6 g of sodium chloride per day. In temperate conditions an intake of 10 to 15 g of sodium chloride per day administered as isotonic saline during the first week after operation leads to a large increase in sodium and water content and body weight, and may cause oedema. To limit loss of sodium by sweating, especially in children and young babies, overheating of patients should be avoided during operations. Even in the case of the newly born, the temperature of the theatre should not exceed 70° F and the humidity 65 per cent. In an operating theatre in which it is comfortable to work, temperature and humidity do not usually exceed these limits. The so-called 'ether' convulsions,

TABLE VII

Daily intake and output of sodium

Intake in food	80 to 100 mEq
Output in urine	70 to 90 mEq
Sweat and faeces	about 10 mEq
Secreted into stomach and intestine and reabsorbed	685 mEq
Filtered by renal glomerulus and reabsorbed up to	24,000 mEq

which were formerly a not uncommon complication of operations on ill and pyrexial children, were probably due largely to the effects of high temperature and humidity in the operating theatre on a child whose water balance was already seriously upset by disease and a raised body temperature.

In hot climates, if an air-conditioned theatre is not available, operations should be performed in the early morning. When sweating is unavoidable, the loss of sodium in sweat should be replaced by the consumption of additional salt according to individual requirements and circumstances, the best indication of an adequate supplement being the taste of the sweat. Ladell (1957) has calculated that the average daily intake of sodium chloride by the Nigerian peasant is probably less than 7 g (119 mEq sodium) and he quotes an estimate by Lange that the daily intake of an Indonesian peasant is only 3 g sodium chloride per day (51 mEq sodium). The dangers of treating such people according to the orthodox principle laid down for certain limited and entirely different environmental conditions is obvious. There is little reliable specific information regarding the range of requirements for either water or sodium of surgical patients under tropical or subtropical conditions. There is wide individual and racial variation in tolerance of heat and humidity, which is complicated by undernutrition and disease, such as chronic dysentery and malaria. There is wide scope for study of these aspects of surgery in tropical countries and also of the metabolic effects of surgical treatment in different races and climates.

Tinckler (1966) is one of the few surgeons who has made any observations on the fluid and electrolyte requirements of the surgical patient in the tropics. He studied the total body water content of the indigenous population, and the insensible loss of water and the loss of electrolytes of hospital patients, during the hot weather of the summer months in Qatar and Bahrein in the Persian Gulf. The patients were in hospital for investigation, were awaiting operation, or were convalescent after operation in wards which were not air-conditioned but opened on to shady verandahs and had good through ventilation and ceiling fans. For about half the 24 hour period the ward atmosphere was very hot and humid, with average dry-bulb temperatures of 90° to 95° F (32° to 35° C) and wet-bulb temperatures of 80° to 85° F (26° to 29° C). Failure to maintain the intake of water and sodium chloride at a level sufficient to prevent water and sodium depletion in such patients impairs their capacity to maintain body temperature by sweating and leads to heat exhaustion and hyperpyrexia. In climatic conditions such as those of the Persian Gulf in summer Tinckler recommends that a minimum of 2000 ml of water is needed for insensible water loss. In some of his apparently normal subjects total body water content was below the normal minimum for temperate climates, and he concluded that these individuals suffered from a chronic water lack due to too small a normal intake. Their sweat contained about 10 mEq of sodium per litre, an indication of good adaption to their environment. He advised that the adult surgical patient who was acclimatised to hot conditions and had not suffered depletion of body fluids should be provided with 2 to 4 litres of fluid per 24 hours after operation, as a 5 per cent solution of dextrose, but that additional sodium was not necessary. For the unacclimatised patient, however, each litre of fluid should contain 250 ml of 0·9 per cent solution (37·5 mEq sodium) to allow for the larger losses of sodium in sweat.

Badoe (1968) studied the pulmonary and cutaneous fluid losses in Ghanian males in hospital in Accra. He measured the changes in body weight and the urinary volume in three 4 hour periods between 8 a.m. and 10 p.m. with 1 hour intervals for two meals, at four different times of the year. The average weight of his 39 subjects was 59 kg; some were volunteers but the rest were male hospital patients of various ages. The ward temperature ranged from a minimum of 68° to 78° F (20° to 25° C) to a maximum of 76° to 88° F (25° to 31° C) but was seldom more than 86° F (30° C), the temperature at which sweating usually starts. The relative humidity ranged from 78 to 89 per cent. The average pulmonary and cutaneous fluid loss in 24 hours was 1·70 kg (range 0·9 to 2·9 kg). Badoe suggested that after operation or accidental injury, when the urine volume is likely to be about 500 ml, a total fluid intake of 2500 ml, consisting of 2000 ml of 5 per cent dextrose solution and 500 ml of 0·9 per cent saline, would be adequate. He later increased this to a total of 3 litres by substituting a litre of Ringer's solution for the 0·9 per cent saline. Badoe found that sweating was not common in his patients. The results obtained by Elebute (1969) in a similar study of 35 adult male Nigerians in Lagos are remarkably like those described by Badoe. The average weight (59 kg) and daily fluid loss through the skin and lungs (1·71 l) were the same. The mean daily temperature in Lagos ranged between 75° to 85·5° F (23° to 30° C) and the relative humidity was between 73 and 93 per cent. There was a marked variation, however, between the fluid losses in the hot dry months from November to April of 1·5 to 2·0 litres, and those in the wet cooler months from May to October of about 1 litre. The smaller average body weight of Nigerian males compared with European and North American males contrasts with their larger evaporative water losses, and emphasises the importance of basing treatment on direct measurement rather than on calculation from formulas based on measurements of a different people living in a very different climate and environment. Elebute recommended the water intake in surgical patients should be at least 2 litres per 24 hours (Elebute, personal communication).

DISTURBANCES OF SODIUM EQUILIBRIUM

Disturbance of sodium equilibrium occurs after injury and in association with all forms of inflammation, and is a feature of many diseases. It may result from alteration in the total quantity of sodium in the body, from change in sodium concentration due to alteration in total water content, or from a combination of both these factors. There may also be alterations in the distribution of sodium in the body with or without change in the total body content of sodium. Disturbances of sodium equilibrium can be broadly classified as due to either sodium depletion or sodium excess. Each of these two main types can be further subdivided into those which are real and are caused by a reduction or an increase in the total body content of sodium, and those which are only apparent, the concentration of sodium in extracellular fluid being altered by variations in water content and distribution in the absence of any change in total body content of sodium. In surgical practice the most common disturbances are due to extrarenal losses of sodium and water following the loss of gastrointestinal secretions, or to the excessive administration of solutions of sodium salts or water; this is in contrast to the situation in patients with severe cardiac and renal disease who are now more commonly subjected to operation than formerly and often suffer from excessive content of water and sodium together with various secondary disturbances. In most clinical circumstances, because both sodium and water are lost, the pure forms of the disturbances of sodium equilibrium are rare. In the absence of severe renal disease, renal conservation of sodium is so efficient that only small quantities of sodium are lost in the urine after surgical operations or severe injury, or during even extensive infective inflammatory disease. The normal distribution of sodium in the body is dependent on the normal production of adrenal cortical hormones. The peripheral circulatory failure which may occur when too little cortisone is given to an adrenalectomised patient is completely corrected by the administration of sufficient cortisone without any saline or sodium.

Sodium Depletion

(a) *Real* sodium depletion (so-called 'salt depletion') is usually due to the loss of both sodium and water. When the sodium and water are lost in the same proportion as they occur in extracellular fluid, for example in the loss of plasma after burning, the extracellular sodium concentration may not change. When a large loss of sodium and water is replaced with water alone or with too much water and too little sodium, the extracellular sodium concentration will fall; for example when a large loss of sweat is replaced by the drinking of water, or when too much glucose solution is used in the replacement of large losses of gastrointestinal secretions.

(b) *Apparent* sodium depletion, or 'sodium dilution': in the absence of any appreciable loss of sodium the extracellular sodium concentrations is reduced by the administration of water more rapidly than it can be excreted by the kidneys or lost insensibly or by sweating. This is probably most common in elderly patients to whom excessive quantities of glucose solution are administered after operations (water intoxication).

Sodium Excess

(a) *Real.* The sodium content of the body may be increased by the rapid intravenous administration of solutions of sodium salts. Even a daily intake of sodium which is within the so-called normal limits may increase total sodium content when renal excretion of sodium is delayed after injury or during inflammation, impaired by renal disease or altered by the administration of adrenal cortical hormones or secondary to cardiac disease. Whether the extracellular sodium concentration changes depends on the state of water balance.

(b) *Apparent* The extracellular sodium concentration may rise in true dehydration when the total body water content is reduced but the body sodium content is maintained; or when there is a loss of both water and sodium, but the loss of water is the greater.

Dehydration

This term, which strictly used implies the loss of water alone from the body, is widely and loosely employed to indicate the loss of water and various ions from the body, without any indication being given of the source of the lost water or of the accompanying losses of ions. Kerpel-Fronius (1935, 1938) showed that there are two distinct kinds of so-called 'dehydration'. In one there is a loss of water but not of an equivalent quantity of cation; this loss is accompanied by thirst and the water may be derived from both extracellular and intracellular fluid. In the other kind the loss of water is accompanied by the loss of an equivalent quantity of sodium, the chief source of the water and sodium being the extracellular fluid; if severe enough, this leads to a bodily disturbance characterised by circulatory disturbances but not by thirst.

The confusion associated with the term dehydration has been increased by each new classification of the disturbance which has appeared. Marriott (1947) wisely suggested that the best solution might be to drop the use of the word 'dehydration', and instead to speak in terms of such causes of disturbance as water depletion, salt depletion or combined water and salt depletion. Pure water depletion corresponds to 'primary' or 'simple' dehydration and affects chiefly, though not always entirely, the intracellular fluid. Pure salt depletion corresponds to 'secondary' or 'extracellular' dehydration and indicates a reduction in the volume of extracellular fluid. In the succeeding years as, our knowledge of these disturbances has increased, it has been recognised that sodium depletion is the most important factor in what was formerly called salt depletion (Table VII).

The effects of deprivation of water on normal subjects were described by Nadal *et al.* (1941): when the intake of food and water was stopped for three days the body weight fell steadily; the daily urine volume fell to about 600 ml, but its specific gravity rose to about 1036 (1250 mosmol per litre). There was no change in the concentration of sodium in the plasma or in the packed cell volume, but the plasma non-protein nitrogen content rose, the mouth and throat became very dry and thirst was intense. When water was given, recovery was rapid, the weight rose, there was a diuresis and the urine specific gravity and the plasma non-protein nitrogen concentration fell. The excretion of sodium in the urine fell while the intake of food and water was stopped, but that of potassium continued unchanged. Nadal *et al.* (1941) also produced sodium depletion in two normal subjects by duodenal suction with a Miller-Abbott tube; the intake of food was stopped but they were allowed to drink water freely, and water was also given as glucose solution by intravenous infusion. In three days weight loss amounted to 6 and 8 per cent of body weight in the two subjects respectively, and more than 8 g (348 mEq) of sodium were removed by suction. The serum concentrations of sodium and chloride fell, the packed

TABLE VIII

Classification of dehydration

Pure 'water depletion'	='primary' or 'simple' dehydration affects chiefly intracellular fluid ∴mainly potassium and water lost THIRST OLIGURIA
Pure 'salt depletion'	='secondary' or 'extracellular' dehydration affects chiefly extracellular fluid ∴mainly sodium and water lost CIRCULATORY DISTURBANCES

cell volume and plasma protein concentration rose, but the urine volume remained high at an average of 1430 ml per day. Towards the end of the period of suction both subjects became weak and apathetic, they fainted when they sat up and the systolic blood pressure was only 85 mmHg. There was marked loss of appetite, but they were not thirsty and did not want to drink water when it was offered to them. No change followed the stoppage of suction, but the intravenous infusion of Ringer's solution produced rapid recovery.

Thus, true water lack or loss causes oliguria but may not alter the concentration of sodium in the blood or cause haemoconcentration. The initial hypertonicity of extracellular fluid due to the insensible loss of water leads to the shift of water from the cells and so spreads the disturbance more widely over the body water. Sodium is well conserved by the kidneys and, in the absence of large losses by any other route, this preserves the body content of sodium and maintains the volume of the extracellular fluid. The continued excretion of potassium at an unchanged rate in the urine indicates a loss of cation as an accompaniment to the loss of water. When sodium loss occurs, if the water intake is adequate, there is no thirst and the daily urinary volume is maintained. These experiments show clearly, however, that the loss of sodium cannot be compensated for simply by an intake of water, but leads to a serious reduction in extracellular fluid and plasma volume. The reduction in plasma volume is directly proportional to the reduction in extracellular fluid volume and is indicated by changes in packed cell volume. The plasma volume is not preferentially maintained at the expense of interstitial fluid since the capillaries are freely permeable to sodium and to water.

These experiments have a very important bearing on much current clinical practice. It is all too common for patients to be allowed to drink water, sometimes without any limitation, while their stomach contents are regularly aspirated. This drinking stimulates gastric secretion containing sodium which is then aspirated and so leads to the unnecessary loss of sodium from the body. The volume of fluid aspirated from the stomach in such circumstances bears a close relationship to the quantity of water which is drunk.

That more patients do not suffer ill-effects from this type of treatment is due to their initially good physical state and normal sodium content before operation. The volume of urine produced per day does not indicate in any way the state of sodium balance in the body, or the adequacy of treatment, except so far as concerns water intake. When water is supplied, urine is excreted freely unless the continued extrarenal loss of sodium causes a critical reduction in extracellular fluid volume, blood pressure falls and glomerular filtration is reduced. In water lack the urinary volume is frequently lowest on the first day of deprivation and is not a good index of the degree of water loss. Continued use of gastric aspiration after operation has been justified by many surgeons on the grounds that any sodium which is removed in the aspirations is replaced by the intravenous infusion of isotonic saline. During any period of aspiration which is really necessary because of accumulation of fluid and blood in the gastric remnant, restriction of drinking will reduce the volume of fluid lost to small quantities which do not require replacement by saline infusions. The relief of postoperative thirst is another problem which has already been discussed (see p. 25).

The confusing effects of apparently simple disturbances, and the complications introduced by equally simple remedies, are well illustrated by the effects of excessive sweating. The sodium and chloride concentrations in sweat vary, but, except in fibrocystic disease, are seldom more than half their concentrations in extracellular fluid and may be very low. Sweat therefore removes more water than sodium or chloride, and a single period of sweating leads to a disturbance dominated by the features of water loss. When there are repeated losses of sweat, and these are consistently replaced by water without the addition of any sodium, the accumulated small daily unreplaced sodium losses lead to sodium deficiency, and this may be aggravated by the dilution superimposed by drinking water. Repeated sweating, by causing sufficiently large loss of sodium, thus leads to circulatory collapse instead of simple water depletion. The close resemblance of 'heat exhaustion' and the sodium depletion induced by gastric aspiration combined with the free consumption of water, and the chances of a combination of these effects in surgical patients in hot climates, are evident. Water depletion results from the restriction or stoppage of water intake or when, following the loss of gastric and intestinal secretions, the replacement of sodium is adequate and that of water is not. Sodium depletion results when both sodium and water are lost and water alone is adequately replaced.

The clinical picture of sodium depletion depends first on the rate at which sodium is lost and only secondly on the total quantity which is lost. Slow losses of up to 250 mEq by unaccustomed sweating or dietary restriction may diminsh energy and appetite. From 250 to 500 mEq may be lost acutely in gastrointestinal secretions by vomiting or gastric aspiration and may cause some circulatory disturbance. Large losses of up to 1500 mEq may be due to repeated vomiting or diarrhoea or fluid loss from an alimentary fistula, and will cause severe or even fatal circulatory disturbances.

Sodium Depletion

By far the most important form of sodium depletion in surgical practice is that caused by the rapid loss of large volumes of intestinal secretion, for example in association with acute obstruction high in the small intestine. The lost secretions are initially derived from the blood plasma, which is replenished from the interstitial fluid. The composition of the secretions which may be lost is shown in Table IX, but in acute losses of large volumes the important disturbance is the large reduction in sodium and water which leads to a depletion of extracellular fluid volume. The best and most severe example of such loss is that associated with Asiatic cholera, but very rapid

TABLE IX

Composition of intestinal secretions (mEq/litre)

Secretion	*Na+*	*K+*	*Mg++*	*Cl−*	*HCO₃−*	*Volume per 24 hours (ml)*
Saliva	15	40				1500
Gastric	50	10	1·5	80		2500
Intestinal	140	10		100	25	3000
Biliary	140	5	2·0	100	30	500
Pancreatic	140	5	1·0	70	120	700
Ileostomy:						
New	125	22	6·0	110	30	300
Established	50	5		20	25	450
Cf. plasma	140	5	1·9	103	25	

reduction of extracellular fluid volume also occurs in acute dilatation of the stomach, acute obstruction of the small intestine, from fistulas of the small intestine, in enterocolitis or from an ileostomy. Less rapid but equally severe loss may follow repeated gastric aspiration after partial gastrectomy.

Reduction in sodium intake is rarely the cause of sodium depletion in normal people because renal conservation of sodium is so effective. A low sodium intake may be an important contributory factor in fever, or in patients who for prolonged periods lose sodium in discharges from extensive wounds or granulating surfaces. The combination of a low sodium diet with the use of mercurial diuretics is dangerous in liver and cardiac disease and in ulcerative colitis with oedema, and is liable to cause acute sodium deficiency. In chronic loss of sodium the sequence of events may be obscured and the onset of clinical disturbances may be delayed by the mobilisation of sodium from bone. Chronic sodium loss also causes more complete reabsorption of sodium by the renal tubules and the urinary output of sodium falls. In sodium depletion of normal subjects, McCance (1936) found the sodium deficit was at first parallel to the weight loss, indicating the maintenance of the sodium concentration in extracellular fluid at the expense of the volume of that fluid. Later the loss of weight was slower than that of sodium, indicating that extracellular fluid volume was being maintained at the expense of extracellular sodium concentration.

Clinical Features

The loss of sodium and water reduces the volume of extracellular fluid and plasma volume, but direct measurement of these reductions is not always practicable and diagnosis depends on observations of the characteristic clinical features. A detailed history of the nature and quantity of fluid lost is of first importance. The reduced plasma volume is accompanied by increases in plasma protein and haemoglobin concentrations, and in packed cell volume and blood viscosity, which may mask pre-existing anaemia or reduction in plasma protein concentration. Peripheral vasoconstriction compensates for reduction in the circulating volume of blood, but the systolic and diastolic blood pressures may be lowered and the pulse rate may be fast. The peripheral veins are small and constricted and poorly filled with sluggishly flowing dark blood. The tongue is dry, hard and reddish brown in colour, but the patient is usually not thirsty. The eyes are sunken in deep dark sockets, the face is drawn and the expression may be anxious. The skin is wrinkled and dry and the subcutaneous tissues feel lax. The patient often appears to have aged by many years in a few hours. The urine is scanty, dark in colour and of high specific gravity. This is the state frequently called 'dehydration', but it is most important to recognise that it is due to the loss of extracellular fluid and in particular of sodium and water.

The chemical changes in the blood are subject to wide variation and are seldom of much immediate value in determining treatment, but may be of assistance later in judging the success of treatment. The plasma sodium concentration may not be altered by an acute loss of intestinal secretions, and the body deficit of sodium may become obvious only when lost fluid is replaced with solutions containing small concentrations of sodium. The plasma concentrations of chloride and bicarbonate should be measured, as well as that of sodium, since the losses of these radicles vary according to the level in the alimentary tract which is involved.

Treatment

No matter what the cause, the first step in the treatment of severe extracellular dehydration must be to ensure survival by immediately restoring the circulating blood volume by the rapid infusion of 0·9 per cent saline.

As soon as possible the fluid loss must be stopped or reduced to a safe rate, if necessary by operation. It is often difficult to decide how much of the fluid loss should be replaced before operative treatment is carried out, and to a large extent this must depend on individual circumstances. In acute intestinal obstruction the bowel above the point of obstruction is usually distended and inflamed. When circulating volume is restored by the rapid injection of saline, there is often a visible and measurable increase in abdominal distension. This is due to the rapid loss of much of the saline into the lumen of the inflamed obstructed bowel, and the resulting increase in intestinal contents hampers subsequent operative manipulations of the bowel. In most cases of acute intestinal obstruction restoration of the circulating blood volume is all that should be done before operation. The management of more chronic losses of intestinal secretions involves consideration of losses of potassium, chloride and bicarbonate, and is dealt with in detail later (see p. 97).

When operation is not required, treatment should be directed to replacing the lost fluid as accurately as possible. The most important part is the replacement of sodium and water, and ideally this should be accompanied by appropriate proportions of anions. In general, however, acute losses can be satisfactorily replaced by 0·9 per cent saline, and provided renal function is satisfactory and the water intake is adequate, renal compensation will remove any excess of chloride which is administered. In controlling such replacement the best guide is its effect on the general state of the patient and the subsidence of the clinical features which have been described The most valuable indications are the systolic and diastolic blood pressures, the filling of the peripheral veins, the state of the peripheral circulation in the finger tips and nail beds as indicated by the quality and the rate of return of colour after compression, and the packed cell volume.

It has been suggested that the fluid requirements can be calculated from the alteration in plasma specific gravity, packed cell volume or haemoglobin concentration (Phillips *et al.*, 1950). It is probably wiser, however, to judge the volume of fluid directly from the response which is obtained in the individual patient rather than to administer an arbitrarily calculated volume which does not allow for variation in fatness and lean tissue mass. It is unwise to try to judge the quantity of sodium or chloride which should be administered from the combination of measurements of their concentrations in the plasma and estimates of the normal extracellular fluid volume of the patient calculated from body weight. The concentration of these ions in extracellular fluid is preserved by several mechanisms at the expense of the volume of the extracellular fluid, and an altered concentration is of most value as an indication either of failure of these compensatory mechanisms or of dilution by excessive administration of water. The degree to which movement of sodium out of bone compensates for losses of sodium from extracellular fluid is unknown. The large quantity of exchangeable, and therefore available, bone sodium and the surprising constancy of extracellular fluid sodium concentration in spite of large losses of sodium in intestinal secretions, suggests that bone sodium is an important second line of defence in the maintenance of the constancy of the composition of the extracellular fluid.

Water Intoxication

The wider recognition of the sodium retention which normally occurs during the early postoperative period led to a tendency to administer isotonic glucose solutions instead of saline at this time. Even this is not without danger because, during the first week after operation, the excretion of water is slower than normal, and when large volumes of glucose solution are injected rapidly a large proportion of the injected water may be retained and may cause a state of water intoxication. This adverse effect of the excessive administration of water is not confined to surgical patients. In chronic disturbances the concentration of sodium may be much more markedly depressed than in water intoxication, without causing any obvious ill-effects. Water intoxication has been described after rectal administration of water (de Takats, 1931) and after excessive drinking of water in the immediate postoperative period. A similar disturbance may follow when sodium depletion by vomiting or diarrhoea is treated by infusions of sodium-free solutions or when vomiting patients are allowed to drink water too freely (salt depletion syndrome: Peters, 1948). It may also follow the administration of dried plasma which has been reconstituted with an excessive volume of water. In cardiac disease it may be associated with the use of mercurial diuretics and a low salt diet combined with an excessive fluid intake (low salt syndrome: Schroeder, 1949). The rate at which water is consumed or injected seems to be the critical factor in causing a rapid dilution of the extracellular fluid and its sodium concentration, especially when combined with an inability of the kidneys to remove the added water by a rapid diuresis.

Clinical Features

This disturbance may occur without sodium loss, especially if water intake is rapid. It is commoner after the age of 50 years and when renal function is impaired; it has also been observed in the neonatal period in severe infections and after operation. There may be a gain in body weight at a time when normally weight would be lost. Symptoms and signs usually appear within 48 hours, often after only 24 hours, and may follow the administration of as little as 3 or 4 litres of glucose solution to an adult in 24 hours (Zimmermann and Wangensteen, 1952). In the early stages there are anorexia, weakness and apathy; later there may be nausea and vomiting or diarrhoea, rapid and stertorous respiration, mental confusion and irritability, twitching of the limbs, epileptiform seizures and coma which may last an hour or two or for days. There are no constant neurological disturbances, but amnesia is usual. The plasma sodium, bicarbonate and chloride concentrations are depressed, potassium also is usually reduced, but may be high when renal function is severely affected; the hemoglobin and plasma protein concentrations and packed cell volume are markedly lowered. At first there is a diuresis and a large volume of dilute urine is passed, but this is followed by oliguria or even anuria, and sweating stops. Oedema is not common and is often most noticeable in the eyelids (Brown *et al.*, 1943).

Diagnosis

The recognition of water intoxication depends mainly on being aware that it may occur, for example when water is being administered by intravenous infusion especially after operation, or when the bowel has been repeatedly washed out. Sudden alteration in behaviour or onset of coma should always arouse suspicion, especially in patients who may have previously suffered sodium depletion. The serum sodium concentration is not always reduced but if it is the slow injection of up to 50 ml of hypertonic saline (5·85 per cent) may produce a remarkable improvement and confirmation of the diagnosis.

Treatment

During spontaneous recovery the waterlogged patient may lie in an irritable confused state for a week or more, while the excess water is removed by vaporisation and excreted as urine; recovery is slow when urinary excretion is reduced by functional changes in the kidneys and may then be accelerated by the intravenous injection of hypertonic saline (5·85 per cent). Only a small volume (200 to

400 ml) should be slowly administered and the injection should be stopped as soon as symptoms are relieved, if urinary output increases before all the fluid has been given or when the serum sodium concentration reaches 130 mEq litre. A too rapid injection of hypertonic saline may cause sudden cardiac arrest or circulatory over loading. It is thought that hypertonic saline acts by increasing the extracellular sodium concentration, thus restoring the original cation equilibrium at the cell membrane and leading to the extrusion of water from the cells and to the restoration of normal water equilibrium and cellular function.

Oedema

There is now some support for the belief that the water of the interstitial fluid and of connective tissue is normally in the gel phase of a gel–sol state. If this normal interstitial gel structure becomes supersaturated, the breaking up of the gel phase to a sol leads to the appearance of recognisable pitting oedema. This idea of a gel–sol structure in the interstitial fluid may seem to impose a limitation on the free movement of fluid in this area; this is likely to be apparent rather than real because changes in saturation are constant and lead to the undetectable but repeated breaking up and reformation of the gell on a minute individual scale but in a vast number of places.

In oedema there is usually also an accumulation of an abnormally large amount of fluid in the tissue spaces which may be due to various disturbances of the mechanism of fluid exchange Oedema may appear when the movement of fluid into the interstitial space exceeds the removal of this fluid back into the venous capillaries or or by the lymph channels; or it may be due to the widespread blockage of lymph channels. It is often difficult to explain the occurrence of oedema in surgical patients. Low concentration of the plasma proteins, especially of albumin, should always be considered; this may be the result of malnutrition before operation, or of protein depletion by prolonged losses of exudate from extensive granulating surfaces after burns or other injuries, from large abscess cavities or from the alimentary tract in protein-losing enteropathy (Dawson, 1965). Reduction in plasma protein concentration may also be due to dilution of the protein by an increase in extracellular fluid volume. This is often due to an increase in the quantity of sodium in the body accompanied by water retention, without alteration in the extracellular sodium concentration .

Retention of sodium may be caused by inadequate renal function following renal disease or by the administration of steroids. It may also, and more commonly, be due to the excessive administration of saline during the immediate postoperative period, when the renal excretion of administered sodium is delayed by the normal post-traumatic conservation of sodium. Stewart and Rourke (1942) found that after even minor gynaecological operations there was retention of a large proportion of the sodium administered intravenously as saline, with expansion of the extracellular fluid volume and reduction in the plasma protein concentration. Moyer *et al.* (1947) studied the effects of the rapid intravenous infusion of large volumes of isotonic glucose solution and saline in two normal men. Five per cent glucose solution equal in volume to 1 per cent of body weight was infused at a rate of 740 or 800 ml per hour; within three hours the rate of excretion exceeded the rate of infusion, which lasted for five hours; a volume of urine equal to the total volume infused had been excreted within one hour of stopping the infusion. When similar quantities of saline were administered to the same subjects, the urine flow rose slowly to a peak of 200 to 300 ml per hour at two hours, and then fell towards the initial rate; at the end of the infusion 75 per cent of the infused volume had not been excreted.

So-called 'starvation oedema' may occasionally be found in surgical patients, especially in those with slowly progressive obstructions of the oesophagus or intestines, or ulcerative colitis; in the latter disease it may be exaggerated by treatment with steroids. It is due to the close conservation of sodium by the kidneys with consequent maintenance of a nearly normal total body content of sodium and volume of extracellular fluid in spite of large reductions in cell mass due to starvation and disease.

Excessive accumulation of extracellular fluid does not always cause recognisable oedema; large quantities of fluid may accumulate before there is pitting on pressure even in dependent parts such as the sacral region, the scrotum, or the feet and legs. Crepitations in the basal regions of the lungs are probably more often due to retention of bronchial secretions than to hydrostatic oedema of the lungs. Provision must be made for the continuing insensible loss of water and for urine formation. It is important to remember that although oedematous patients have an excessive quantity of extracellular fluid, they may at the same time be losing intracellular fluid and potassium. The intracellular dehydration causes thirst and a dry tongue; sufficient water to relieve thirst should always be provided.

This water is unlikely to increase the oedema which is due to retention of sodium, but by maintaining urinary output will help to remove sodium if this is within the capacity of the kidneys. Sodium excretion may also be promoted by the use of a mercurial diuretic. The intake of sodium should be reduced, but the value of a low sodium diet is doubtful, especially in convalescent surgical patients; this diet is tasteless and many patients find it unattractive and difficult to consume. The resulting inadequate calorie intake prolongs the catabolism of protein tissues and accentuates existing protein deficiency. Some reduction in body sodium content may be achieved by the use of a resin in the ammonium and potassium cycle but this may cause depletion of calcium, iron or magnesium. The mercurial diuretics given by intramuscular injection are rapid and effective but should be combined with the administration of potassium chloride to prevent alkalosis or potassium depletion. For long-term use one of the thiazide drugs is probably preferable.

CHAPTER THREE

Potassium

NORMAL CONTENT AND DISTRIBUTION

Nearly 98 per cent (3360 mEq) of the 130 g potassium in the body is in the cells, three-quarters in the skeletal muscles, and only about 2 per cent of the total (60 mEq) in the extracellular fluid. Whereas sodium forms 90 per cent of the total cations of the extracellular fluid, potassium, although the predominant cation of intracellular fluid, accounts for only two-thirds of the total active intracellular cations, the remainder being magnesium (Fig. 3). For many years potassium has been used in metabolic experiments as an index of change in intracellular fluid volume.

INTAKE AND OUTPUT

Each day a healthy adult consumes about 2 to 3 g (52 to 78 mEq) of potassium and about 2 to 3 g are excreted in the urine and a very small quantity in the faeces and sweat. In addition, from 2 to 5 g (52 to 130 mEq) are secreted into and reabsorbed from the alimentary tract every day (Table X).

TABLE X

The daily potassium cycle

Consumed in ordinary diet	2 to 3 g (52 to 78 mEq)
Excreted in urine	2 to 3 g (52 to 78 mEq)
Secreted into and reabsorbed from gastro-intestinal tract	2 to 5 g (52 to 130 mEq)
Lost in sweat	trace
Lost in faeces	less than 10 mEq

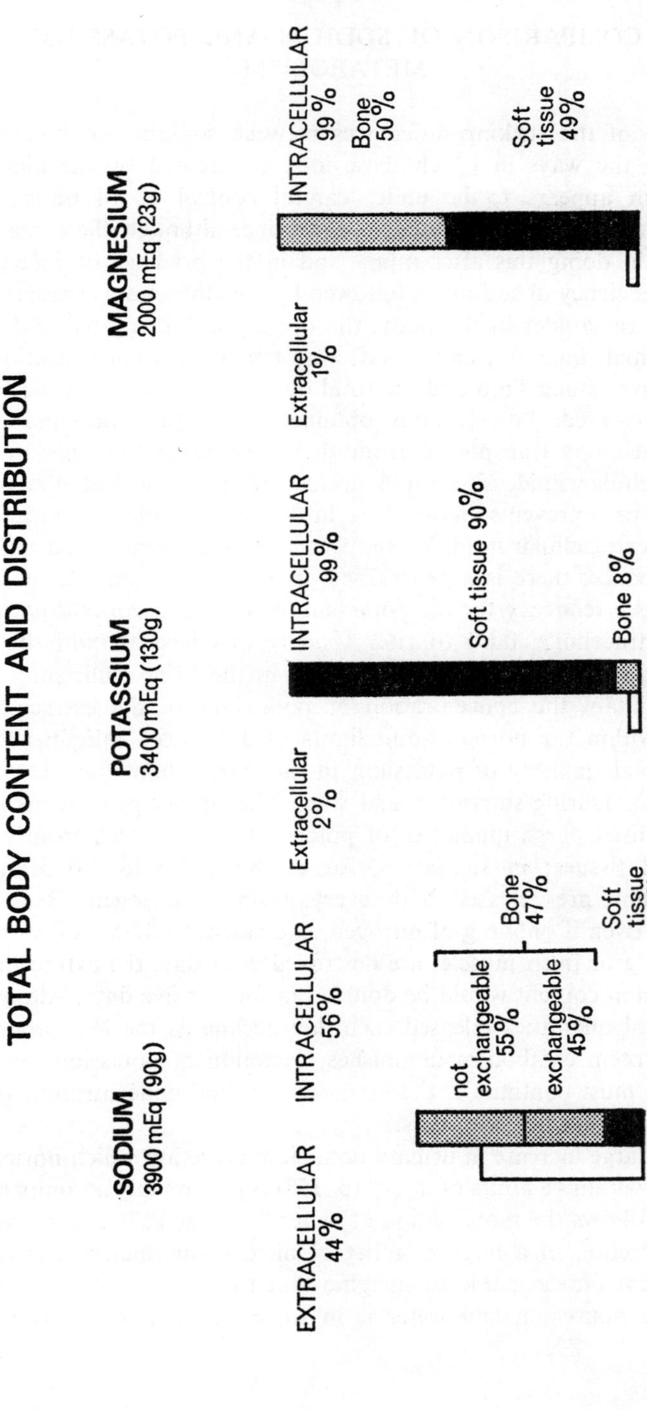

FIGURE 3. Comparison of distribution of sodium, potassium and magnesium.

COMPARISON OF SODIUM AND POTASSIUM METABOLISM

One of the striking differences between sodium and potassium lies in the ways in which these ions are treated by the kidneys. Sodium appears to be under careful control at all times; any excess of intake is excreted in the urine, although there may be delay in doing this after injury and in the presence of infection; any deficiency of sodium is followed by the close renal conservation of the remainder in the body, the urinary loss being reduced to a very small quantity, and in this way the sodium concentration in the extracellular fluid and the total quantity of sodium in the body are preserved. Potassium is obtained from the food, and after absorption is transported from the intestine to the cells by the extracellular fluid. The rapid uptake of this absorbed potassium by the cells prevents any increase in the concentration of potassium in the extracellular fluid. When, because of some generalised cellular disturbance, there is a generalised shift of potassium out of cells, there is a tendency for the potassium content and concentration of the extracellular fluid to rise. Usually this is dealt with by the kidneys, which excrete the potassium in the urine sufficiently fast to maintain the concentration of potassium in the extracellular fluid within the normal adult limits of 3·8 to 5·1 mEq per litre. The total quantity of potassium in the extracellular fluid is about 60 mEq. During starvation and when after injury protein tissue is catabolised, large quantities of potassium are released from catabolised tissues; in starvation, for example, 2·5 to 3·0 mEq of potassium are released with every gram of nitrogen (Benedict, 1915). Even if only 6 g of nitrogen, equivalent to 37·5 g of protein, or 180 g of fresh muscle, are destroyed each day, the extracellular potassium content would be doubled in four or five days. Although the total quantities released each day decline as the fast proceeds and protein catabolism diminishes, excretion of potassium by the kidney must continue if the extracellular fluid concentration is to be kept within normal limits.

The large increase in urinary potassium excretion which normally occurs within 48 hours of injury (p. 158) is presumably accompanied by or follows the mobilisation of water from the cells and precedes the excretion of a large quantity of nitrogenous material. It does not seem unreasonable to imagine that this large mobilisation of cellular potassium and water is in some way connected with the capacity of the organism to survive injury without external aid, especially as this response to injury is not modified by the administration of water. Yet survival also depends on the ability of the kidneys to conserve sodium and thus preserve a sufficient volume of extracellular fluid to allow the transport of oxygen and sources of energy to the cells and the removal of the products of cellular metabolism and destruction. In patients with anuria the accumulation of potassium in the extracellular fluid raises its concentration to a toxic level, which is probably the commonest cause of death in this condition. Thus survival depends jointly on the ability of the kidneys to conserve sodium and to excrete potassium. Because of this continuing loss of potassium in the urine, the body content of potassium falls when the intake is reduced or stopped by starvation or restriction of the diet, or by vomiting, and also when the output is largely increased by the loss of intestinal secretions. Potassium excretion in the urine is increased by the administration of ACTH, cortisone, desoxycorticosterone, aldosterone, PAS and mercurial and other diuretics such as chlorthiazide, and by the intravenous administration of solutions containing sodium salts, glucose or ammonium chloride.

The normal daily output of potassium in the urine ranges up to 2 to 3 g (52 to 78 mEq) and is related closely to the dietary intake. It is impossible to say what proportion of the urinary potassium is derived from unabsorbed filtrate and how much is due to tubular secretion. Berliner *et al.* (1950) came to the conclusion that the excretion of potassium in the urine was largely independent of its plasma concentration and the glomerular filtration rate, which accords well with the large urinary output of potassium in high concentration so often found after even very severe injury. The independence of potassium excretion of any relationship with that of sodium can be illustrated in many ways; Stanbury and Thomson (1951) found on a rice diet that not only was potassium excretion independent of large changes in glomerular filtration rate but that the usual morning rise in potassium excretion occurred when sodium excretion was negligible. In some way the urinary excretion of potassium is related to the state of cellular economy as that of sodium is related to extracellular fluid economy.

Evidence from depletion experiments in normal subjects led Fourman (1952) to suggest that there is some renal conservation when large quantities of potassium are lost from the body. When Lowe (1953) fed to normal subjects an electrolyte-free diet consisting of 300 g glucose and 150 g arachis oil, emulsified in a total volume of one litre, and containing an adequate vitamin supplement the urinary excretion of potassium fell from 65 mEq per day to under 10 mEq per day and remained thereafter at a low level. Urinary sodium and chloride also fell, but the plasma chemistry remained within normal limits. This mixture provided an adequate intake of energy, and the low urinary urea output indicated that tissue protein was not catabolised to any great extent. It might be inferred from these results that renal conservation of potassium was good because the urinary output of potassium, like that of sodium fell markedly when the intake was reduced. It seems as reasonable to conclude, however, that since the intake of potassium was stopped and tissue catabolism was almost completely prevented by the high calorie intake, there was little potassium to be excreted. This does not mean that renal conservation of potassium is good in these circumstances but bad when, following severe injury and in the absence of a supply of calories and water, the kidneys excrete large quantities of potassium at a high concentration in the urine.

Whether potassium is excreted in the urine seems to be determined by how much there is available for excretion in the extracellular fluid; and on whether cells are shedding or retaining potassium, which depends in part on the events to which the body has recently been subjected and their effect on cellular and whole body metabolism. Restriction of water intake does not alter the total daily requirements of water for insensible loss, although it does affect urinary volumes. At least part of the obligatory water expenditure is derived from intracellular fluid and may lead to the mobilisation of potassium from the cells and to its transfer to the extracellular fluid before it is excreted in the urine.

Starvation for food leads to catabolism of tissue protein and fat to provide energy for continuing metabolism. Injury induces a complex chain of circumstances which include tissue catabolism whether food is supplied or not. Tissue catabolism releases potassium from cells into extracellular fluid. Clearly it must be an important function of the kidneys to get rid of potassium from the body when there is any tendency for the potassium content of the extracellular fluid to rise. The rate of urinary excretion of potassium seems to depend partly on the effect of external agencies (injury, starvation, water restriction) on cellular and whole body economy, and partly on the efficiency with which the kidneys can maintain the extracellular fluid as an environment fit for cells to live in; if these views are sound, then the term conservation cannot be applied to the renal treatment of potassium in the same sense as for sodium.

Because the measurement of the total body content of potassium with ^{42}K or by whole body counting is seldom possible it has been suggested that the potassium content of the red blood corpuscle would serve as an index of the intracellular potassium; however, the red cell potassium content does not reflect the general cell state, and under circumstances of acute alteration in potassium content change in the red cells lags behind the rest of the body (Corsa *et al.*, 1950). The potassium content of skeletal muscle biopsies can be readily measured, but it is necessary to apply corrections for the quantity of extracellular fluid in the muscle; this is most difficult and unreliable in just those circumstances of body fluid disorder in which the estimation would be of most value. It is possible to compared the potassium and sodium contents of fat-free dried biopsy specimens of skeletal muscle with those of normal muscle and so to get some idea of whether the values lie within the normal limits and ratios, but the total body content of potassium cannot be measured in this way. The only really practicable means of measuring potassium deficiency is by measuring the degree of retention of administered potassium when a deficiency is being replaced. In this connection it is well known that during the administration of potassium salts after depletion the urinary output of potassium may not rise and may even fall, in spite of an elevation in the potassium concentration of the plasma.

PLASMA POTASSIUM CONCENTRATION

The normal range of potassium concentration in the plasma is from 3·8 to 5·1 mEq per litre and values of less than 3·5 mEq or more than 7 mEq per litre are usually considered to be abnormal. The concentration at a particular moment depends on the rate at which potassium is being mobilised from or deposited in cells or excreted in the urine, and also on changes in the volume of the extracellular fluid. Although the total body content is normal, the serum potassium concentration may be reduced when the extracellular fluid volume is rapidly increased by intravenous infusions, or by the rapid deposition of glycogen after the administration of glucose and insulin, or in patients who are being treated with adrenal cortical hormones and are excreting potassium in the urine more rapidly than it is being mobilised from the cells. The serum potassium concentration may be raised in spite of a large body deficit of potassium when the extracellular fluid volume is reduced, especially if renal function is impaired or the output of urine is reduced. Persistent depression of the serum concentration is usually a feature of severe and prolonged potassium deficiency, whereas elevation of the concentration is most often found in association with renal failure or anuria.

The interpretation of the serum potassium concentration is difficult. The typical 70 kg adult male with a total potassium content of 3400 mEq would have only 60 mEq of potassium in his 12 litres of extracellular fluid and 15 mEq in 3 litres of plasma (equivalent to the potassium in only 1·2 g potassium chloride). The plasma concentration can be raised by 50 per cent from 5 to 7·5 mEq per litre by altering the distribution of only 30 mEq of potassium, less than 1 per cent of the total body content and roughly equivalent to the potassium content of half a pound of beef. When an abnormal serum concentration is found, the measurement should be repeated and the daily intake and urinary and other outputs or losses of potassium should be measured, and if possible sodium and water exchanges also should be measured. When it has been possible in adults to measure the total exchangeable potassium by the isotope dilution method, deficiencies of up to 1000 mEq of potassium, one-third of the normal body content, have been found in chronic malnutrition and in prolonged pyloric stenosis; such huge deficiencies are not always accompanied by low serum potassium concentrations. In children suffering from severe malnutrition Garrow (1965) found by whole body counting, that the deficit of potassium might be as much as 40 per cent of the normal total body content.

POTASSIUM DEFICIENCY

The maintenance of a normal content of potassium in the body depends on the steady daily intake of a sufficient quantity of potassium in food. Because the kidneys do not deal with potassium in the same way as sodium, excretion of potassium in the urine continues under all circumstances save anuria, and when the intake of food is restricted or ceases this continuing urinary loss leads to slow depletion of the body content of potassium.

Types of Potassium Loss

Broadly speaking, there are two main modes of loss of potassium from the body:

1. *Proportionate loss of potassium and nitrogen occurs* in starvation without restriction of water intake. As the result of the catabolism of protein tissue, potassium and nitrogen are excreted in the urine in proportions closely resembling those in which they are found in a typical protein such as skeletal muscle (2·5 to 3·0 mEq potassium per gram of nitrogen). In recovery from starvation, nitrogen and potassium are retained in the body in the same proportions.

2. *Disproportionate loss of potassium in comparison with nitrogen* occurs in intracellular dehydration. This consists in the outward movement of potassium and water from the cell into the extracellular fluid and then into the plasma, from which potassium is excreted in the urine. The result is a loss of water and potassium from the body. This type of loss provides a means of supplying limited quantities of water for various purposes. Gamble (1954) has shown that when the intake of water as well as of food is stopped, within 48 to 72 hours renal conservation reduces to a very low level the urinary loss of sodium and thus of extracellular fluid, and thereafter the main endogenous source of water is the intracellular fluid, as is shown by the steady excretion of potassium in the urine. A disproportionate loss of potassium also occurs when gastrointestinal secretions are lost from the body, and this type of fluid loss also leads to intracellular dehydration.

The intravenous administration of 0·9 per cent saline or of 5 per cent glucose solution, even to normal subjects, leads to an increased output of potassium in the urine; the administration of these fluids to surgical patients is an important factor in increasing potassium depletion. When a large volume of glucose solution is rapidly infused, the resulting water diuresis usually continues longer than is necessary to excrete all the added water, and some degree of water depletion occurs; this in turn leads to the movement of water out of cells with the transfer of potassium from cells to extracellular fluid. When saline is infused, it makes little contribution to the water requirements of the body, since even normal kidneys can concentrate sodium and free water from it only to a limited extent; water is then obtained by the mobilisation of intracellular fluid with excretion of potassium in the urine.

The concentration of potassium in the gastrointestinal secretions may be up to twice that in the plasma, whereas the concentration of sodium never exceeds and may be less than that in plasma. In acute losses of gastrointestinal secretions the lost fluid resembles in composition and is derived from the plasma and extracellular fluid, but usually contains more potassium than these fluids. This loss of potassium is replenished from the intracellular fluid. In acute losses of short duration, because of the low extracellular fluid concentration of potassium, only about 4 per cent of the total body potassium may be lost, but up to 25 per cent of the total available extraskeletal sodium may be lost as well as an unknown quantity from the bones. In the treatment of such acute losses of gastro-intestinal fluids the initial emphasis is rightly on the replacement of extracellular fluid, and is satisfactorily achieved by the intravenous administration of sodium and water as 0·9 per cent saline. Provided that the consumption of a normal diet is then resumed, the relatively small loss of potassium will be made good from dietary potassium. However, when there is prolonged vomiting with restricted food intake, or when in gastroenteritis there is loss by vomiting and in fluid stools together with restriction of intake, the losses of potassium are repeated. There may be replacement of the sodium and water by saline infusion, but if potassium is not also replaced the total loss may eventually amount to as much as 25 per cent of the original potassium content of the body. The importance of replacing this potassium loss was first shown by Darrow (1946). By adding the administration of potassium chloride to the previous treatment he reduced the mortality in infants suffering from gastroenteritis from 17 deaths in 53 patients to only 3 in 50 patients. He showed also, by carrying out nitrogen and potassium balance estimations during treatment and the recovery period, that these young children retained more potassium than would have been expected from the nitrogen balance. This means that more potassium was retained in the body than the quantity required in combination with nitrogen (2·5 to 3·0 mEq potassium per gram of nitrogen) to reform the catabolised tissue protein. In other words, potassium lost in the intestinal secretions during the period of vomiting and diarrhoea, and in the urine, was derived from intracellular fluid. Only very small quantities of potassium and sodium are lost in normal formed stools and usually more potassium than sodium is lost. Darrow found that in watery stools the loss of both sodium and potassium was large and that that of sodium was the greater.

Darrow and his colleagues (Darrow and Pratt, 1950; Cooke

et al., 1952) have produced evidence that when potassium is lost from the cells it is replaced in part by sodium and hydrogen ions in the proportion of two sodium ions and one hydrogen ion for three potassium ions. When potassium is replaced in the cells, the sodium and hydrogen ions are equivalently displaced by the potassium. This substitution of sodium and hydrogen for intracellular potassium reduces the otherwise great disturbance in cellular function which would result from the loss of up to 25 per cent of the body potassium and its associated water from the cells, but does not entirely prevent distortion of the normal equilibrium between intracellular and extracellular fluid. At the same time the transfer of sodium into the cells may reduce the total extracellular cation and the volume of extracellular fluid, especially if the intake of sodium is restricted or the output or loss is excessive. The shift of hydrogen ion from extracellular to intracellular fluid leads to an extracellular alkalosis and intracellular acidosis which are corrected only when the primary disturbance, the loss of potassium from the cells, is overcome by the replenishment of the body content of potassium. This alteration in the content and distribution in the body of both sodium and potassium causes disturbances of function which it is probably wrong to ascribe particularly to the primary loss of potassium although it is probably correct to emphasise the potassium factor in the design of suitable treatment.

Causes of Potassium Deficiency

In the production of potassium deficiency in surgical patients, any or all of the following factors may be concerned:

1. Restriction or stoppage of intake of food, with cessation of potassium intake combined with continued loss of potassium in the urine;

2. Proportionate loss with nitrogen and other constituents of cellular protoplasm due to tissue catabolism because of starvation or in response to injury;

3. Disproportionate loss (*a*) from cells due to intracellular fluid loss because of inadequate water intake; (*b*) in gastrointestinal secretions by vomiting, diarrhoea or in fluid lost from intestinal fistula.

Clinical Features of Potassium Deficiency

Apart from the continuing daily loss of potassium in the urine, the losses of potassium in intestinal secretions are small compared with those of sodium and water. There is therefore in most cases of severe potassium deficiency a long history of loss of secretions, and this is by far the most important stimulus of the suspicions which lead to accurate diagnosis. The clinical picture varies greatly and is commonly obscured by associated disturbances of sodium and water. Black (1953) voiced a widely held opinion when he said that many of the symptoms of potassium deficiency may be found in any severe prolonged illness, and this may be because any severe prolonged illness may cause some degree of potassium depletion. The most effective combination is severe and prolonged illness with repeated and large losses of gastrointestinal secretions.

The most striking feature of severe deficiency is the gradual onset of an intense drowsiness or even coma. The patient lies slumped in bed, the head drooping down on one shoulder and the jaw and cheeks hanging slackly; he is roused with difficulty and opens his eyes slowly and with obvious effort, blinking and screwing up his face, then, apparently too tired to go on looking, the eyelids drop and he seems to go to sleep again. Speech is slow and slurred and he may break off in the middle of a sentence. These patients are often irritable and may suffer much change in personality, but after recovery there is commonly amnesia for several days during the most severe part of the disturbance. One patient had been seen by a pyschiatrist, so prominent were the mental changes; in another, potassium deficiency was recognised after a physiotherapist had complained that the patient was always going to sleep during her exercises; a third when asked to put out her tongue did so, but drowsed away again with her tongue still protruding.

As well as such profound apathy there may be muscular weakness and rarely even neuromuscular inco-ordination. The deep reflexes may be absent. There may be difficulty in swallowing with inhalation of food or drinks. Incontinence of urine is common, perhaps because the sensation of fullness of the bladder is impaired.

Abdominal distension due to chronic ileus is a common feature of postoperative potassium deficiency, but is uncommon before operation. The potassium depletion causes diminished motility of the intestinal musculature which results in the accumulation of intestinal secretions; this in turn stimulates further secretion, and more potassium is thereby lost into the lumen of the intestine. In pyloric stenosis there is accumulation of secretions in the dilated, oedematous and hypertrophied stomach, but the intestines are usually empty and contracted. Part at least of the stenosis may be due to muscular inco-ordination or spasm of the pylorus, and although this may be due to sodium deficiency it may persist in spite of the infusion of large volumes of saline and be relieved only when potassium chloride is administered.

The peripheral blood pressure is lowered, the pulse rate is slow and the superficial veins are well filled, the skin is warm and dry, but there may be a reddish flush of the face and the backs of the hands. The blood pressure is reduced also in sodium depletion, with reduction in the extracellular fluid volume, but there is then usually acceleration of the pulse rate and the peripheral veins are poorly filled. The heart may be enlarged and there may be changes in the electrocardiographic tracing, but these vary widely and are not always present even in severe deficiency and do not seem to be closely related either to the severity of the deficiency or to the serum potassium concentration. A large number of changes have been described, including reduction in the magnitude of all waves, increased QT interval, decreased height and inversion or rounding and prolongation of T wave, depression of ST or inversion of P wave. These changes may be produced by alkalosis and changes in blood pH as well as by potassium deficiency (Nadler *et al.*, 1948). When they are due to potassium deficiency, there is usually improvement after the administration of potassium salts.

The plasma potassium concentration is not always reduced and may sometimes be raised.

Potassium-depleted patients are often very thirsty and may drink large volumes of fluid; although the osmolality of the urine is low and cannot be raised much, a water load is usually excreted promptly. It is still uncertain whether the thirst is due directly to the potassium depletion as was suggested by Welt *et al.* (1960). These functional disturbances can be related to the histological appearances of vacuolation of the epithelium of the proximal tubules. In young subjects these changes disappear when the potassium deficiency is corrected but they may persist longer in old people who have been deficient for a longer time (Schwartz and Relman, 1967). The changes they have observed in biopsies of human kidneys are similar to those first described in the kidneys of potassium-deficient rats by Schrader *et al.*, (1937).

Diagnosis of Potassium Deficiency

Potassium deficiency should be suspected and looked for whenever there has been prolonged loss of gastrointestinal secretions and severe restriction of food intake, and especially when there is severe alkalosis. In these circumstances it is also predisposed to by the intravenous administration of fluids which do not contain potassium, especially when such treatment is the only source of water and calories. The history and the clinical appearance are the most certain means of making the diagnosis; a low plasma potassium concentration and typical alterations in the electrocardiographic tracing are valuable confirmatory evidence but are seldom the only signs of deficiency, nor should great emphasis be laid on these investigations. It is important to remember that the plasma potassium concentration may be low in the absence of the characteristic symptoms and signs of deficiency, and that not all cases of severe deficiency are consistently associated with depression of the potassium concentration in the extracellular fluid. Sometimes potassium deficiency becomes evident only when fluid losses are replaced by solutions which do not contain potassium. In the resulting expansion of the volume of extracellular fluid the concentration of the depleted extracellular potassium falls from what, in the previously haemoconcentrated state of the blood, had appeared to be a normal level. In slowly advancing depletion the plasma concentration usually falls only when the total loss is very large. The very rapid loss of intestinal secretions, containing two or three times as much potassium as the extracellular fluid, may cause acute depression of the plasma potassium concentration which is rapidly restored from the cells when the fluid loss diminished or ceases. In chronic severe potassium depletion only 10 mEq or less of potassium may be excreted in the urine each day.

Treatment of Potassium Deficiency

The replacement of a large deficit of potassium involves the administration of sufficient potassium and its transfer into the depleted cells. The common coexistence of alkalosis or acidosis with potassium deficiency also requires that a suitable potassium salt should be chosen. In advanced potassium deficiency, sodium and hydrogen which have replaced the lost potassium in the cells are displaced when potassium is once more made available in sufficiently large quantities.

The proportion of the total original content of potassium which must be lost before clinical signs of deficiency arise has not been accurately estimated and probably varies to some extent in different people. It is related to the general state of nutrition and to the size of the muscle mass, which contains over 75 per cent of the total potassium in the body. The loss of 200 mEq in 2 or 3 days is well tolerated by most patients and is a common event after many major operations such as partial gastrectomy. It seems probable that, in adults, losses of up to 500 mEq (19·5 g) do not cause any ill-effects. Elkinton and Tarail (1950) concluded that the potassium deficit may range from 3·8 to 15·6 mEq per kg body weight (286 to 1092 mEq in a 70 kg patient) after loss of gastrointestinal secretions combined with a low potassium intake, and from 5·8 to 17·3 mEq per kg in infantile diarrhoea. Martin *et al.* (1951) measured the retention of potassium during replenishment of patients depleted of potassium, and concluded that in chronic types of potassium depletion the deficiency amounts to about 1000 mEq. A typical adult weighing 70 kg (11 stones) contains about 3400 mEq potassium 25 per cent of which is 850 mEq (33·15 g) potassium. The loss of a quarter of the body potassium implies the loss also of about a quarter of the intracellular water equal to about 7·5 litres. This water may be lost before or at the same time as potassium is lost but may be in part replaced by the subsequent transfer of water with sodium and hydrogen into the cells. The final result is the loss with potassium of some of the original water content of the body, although this may be masked later by the excessive retention and abnormal distribution of administered water and sodium.

Whenever possible, potassium salts should be administered by mouth because of the danger of rapid increase in potassium concentration in the extracellular fluid which is inseparable from the intravenous administration of solutions of potassium salts; this danger is particularly great when the extracellular fluid volume is reduced by rapid loss of intestinal secretions and when urine output is low. If there is peripheral circulatory failure, the blood volume must first be rapidly restored by the infusion of dextran. It may sometimes be necessary also to administer saline to restore the extracellular fluid volume in general, but in view of the known tendency of sodium to be transferred into the potassium-deficient cells, only a minimum of sodium should be given to patients who exhibit the clinical signs of potassium deficiency.

When the patient is comatose, has difficulty in swallowing or is nauseated, intravenous administration is often unavoidable, and it is fortunate that in many cases the infusion of as little as 1 g of potassium chloride (containing 13·5 mEq potassium) may lead to the recovery of consciousness; there may also be an equally rapid improvement in the mental state of irritable and drowsy patients. Because of the risk of raising the extracellular potassium concentration to a toxic level (above 7 mEq per litre) and thus causing cardiac arrest, it is essential to ensure if possible an adequate flow of urine equivalent to 500 ml per 24 hours (or 20 ml per hour). If necessary, therefore, 500 ml of 5 per cent glucose solution should be administered before the infusion of a solution of a potassium salt is started. In severe potassium depletion the kidneys are less able either to reduce the urinary sodium concentration to a very low level or to excrete promptly a large load of sodium, and especially in depletion due to loose stools, sodium replacements are more than usually liable to cause oedema.

Potassium deficiency is usually accompanied by extracellular alkalosis when the disturbance is due to vomiting or to high small intestinal fistulas, or by acidosis when it is due to diarrhoea or to a low intestinal fistula.

When alkalosis is present, potassium chloride should be employed, and provided that the urinary volume is adequate, up to 2 g (containing 27 mEq potassium) should be administered over a period of 4 hours by the intravenous route, using a solution containing 0·55 per cent potassium chloride (74 mEq per litre). Depending on the clinical state of the patient, a further 2 g potassium chloride may then be given, preceded if necessary by 500 to 1000 ml of 5 per cent glucose solution to maintain urinary volume and prevent intracellular dehydration. Alternatively, the potassium chloride may be administered dissolved in glucose solution, by having available small bottles containing a sterile 10 per cent. solution of potassium chloride, 20 ml of which are added to 500 ml of 5 per cent glucose solution. In the early stages of treatment, up to 12 g of potassium chloride (162 mEq potassium) per day, in doses of 2 g every 4 hours, may be administered orally to co-operative patients whose daily output of urine exceeds 500 ml.

When there is associated acidosis, the intravenous solution should contain sodium acetate in addition to potassium chloride; when the patient is able to swallow, potassium citrate should be administered by mouth in 2 g doses every 4 hours. Alternatively, the mixture proposed by Leonsins (1951) may be used; 1 g each of potassium bicarbonate, acetate and citrate dissolved in 8 ml of water and flavoured with fruit juice being given every 6 hours, providing 116 mEq potassium per day. In fluids for intravenous administration the potassium concentration should not exceed 70 to 80 mEq per litre, equivalent to 0·5 to 0·6 per cent solution of potassium chloride and the rate of infusion should not exceed 20 mEq potassium per hour, equivalent to 1·5 g potassium chloride per hour, which may be rather too fast to be safe in patients whose extracellular fluid volume is reduced.

The total quantity of potassium which is required to overcome the potassium deficiency in any particular patient must be judged by the individual response to treatment. The serum potassium concentration commonly falls a day or so after treatment has begun, even when saline has not been administered by infusion, and may drop to a very low level during replacement before slowly rising to within normal limits. It is usual for correction of the alkalosis to be achieved some days before potassium replacement is complete. The administration of potassium salts should be continued for at least three days after the plasma potassium concentration has returned to within normal limits, and no harm is likely to result from persisting even longer. If treatment is stopped too soon, the disturbance is liable to recur, especially after a subsequent operation. During the period of intravenous treatment up to 6 g of potassium chloride (81 mEq potassium) should be given in the first 24 hours. Up to 12 g potassium chloride per day (162 mEq potassium) in 6 doses of 2 g at intervals of 4 hours should be given by mouth until the plasma potassium concentration returns to within the normal limits; the total may then be reduced to 8 g per day (4 doses of 2 g at intervals of 6 hours) for at least another 3 days, or until a full diet is being consumed. If the patient continues to lose fluid by vomiting, fistula or diarrhoea, more prolonged intravenous administration may be needed. Such continuing losses should be stopped by suitable surgical treatment as soon as possible.

The intravenous administration of potassium salts is dangerous and should never be treated as a matter of routine. The decision to start an infusion containing an effective concentration of a potassium salt should be taken only after the most careful consideration of the history and clinical state of the patient. The quantity to be given and the rate of its administration should be stated in writing, and the infusion should be closely supervised by a house surgeon. When, for example, 2 g potassium chloride have been infused, the patient should be re-examined before more is administered. Rarely, signs of improvement may then justify cessation of intravenous administration, but usually it is necessary to give 4 to 6 g by the intravenous route. The best indication of a dangerous rise in extracellular potassium concentration is slowing of the heart and pulse rates; the solution of potassium chloride should at once be replaced by 5 per cent glucose solution. With care and close observation, serious complications can be avoided, but the risk of intravenous administration should always be borne in mind and balanced carefully against that of failing to replace sufficiently rapidly, by oral administration alone, the continuing losses of potassium.

A few patients are in such an advanced state of potassium depletion when first seen that nothing but the rapid intravenous administration of potassium can save their lives; in some of these the administration of potassium appears to be necessary to restart urine formation. On the other hand there does not seem to be any indication for the administration of potassium salts during the first week after operation. There is good evidence that for at least three days after operation the body is so constituted that the emphasis is on potassium excretion and that infusions of potassium are not of any use. There is no evidence that the administration of potassium during the first week after an operation does any good and when renal function is impaired it may be dangerous. Potassium salts should be administered only when there is a clear history of severe loss or prolonged deficiency of potassium, or in the presence of clinical signs of deficiency.

The remission of symptoms after the administration of potassium salts is not conclusive proof that they were due solely to potassium deficiency, because the restoration of the potassium content of the body has effects on other associated abnormalities such as alkalosis. The only certain way of judging when a deficit has been fully replaced is by carrying out a potassium balance study during replacement, measuring and comparing the daily intake and the output in the urine and any other losses which occur. The urinary output usually remains low until replenishment is almost complete, when it rises. When the plasma concentration of potassium is low initially it also usually remains low until replacement is nearly complete. Unless a potassium deficit is corrected before operation, the normal postoperative urinary loss of potassium may be sufficient to convert an occult into a manifest acute clinical deficiency state. When there is a history of prolonged loss of potassium it is important to try to replace as much as possible of the lost potassium before operation is undertaken. In normal circumstances potassium requirements are fully satisfied by the consumption of a good mixed diet. When only a limited diet is being consumed during convalescence from operations, severe injuries and other extensive inflammations, it is at least theoretically desirable to increase the consumption of potassium. Such well recognised 'invalid foods' as chicken and beef tea, broth, meat extracts, fruit and fruit juices are good natural sources of potassium in palatable forms; the richest natural source is black treacle. The addition of dried milk powder to soups, sauces and custards also increases their potassium content.

Drugs of the thiazide group are often used in the treatment of oedema and hypertension and are liable to cause potassium depletion. Even in the absence of obvious clinical signs of such depletion it should be suspected and treated before operation. The rapid release of potassium chloride from enteric-coated tablets may lead to intestinal ulceration, stenosis, obstruction or perforation. Tablets are now available from which the release of potassium chloride is delayed for up to 4 hours by a coating of inert wax and sugar.

Potassium Retention

In the healthy subject it appears to be impossible to increase the potassium content of the body to such a degree that the plasma potassium concentration rises above the normal limits. This depends on the ability of the kidneys rapidly to excrete excessive added potassium. Elevation of the plasma potassium concentration is not uncommon late in many diseases, and, as food intake is then often reduced or has been stopped, is due to the incomplete excretion of potassium derived from cellular breakdown; this is usually associated with severe oliguria or anuria. It may also be due to the intravenous infusion of potassium salts in excessive quantities or at too fast a rate when urinary volume is low. In many reported cases the serum sodium concentration was low. This suggests that reduction in the volume of extracellular fluid is also an important factor in raising the potassium concentration, and that although the plasma and extracellular fluid concentration of potassium may be high, the total body content may be reduced.

Clinical Features

It is difficult and perhaps not justifiable to associate any particular clinical features specifically with a raised plasma potassium concentration. Attention is focused in most cases on the condition underlying the potassium retention, for example anuria or an acute loss of extracellular fluid, and in the latter particularly the raised potassium concentration is often only an incidental discovery. In anuria, progressive increase in extracellular potassium concentration appears to be the commonest cause of death. Electrocardiographic changes are more common with a high than with a low plasma potassium concentration, and are likely to be found when this reaches 7 mEq per litre. The T wave is peaked, and the duration of the QRS complex and the P–R interval are increased. There may also be some mental confusion and apathy, sensory disturbances and weakness of the limbs. The peripheral circulation is poor with cold, pale, cyanosed skin and low blood pressure; the heart rate is slow, the beats are irregular and cardiac arrest may follow.

Treatment

Success in treatment depends first on preventing any further increase in extracellular potassium concentration, and secondly on the elimination of the accumulated potassium. If the accumulation is due to the excessive intravenous administration of potassium salts, this must be stopped, and the urinary volume and excretion of potassium promoted by the rapid infusion of 5 per cent glucose solution. When associated with oliguria due to water intoxication or sodium depletion, urinary output may be increased by the infusion of hypertonic saline. The treatment of potassium retention in anuria is discussed in detail on p. 142

CHAPTER FOUR

Magnesium

Magnesium is an important factor in the maintenance of normal contractility in muscle and excitability in neural tissue, and is necessary for the catalysis of many of the enzymic processes concerned with the storage, transfer and utilisation of energy.

The total magnesium content of the typical 70 kg adult man is about 2000 mEq (21 to 28 g or 1750 to 2333 mEq; Widdowson *et al.*, 1951) compared with 3400 mEq of potassium and 3900 mEq of sodium. About half the magnesium is in bone, nearly all the rest is in the cells of the soft tissues and less than 1 per cent is in the extracellular fluid. The average daily British diet contains about 20 to 25 mEq of magnesium, of which about 8 mEq are absorbed and the same quantity is excreted daily in the urine by adults (Macintyre, 1963). From a nutritional standpoint magnesium is usually considered with calcium and phosphorus because calcium and magnesium constitute the major part of the mineral content of bone. The absorption of both calcium and magnesium may be impaired by an excess of phosphate, with which insoluble complexes may be formed. More calcium is absorbed by magnesium deficient rats than by normal controls, and more magnesium may be absorbed by calcium deficient rats than by normal controls, and both these observations suggest that there may be a common absorptive pathway for calcium and magnesium in the intestine and perhaps also in the kidneys (Schachter and Rosen, 1959).

Until recently little was known of changes in the content and distribution of magnesium in the body during health or disease, mainly because of the difficulties formerly associated with its chemical estimation. Since the introduction of the atomic absorption spectrophotometer magnesium metabolism has become much better understood and it is now realised that magnesium deficiency is much more common than was formerly believed. Such deficiency should be suspected in those circumstances which are known to cause potassium depletion, especially when after apparently adequate replacement of potassium the patient remains ill.

Amongst the intracellular cations, magnesium is next in importance to potassium. Baldwin *et al.* (1952) studied the interrelationship of magnesium, potassium, phosphorus and creatinine in human skeletal muscle, and concluded that there is a constant potassium magnesium ratio of 5·67:1 in all muscle, regardless of the physical state of the subject or the serum potassium concentration. In muscle the average content of magnesium was 16·4 mEq per kg wet muscle compared with 94·6 mEq of potassium and they found a proportional loss of nitrogen, potassium, phosphorous and magnesium when muscles atrophied. There was as little relationship between the intracellular and serum concentrations of magnesium as there was for potassium. The range of concentration of magnesium in the serum of normal subjects has been variously stated, from 1·7 to 2·2 mEq per litre (Baldwin *et al.*, 1952), 1·45 to 1·85 mEq per litre (Alcock *et al.*, 1960) and 1·43 to 1·93 mEq per litre (Thoren, 1963).

Another important similarity between potassium and magnesium is the continued urinary excretion of magnesium even when the serum concentration of magnesium is reduced (Martin *et al.*, 1952). Conway (1956) believed that the behaviour of magnesium is influenced by the adrenal cortical hormones in a similar way to potassium.

Magnesium Deficiency

The normal daily requirement of magnesium during growth has been estimated at up to 10 mg (0·85 mEq) per day, and since, like potassium, ordinary foodstuffs contain an abundance of magnesium, in health magnesium deficiency must be very rare. Balance studies in children have shown intakes of 200 to 300 mg (17 to 25 mEq) per day, of which only 20 mg (1·7 mEq) may be retained (Duckworth and Warnock, 1942). The magnesium content of cow's milk is 12 mg (1·0 mEq) per 100 ml (12 per cent of calcium content) and of human milk is 4 mg (0·3 mEq) per 100 ml (10 per cent of calcium content). Thoren (1963) also found that the normal daily average urinary magnesium output of an adult was 5·6 mEq per day, and that in the normal subject 90 per cent of a parenteral loading dose of magnesium was rapidly excreted in the urine.

Watchorn and McCance (1937) showed that the magnesium-deficient rat lost a lot of magnesium from the bones, teeth and serum and little from the soft tissues. According to Duckworth and Godden (1943), some of the skeletal magnesium is very labile, and is readily withdrawn from bone to replenish losses of magnesium from the soft tissues; the subsequent restoration of magnesium to the skeleton is much slower than its removal, perhaps because of the prior replacement of magnesium in the soft tissues. Deficiency of magnesium disturbs calcium equilibrium, and it appears as if magnesium can replace calcium when this is deficient and magnesium is readily available. Smith (1959) showed, by analysis of the magnesium content of serum and the vertebrae of the tails of magnesium-deficient cows, that in fatal magnesium deficiency about a third of the total body content was lost, most of it from the bones, and that the magnesium contents of bone and serum were closely related. Booth *et al.*, (1963) found the magnesium–calcium ratio in bone was reduced in patients with low serum magnesium concentrations and that there might also be a reduction in the muscle magnesium content.

Causes

The most likely factors seem to be reduction of intake, especially in chronic alcoholics; the excretion of magnesium in the urine is increased by the ingestion of alcohol but the poor diet of most alcoholics is an even more important factor. Depletion is most common in association with the prolonged loss of gastrointestinal secretions due to a postoperative intestinal fistula or to the resection of large parts of the small intestine. Barker *et al.* (1959) made the important observation that there was a large increase in the urinary excretion of magnesium after an injection of a solution containing sodium lactate, but not after one containing a similar amount of sodium bicarbonate. Depletion of magnesium is particularly likely to result from the combination of starvation and large repeated losses of lower intestinal secretions, which are replaced by the administration of adequate quantities of sodium and potassium, but not of magnesium; and lactate is commonly used rather than bicarbonate in such intravenous replacements. During the aspiration of gastric and upper intestinal secretions there is a close relationship between the volume of fluid removed and the loss of magnesium from the body (Levey *et al.*, 1956).

Clinical Features

Pure primary magnesium deficiency is extremely rare. In most patients a deficit becomes evident only when the coexisting disturbance of potassium metabolism has been corrected, or when in an infant convulsions and tetany are not relieved by intravenous injections of calcium salts. It is difficult therefore to describe the features which are typical of magnesium depletion alone. The total picture of the combination of magnesium, potassium and calcium depletions is mainly one of mental apathy and profound weakness, becoming evident after prolonged partial or complete starvation. This has usually followed a complicated abdominal operation which itself may have been preceded by a period of chronic diarrhoea and malnutrition. It has also been described in both infants and adults after resection of large parts of the small bowel in association with malabsorption and large losses of faecal fluids. Adults with magnesium deficiency may be confused, irritable, aggressive, anxious and restless, with athetoid movements, and look pale and ill.

After operation there is usually no change in the urinary output of magnesium (Levey *et al.*, 1956; Macbeth and Mabbott, 1964). Only small quantities are lost in fluid aspirated from the stomach but the fluid lost in diarrhoeal stools or in the discharges from an intestinal fistula or an ileostomy may contain 6 mEq per litre (Thoren, 1963). It seems likely that large losses of intestinal secretions or a poor intake for a long time are necessary to produce clinical signs of deficiency. When tetany is not relieved by the injection of a calcium supplement magnesium depletion is the next most likely cause. Macintyre (1963) stated that the most serious feature of marked magnesium deficiency was a liability to severe and possibly fatal epileptiform seizures. Most patients who have suffered from the combination of potassium and magnesium depletion have no memory for anything during the time of most profound clinical disturbance.

Diagnosis

This depends mainly on being aware of the possibility that magnesium depletion may exist and in looking for it. The serum magnesium level is of little value in diagnosis (Harris and Wilkinson, 1971). A low serum magnesium concentration does not always indicate depletion, and conversely there may be severe reduction in tissue magnesium content without reduction of the serum concentration. Thoren (1963) has pointed out that in normal subjects the equivalent of 90 per cent of a loading dose of magnesium administered by intravenous infusion is excreted promptly in the urine, whereas in a depleted subject, who may be excreting only 1 mEq magnesium per day, 40 to 80 per cent of the dose may be retained. The complete collection of the urine for 24 hours before and after 0·5 mEq per kg body weight of magnesium chloride or sulphate has been administered by slow intravenous infusion, with comparison of the urinary magnesium output in the two urine collections and with the loading dose, is the best method of confirming the clinical diagnosis.

Treatment

Just as in severe potassium depletion, clinical signs of magnesium depletion are associated with large losses, and replacement must be lavish, prolonged and complete. Booth *et al.* (1963) recommended that 0·5 mEq magnesium per kg body weight per day should be given as magnesium chloride. Fletcher *et al.* (1960) gave a patient with magnesium deficiency, which followed the excision of most of the small intestine, 60 mEq of magnesium per day as 20 ml of the B.P. mixture of magnesium hydroxide, in addition to a normal diet which contained 15 to 20 mEq magnesium per day and also maintained a supplementary daily intake of 50 mEq potassium as potassium chloride. They found that the volume and number of stools passed by the patient rapidly diminished after the magnesium supplement was started.

In severe depletion, which is sometimes associated with generalised convulsions when the serum magnesium concentration is very low, 0·5 ml of a 10 per cent solution of magnesium sulphate per kg body weight may be given by intravenous infusion with rapid arrest of the seizures. It is important to remember that because there is probably a common transport mechanism for calcium and magnesium (Schachter and Rosen, 1959), in patients with steatorrhoea magnesium deficiency may be due at least in part to the use of excessively large supplements of calcium salts (Hanna *et al.*, 1960). It is almost certainly unwise to give calcium supplements to patients with steatorrhoea or chronic severe diarrhoea unless they are given supplements of magnesium salts as well.

Baldwin suggested that because of the close proportional association between potassium, magnesium and phosphate, it would be reasonable when trying to replace deficits of potassium to add magnesium and phosphate to the repair solutions. This suggestion receives support from the observations of Flink *et al.* (1953), who found a serum magnesium concentration of 1·19 mEq per litre in a patient with severe potassium deficiency associated with alkalosis and phosphorus deficiency. While this patient was receiving treatment for the potassium deficiency and alkalosis, she developed fibrillary twitchings, gross muscle tremors and choreiform movements of the limbs, jaw, tongue and facial muscles, and she was unable to eat or talk. When magnesium sulphate was administered by intramuscular injection the twitchings promptly stopped and within 24 hours she was able to eat and talk. Low serum magnesium concentrations were subsequently found in 19 other patients suffering from delirium tremens of whom 15 improved after the intramuscular administration of magnesium sulphate. Flink *et al.* mention that magnesium deficiency causes 'grass staggers' in horses and cattle; this can often be cured by the rapid intravenous injection of a solution containing magnesium. It is better, however, to give a mixture of magnesium acetate and molasses in spring and autumn when the risk of magnesium deficiency is highest. Molasses is also a very rich source of potassium.

Magnesium Excess

An excessive body content of magnesium has been reported when renal dialysis has been carried out with a dialysate which was made up with hard water, and when toxaemia of pregnancy has been treated with magnesium sulphate. Lipsitz and English (1967) studied 16 babies whose mothers had suffered from toxaemia of pregnancy for which they had been given 16 to 60 g of magnesium sulphate by intravenous infusion during 8 to 33 hours before delivery at rates of 0·16 to 0·68 g magnesium per hour; these doses were equivalent to one-eighth to one-half of an assumed normal total body magnesium content of 25 g. Compared with the normal serum magnesium concentrations of 1·8 mEq per litre in the mother and 1·9 mEq per litre in cord blood, Lipsitz and English found concentrations of 3 to 14 and 3·1 to 11·5 mEq per litre respectively in the mother's serum and cord blood. Three of the 16 babies were flaccid with poor reflexes and depression of respiration, and died. The others were affected less severely for a varying number of days as the serum magnesium slowly fell to within the normal range. In both man and animals the symptoms and signs of magnesium intoxication are closely related to the serum concentration of magnesium. At concentrations of 3 to 8 mEq per litre, hypotension, drowsiness and changes in the electrocardiographic tracing are seen;

loss of tendon reflexes, respiratory depression, weakness and coma are associated with concentrations of 5 to 15 mEq per litre and cardiac arrest occurs when the concentration rises to 20 to 30 mEq per litre (Engback, 1951; Randal *et al.*, 1964).

CHAPTER FIVE

The Maintenance of Chemical Neutrality in the Body

'ACID-BASE BALANCE'

Normal cellular function depends on the preservation of a suitable environment for the cells by the maintenance of a large enough volume of extracellular fluid at a suitable pH and concentration (or tonicity or osmotic pressure). This mainly depends in turn on the total quantity and concentration in the extracellular fluid of sodium and its principal associated anions, chloride and bicarbonate; normal cell function is also dependent on the maintenance of normal contents of calcium, magnesium and potassium within a narrow range of concentration in extracellular fluid. But the composition of extracellular fluid is subject to repeated disturbances by the addition of the products of digestion of food and of cellular metabolism, and by the removal of the components of the intestinal secretions, urine, insensible water loss and sweat. These various chemical surges of secretion, absorption and excretion, as well as the general tendency of the body by the accumulation of the products of metabolism to become more and more acid, are damped and resisted by various processes.

The difficulty which many clinicians experience in understanding the processes involved in the regulation of chemical neutrality in the body is probably largely due to the terminology which is used. The loose and inconsistent use of the terms 'acid' and 'base' has caused clinical confusion, which is the greater because the meanings of these terms are so completely different to chemists and to doctors. The increasing use of the biochemical convention of milliequivalents has made essential the revision of the chemical uses of the terms acid and base. The name 'acid' was originally applied to substances which tasted sour and dissolved 'bases' (alkalis, earths or metals) to form salts. Subsequently the theory of ionisation led to more precise definitions and the term acid was limited to a substance which could yield hydrogen ions and a base was one which could produce hydroxyl ions. In 1923 Bronsted and Lowry further modified the conception and defined acids as donors of protons and bases as acceptors of protons. Thus an acid is a substance which yields hydrogen ions and a base, whereas a base is a substance which combines with hydrogen ions to form an acid. This is shown in Table XI, which also makes it clear that in this convention a base is

TABLE XI

Acid	$\rightleftharpoons$	Hydrogen ion	+anion (base)
HA	$\rightleftharpoons$	H^+	$+A^-$
HCl	$\rightleftharpoons$	H^+	$+Cl^-$
a salt	$\rightleftharpoons$	a cation	+an anion
NaCl	$\rightleftharpoons$	Na^+	$+Cl^-$

usually an anion and that cations can combine with bases or anions to form acids or salts. Moreover, some substances such as ammonium ions which would not otherwise be thought of as acids can yield hydrogen ions and can therefore be considered as acids; other substances such as the dihydrogen phosphate ion can, like protein molecules, act as either acid or base according to the pH of the solution. When these chemical terms are applied to the constituents of the body it is obvious that sodium and potassium ions are neither acids (since they cannot yield hydrogen ions) nor bases (since they cannot combine with hydrogen ions), and that they do not play any direct part in acid-base regulation.

The strongest acids are those which ionise most freely and therefore liberate more hydrogen ions. The anions of acids which are poorly ionised accept hydrogen ions more readily than do those of strong acids and therefore act more strongly as bases; thus the strength of a base is inversely proportional to the readiness with which its corresponding acid is ionised. Bicarbonate is a strong base, but chloride has almost no physiological activity as a base. Even a small amount of a strong acid will produce a large increase in the number of free hydrogen ions when added to a solution. If the solution contains the salt of a weak acid such as sodium bicarbonate which is also ionised, the bicarbonate accepts as many of the free hydrogen ions as it can, substituting for a highly dissociated strong free acid a much less dissociated weak acid. If a solution contains a weak acid and its salt, it can act in either direction and accept added hydrogen ions or basic ions; such a solution is known as a buffer. In alkalosis the hydrogen ion concentration decreases and pH rises, while in acidosis the hydrogen ion concentration is increased and pH falls.

Buffer Systems of the Blood

The buffer systems of the blood consist mainly of the sodium salts in the plasma, and in the cells the potassium salts of carbonic acid, dihydrogen phosphoric acid and protein, in equilibrium with their corresponding acids. Acid-base balance in the body as a whole depends first on the immediate effects of these buffer systems on the body fluids. The buffer systems are of limited capacity and must be reinforced by the excretion of acid or base through the lungs or kidneys. The maintenance of pH within narrow limits thus depends primarily on the maintenance of suitable proportions of buffer acids to buffer bases, and the capacity of the buffer systems is clearly related to the quantities of buffer base or acid which are available. The mutual assistance which the buffering systems may provide is well illustrated by the amphoteric haemoglobin and oxyhaemoglobin. Their reversible combinations with carbon dioxide to form carbamino complexes differ because oxyhaemoglobin is a stronger acid than haemoglobin and can release more hydrogen ions. When therefore the breakdown of carbonic acid in the tissues tends to raise the concentration of hydrogen ions the conversion of oxyhaemoglobin to haemoglobin tends to reduce it. Moreover, haemoglobin has a much greater affinity for carbon dioxide than has oxyhaemoglobin.

The Bicarbonate–Carbon Dioxide System

About a kilogram of carbon dioxide enters the capillary blood of a large adult each day. Some of this carbon dioxide dissolves in the plasma and forms carbonic acid which dissociates to liberate hydrogen and bicarbonate ions. About a quarter of the carbon dioxide combines, mainly with haemoglobin inside the red cell, to form carbaminohaemoglobin. The rest of the carbon dioxide is converted by the action of carbonic anhydrase in the red cell to carbonic acid which dissociates to hydrogen and bicarbonate ions. The hydrogen ions combine with haemoglobin, which prevents a change in pH (the isohydric shift). The bicarbonate ions diffuse out of the cell and their place is taken by chloride ions moving in (the chloride shift). In the lungs these changes are reversed when the equilibrium is disturbed by the loss of carbon dioxide from the blood as it passes through the pulmonary capillaries. The concentration of carbonic acid in extracellular fluid is related to the carbon dioxide tension in the alveolar air, which in turn depends on respiratory exchange; the plasma carbonic acid concentration is normally held at between 1·25 and 1·35 mEq per litre. The concentration of bicarbonate in extracellular fluid is controlled by the total quantity of cation, the 'alkali reserve', which is available to combine with it. This quantity of cation, which in the past was often called 'the total available base', is indicated by the amount by which the sum of the cations in extracellular fluid or plasma (sodium, potassium, magnesium and calcium) exceeds the sum of the anions (chloride, phosphate, sulphate, keto acids and plasma proteins). This difference is equal to the quantity of carbonic acid which must enter into combination with cation to form bicarbonate in order to maintain the neutrality of reaction of the blood—the 'carbon dioxide combining power'. The normal amount of cation which is combined with bicarbonate is 25 to 27 mEq per litre. The plasma carbonic acid and bicarbonate concentrations together determine the pH of the plasma; under ordinary circumstances this is held with remarkable constancy at 7·4.

Sodium is the most important extracellular cation, and when large quantities of it are lost by vomiting or diarrhoea the reduction of total available cation disturbs the normal equilibrium between cations and anions. Unless the accompanying loss of anion exactly balances that of cation, and in the absence of rapid and accurate compensation, the loss of sodium leads to reduction in the alkali reserve and therefore of bicarbonate and a tendency to an alteration in extracellular pH. An increase in anion content without a balancing rise in cation content also reduces the cation available to combine with bicarbonate and will lead to a compensatory reduction in bicarbonate and a tendency to a shift in pH.

When acid is produced by metabolism, or is absorbed from the intestine, it displaces bicarbonate from combination with cations in plasma or extracellular fluid, and carbonic acid is formed from which carbon dioxide is liberated and excreted in the lungs. Conversely, when acid is lost from the body its place in the chemical equilibrium with cations can be taken by bicarbonate, carbon dioxide being retained in the body to form the necessary carbonic acid. The total quantity of anions which can be held in the body is dependent on the total quantity of cations present in the body. The efficiency of the buffering of strong acids such as phosphoric, sulphuric or lactic by bicarbonate depends on the formation of a weak acid, carbonic, from which carbon dioxide is removed in the lungs. The most active cations, at least in the regulatory processes, are sodium and potassium, but much remains to be learned about the parts played by other ions and also by the sodium, and perhaps the calcium, in bone.

The Kidneys

The kidneys are probably the most important agents in the regulation of the composition of body fluid, since they are the chief means of conservation of sodium when this is deficient, and of excretion of acid when this is excessive. The kidneys are so efficient in chemical regulation that disturbances of pH seldom occur unless renal function is impaired. Such alterations of pH are very rare in surgical patients and are usually due to marked reduction or increase in pulmonary ventilation, or severe disturbance of renal function.

The concentrations of sodium and bicarbonate in extracellular fluid are liable to disturbance by many factors. Sulphate and phosphate, produced by the oxidation of foodstuffs or by catabolism of body tissues, displace bicarbonate, combine with sodium and are filtered out in the glomeruli. On an ordinary mixed diet metabolism leads to the production of a urine of pH 5·0 to 6·0 and there is a diurnal rhythm of acid secretion which is related reciprocally to the output of sodium in the urine. If the renal tubules are unable to substitute another cation, such as ammonium, for the sodium and to recombine the latter with bicarbonate, sodium will be lost in the urine and extracellular fluid volume will fall. In one sense the kidneys may be regarded as the most important factors in chemical regulation, because they maintain in the extracellular fluid a stable concentration of cations 25 to 27 mEq per litre in excess of the anions. This reserve of cations is neutralised, as well as indicated, by the variable concentration of bicarbonate, and is readily available to combine with and neutralise any strong acid which is formed or introduced into the body.

The kidney may conserve sodium in three ways: first by reabsorbing the filtered sodium and bicarbonate from tubular urine; secondly by acidifying the urinary buffer salts; and thirdly by exchanging ammonium for the sodium combined with anions in the urine. As Gilman and Brazeau (1953) have pointed out, not only do these three processes have a common purpose, the conservation of sodium and bicarbonate, they also share the same mechanism of hydrogen ion–sodium ion exchange in carrying out these varied functions.

It is not now credible that the differences between bladder urine and glomerular filtrate depend solely, or even largely, on modification of glomerular filtrate by selective reabsorption in the tubules, or even that all the eventual constituents of the urine are present

TABLE XII

Sodium and hydrogen ion exchange

Tubular urine		*Tubule cell*		*Extracellular fluid*
	↓	$H^+OH^- + CO_2$		
Na^+A^- ↓		(carbonic anhydrase) ↓		
		H^+		
		HCO_3^-		
Na^+	→			
A^- ↓	←	H^+		
		HCO_3^- ↓		
H^+A^-		$NaHCO_3$	→	$NaHCO_3$

$$NA + H_2CO_3 \longrightarrow NaHCO_3 + HA$$
(reabsorbed) (excreted)

Sodium-hydrogen ion exchange; the sodium ions in the tubular urine are exchanged with hydrogen ions from the carbonic acid formed in the tubule cell by action of carbonic anhydrase. The free acid resulting from the transfer of hydrogen ions into the tubular urine is excreted and sodium is conserved.

in the glomerular filtrate. In 1945 Pitts and Alexander stated that since the quantity of acid in the urine might be far more than that contained in the glomerular filtrate, hydrogen ion must have been added in the tubules. They suggested that carbonic acid was formed in the tubular cells from carbon dioxide and water by the action of carbonic anhydrase (Tables XII and XIII); hydrogen ions from the carbonic acid contained in tubular cells were then exchanged with sodium ions in the tubular urine, which thus became more acid. The sodium, however, was conserved, passed into the extracellular fluid as sodium bicarbonate and reduced a tendency to acidosis. They showed that when the activity of carbonic anhydrase was inhibited by sulphanilamide, the urinary acidity fell.

This complete reabsorption by the tubules of all the filtered sodium bicarbonate preserves sodium as well as preventing the development of acidosis. Most of the sodium bicarbonate is absorbed in the proximal tubules and it used to be thought that the remainder was absorbed as sodium bicarbonate by the distal tubules. However, Berliner (1952) has suggested that this distal absorption also may be

TABLE XIII

Tubular absorption of sodium bicarbonate

Tubular urine		*Tubule cell*		*Extracellular fluid*
$NaHCO_3$	↓	$H+OH^- + CO_2$ (carbonic anhydrase)	↓	
$Na+$ HCO_3^-		$H+$ HCO_3^-		
$Na+$	⟶			
	⟵	$H+$		
HCO_3^-		HCO_3^-	↓	
$H+HCO_3$	↓	$NaHCO_3$	⟶	$NaHCO_3$

$NaHCO_3 + H_3CO_3 \longrightarrow NaHCO_8$ (reabsorbed) $+ H_2CO_3$ (excreted)

due to sodium–hydrogen ion exchange. When tubular carbonic anhydrase was inhibited with Diamox, the urine became alkaline, and nearly half the filtered sodium bicarbonate was excreted in the urine. The excretion of the sodium was due to inhibition of the sodium–hydrogen ion exchange, which depends on the promotion by carbonic anhydrase of the conversion of hydrogen and carbon dioxide to carbonic acid. They suggested that failure of reabsorption of bicarbonate was also due to inhibition of carbonic anhydrase. Thus when the neutral salts of a weak buffer acid, such as disodium hydrogen phosphate, reach the renal tubules in glomerular filtrate, and react with carbonic acid formed in the tubular cells, sodium dihydrogen phosphate and sodium bicarbonate are formed and the reabsorption of the latter promotes the progression of the reaction (Table XIV). Thus half the sodium combined with phosphate may be conserved and the reaction of the tubular urine becomes more acid. The quantity of sodium which is thus conserved can be measured by the volume of 0·1 N alkali which must be added to the urine to return its pH to 7·4 ('titratable acidity').

TABLE XIV

Phosphate excretion

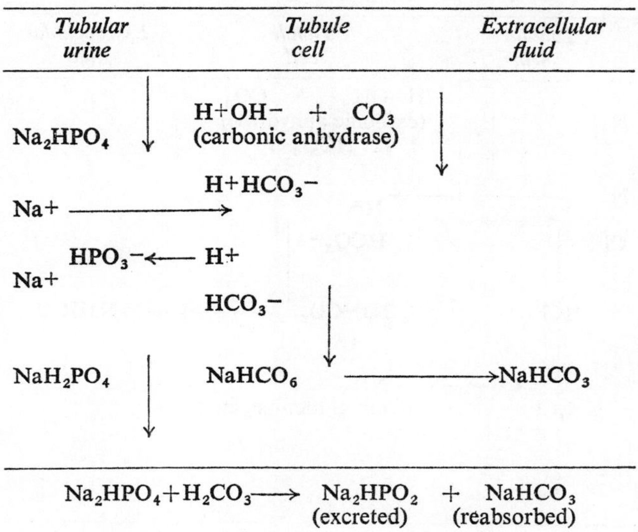

Each day about 173 litres of glomerular filtrate are formed containing (at 25 mEq per litre) 4500 mEq of bicarbonate, but only 1 to 2 mEq of bicarbonate may be excreted in the urine, the remainder having been repeatedly filtered and absorbed. More than 300 litres (about 15 mEq) of carbon dioxide are produced daily in the tissues almost all of which is excreted in the lungs. In addition 50 to 70 mEq of hydrogen ion are produced in the oxidation of sulphur-containing amino acids and by the incomplete catabolism of fat and carbohydrate to organic acids. At the maximum acidity which can be achieved, of pH 4·4, the urine is about a thousand times as acid as the extracellular fluid; this pH would be rapidly reached if the sodium in the tubular fluid were present only as salts of strong acids, for free strong acid would be formed by the sodium–hydrogen ion exchange. The conservation of sodium and the continued excretion of strong acid does not depend solely on the presence and buffering action of phosphate; by the substitution of ammonium for sodium, strong acids are buffered and sodium is conserved, the process being similar to that involved in the acidification of phosphate (Table XV). Ammonia is formed in the tubular cells from glutamine and other amino acids, combines

TABLE XV

Substitution of ammonium for sodium

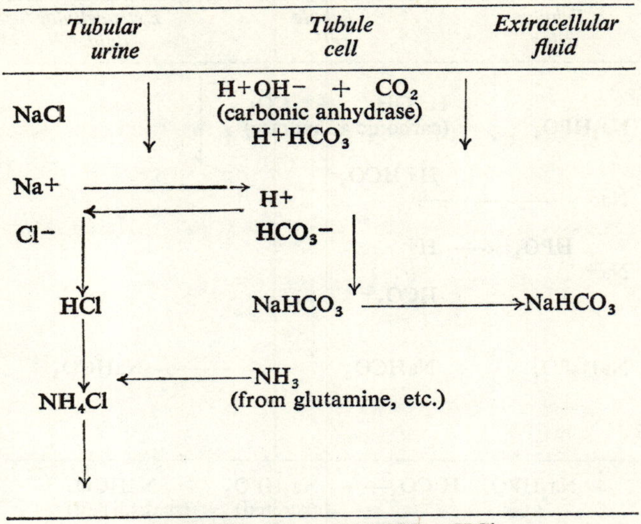

$$NaCl + H_2CO_3 \longrightarrow NaHCO_3 + HCl$$
$$NH_3 + HCl \longrightarrow NH_4Cl \text{ (excreted)}$$

with bicarbonate and diffuses into the tubular urine. This ammonium bicarbonate is then available to react with sodium salts of strong acids, such as sulphate or chloride, to form ammonium sulphate or chloride and sodium bicarbonate; this reaction is promoted by the absorption of the sodium bicarbonate by the tubular cells. According to Pitts (1950), reabsorption of bicarbonate from the tubular urine is complete when plasma bicarbonate lies between 13 and 24 mEq per litre, but only partial at plasma concentrations of 28 mEq and over.

It is possible, however, that changes in the composition of the tubular cells may exert an important influence on tubular function and on what is reabsorbed from tubular urine. The intracellular acidosis of severe potassium deficiency is associated with an extracellular alkalosis. The intracellular acidosis may increase the rate of diffusion of bicarbonate into the cell and so reduce its content in the urine. It is a common observation that in potassium deficiency associated with extracellular alkalosis, for example after prolonged vomiting due to pyloric stenosis, the urine becomes and remains acid and free of bicarbonate even after treatment has begun. There is no proof that potassium deficiency alone is associated with the production of an acid urine; patients who have vomited repeatedly always suffer from some degree of sodium depletion which itself results in renal sodium conservation and the formation of an acid urine, and it has not been proved that the combination of potassium deficiency and an acid urine persists after the complete replacement of earlier sodium losses.

By a combination of these renal mechanisms the normal person excretes the excess of acid produced by metabolism and maintains the reaction of his body fluids and the body content of cations within normal limit. When an excess of acid is produced, for example in diabetic ketosis, in spite of marked increases in ammonium and titratable acidity, compensation may be incomplete and there may be a urinary loss of sodium as well as an increase in the acid content of the body. In severe renal disease the capacity of the renal tubules to conserve sodium by sodium–hydrogen ion exchange and other mechanisms is reduced and again sodium depletion and acidosis result.

DISTURBANCES OF ACID-BASE BALANCE ACIDOSIS AND ALKALOSIS

Acid-base balance is disturbed only by the loss or accumulation of acids or bases in the body, that is to say by variation in the hydrogen ion concentration of the body fluids and the tissues. This specific alteration in hydrogen ion concentration is liable to be forgotten by clinicians who have learned to be concerned with alterations in sodium, potassium, bicarbonate or chloride concentrations which can now be readily measured, rather than with the plasma concentrations of carbon dioxide or hydrogen ion. Buffers cannot completely prevent changes in pH of the body fluids and their capacity is limited both by the quantity of buffer and by the means available to refresh the reactions. Because of its efficiency plasma pH depends mainly on the bicarbonate–carbonic acid buffer pair and pH is indicated by the ratio between these components ($HCO_3 : H_2CO_3$). These two components may fluctuate over a wide range, but so long as they change proportionately pH is not altered. Only when the changes are disproportionate does pH rise or fall. Clinical disturbances of acid-base balance result when the various compensatory reactions to the loss or addition of acid or base can no longer maintain neutrality. Such a disturbance may result from the loss of gastrointestinal secretions containing cations such as sodium, potassium or hydrogen and anions like chloride and bicarbonate, and water; the ensuing compensatory reactions will involve the buffer systems, kidneys and lungs. Although for ease of description simple 'pure' types of disturbance are described and discussed, in nature the interactions between the many components are rapid and continuous and all that chemical analyses of plasma can do is to indicate part of the situation at the time the blood is withdrawn from the vein.

The term acidosis indicates an accumulation of acid or a loss of base, both of which tend to lower pH. Alkalosis or 'baseosis' indicates an accumulation of base or a loss of acid and tends to cause pH to rise. For clinical purposes acidosis and alkalosis are classified according to the predominant causal process into respiratory and metabolic (or non-respiratory) types. The respiratory disturbances are due to failure in the regulation of the carbonic acid content of the body by respiratory exchange, while the metabolic disturbances depend primarily on changes in the non-volatile or 'fixed' acids and bases. A respiratory disturbance may be compensated by a renal response and a metabolic disturbance by a respiratory response. Such compensation may vary greatly in degree and on this depends the size and direction of alterations in pH.

Astrup *et al.* (1960) have shown that for clinical purposes the state of acid base equilibrium can be estimated from the actual pH, carbon dioxide tension ($P\text{CO}_2$), standard bicarbonate and base excess of blood. Sigaard Andersen *et al.* (1960) have described micromethods of analysis suitable for these determinations and Sigaard Andersen and Engel (1960) have revised the original nomogram used in the calculations. The pH of the blood is measured on blood as withdrawn into heparinised capillary tubes and also after equilibration with two different mixtures of oxygen and carbon dioxide. The $P\text{CO}_2$, base excess or standard bicarbonate are then calculated from the nomogram. By means of these measurements the respiratory and metabolic components of a disturbance can be judged, changes in $P\text{CO}_2$ reflect respiratory disturbances and in base a metabolic disturbance. The base content may be expressed as standard bicarbonate or as base excess; the latter is undoubtedly the more useful in the management of patients. 'Standard' bicarbonate means that the bicarbonate content has been measured under the standard conditions of a known $P\text{CO}_2$ of 40 mmHg at 38°C and on fully oxygenated blood, to eliminate the influence of respiration.

From the measured pH of the blood the standard bicarbonate can be calculated from the Henderson-Hasselbalch equation:

$$pH = 6{\cdot}10 + \log \frac{HCO^3}{P\text{CO}_2 \times 0{\cdot}0300}$$

Base excess or deficit expresses in mEq the surplus of strong base or acid per litre of blood when zero is arbitrarily fixed at the normal mean for bicarbonate of 22·9 mEq per litre. The deficit or excess of base in the extracellular fluid is found by multiplying the value for base excess or deficit by 0·3 × the body weight in kg (Mellemgaard and Astrup, 1960). This quantity indicates the amount of sodium bicarbonate or ammonium chloride needed to neutralise the extracellular disturbance, but gives no indication of the total disturbance in the body as a whole.

It is important not to suppose that values for pH or $P\text{CO}_2$ in the blood necessarily reflect changes in the whole body. It is well established that there is a large quantity of available buffer substances in tissues which can be used when the extracellular bicarbonate is reduced by metabolic acidosis. When large quantities of acid substances are administered about half the acid is buffered in the tissues. Relman (1966) has calculated that the extracellular bicarbonate would be exhausted when 10 to 15 mEq per kg of mineral acid had been absorbed by the total body buffers.

Metabolic Acidosis

This is the common clinical type of acidosis and may be due to the loss of bicarbonate in intestinal secretions by vomiting or diarrhoea, to the use of bicarbonate as a buffer against the increased production of keto acids in starvation or in diabetes, or of other organic acids in fever, infection or violent exercise. It may follow the administration of ammonium chloride, or the rapid transfusion of bank blood which has been preserved with acid citrate dextrose and may have a pH of less than 6·8. Acidosis also occurs during cardiac bypass, hypothermia or when pulmonary ventilation is inadequate or during cardiac arrest. It may follow the sudden restoration of an adequate blood flow to any large mass of tissue which has been poorly perfused for some time, for example when an aortic embolus is removed, or a volvulus of the intestine is untwisted. In chronic glomerulonephritis or chronic pyelonephritis it may be due to the diminished absorption of bicarbonate by the renal tubular cells, or to the failure of the renal mechanisms for the transfer of hydrogen ions to the urine.

Clinical Features

In surgical patients the loss of intestinal secretions during prolonged diarrhoea, especially in the absence of vomiting, is probably the most important cause of this type of acidosis and this may be aggravated by the ketosis of starvation, especially in children. The most marked clinical sign is the deep raucous and rapid respiration, the so-called 'air hunger', which is the main compensatory mechanism; the respiratory rate may rise to as fast as 50 per minute, but there are moments when the patient stops breathing and tries unsuccessfully to moisten his lips with a hard, brown, parched tongue. The respiratory centre is stimulated by the lowered pH, and by increased pulmonary exchange the plasma concentrations of carbon dioxide and of carbonic acid are reduced and the disturbed ratio between bicarbonate and carbonic acid tends to return towards normal. When renal function is good, and is not impaired by the loss of fluid in the discharges from the body, an increase in ammonium excretion and if possible more complete sodium conservation will also help to reduce the acidosis and raise the pH.

Diagnosis

A history may be obtained of the loss of intestinal secretions or of an operation such as transplantation of the ureters to the colon. Rarely the patient may be comatose when first seen, and this combined with stertorous respiration and what information can be obtained from relatives may be enough evidence on which to start treatment. Coma may be due to potassium depletion, or to the excessive loss of extracellular fluid (sodium and water depletion), and diabetic coma may also confuse the diagnosis and may be accompanied by changes in respiratory rhythm. The precise diagnosis of the degree of acidosis depends on the measurement of pH, standard bicarbonate and base excess.

Treatment

This depends chiefly on reversing the causal disturbance as completely as possible and in assisting compensation as far as this can be done. Fortunately acidosis due to the loss of intestinal secretions is not only the commonest type found in surgical patients but also the one most susceptible to treatment; the administration of a balanced electrolyte solution which contains sodium acetate and some potassium chloride, as well as sodium chloride, provides bicarbonate and potassium as well as the sodium and water which are the most important components of the lost secretions. When there is a marked reduction of the extracellular fluid and plasma volumes, sufficient 0·9 per cent. saline should first be rapidly infused to restore extracellular fluid volume and an adequate circulation before any attempt is made to correct the accompanying acidosis. Sodium bicarbonate may be administered as a 4·2 per cent solution which contains 0·5 mEq bicarbonate per ml; this solution is hypertonic and is usually mixed with other solutions and it should be remembered that repeated use of it may lead to the retention of undesirably large amounts of sodium. The normal range of base excess is $\pm$2·3 mEq. A negative base excess of 15 mEq is not uncommon even in normal subjects after 48 hours starvation but is soon corrected when the consumption of food is resumed. Except in patients with cardiac lesions or dysfunction there is probably no real need to correct variations in base excess of less than 15 mEq. Acidosis due to renal failure does not respond well to the administration of sodium acetate or bicarbonate but remarkable improvement may follow dialysis; solutions containing potassium salts should usually be avoided in the treatment of acidosis due to renal failure. Acidosis sometimes accompanies severe infections, but this type is seldom improved by the infusion of sodium acetate or bicarbonate.

Respiratory Acidosis

This is less common than the metabolic type and is normally caused by interference with gaseous exchange in the lungs leading to the retention of carbon dioxide. Poor pulmonary ventilation may be due to crushing or other injury of the chest, peritonitis, emphysema, pulmonary oedema or bronchopneumonia especially when accompanied by cardiac failure. During anaesthesia, when muscle relaxants have paralysed the respiratory muscles, artificial ventilation may be inadequate, and in other types of closed-circuit anaesthesia the removal of carbon dioxide from the circulating gases may be inefficient; poliomyelitis also may reduce respiratory efficiency. The respiratory centre may be depressed by brain injury or by poisoning with morphine, alcohol or the barbiturate drugs. In such circumstances compensation largely depends on the increased reabsorption in the renal tubules of sodium and bicarbonate and the increased renal excretion of hydrogen and ammonium ions.

Clinical Features

These depend on the cause and the degree to which compensation is effective. During anaesthesia there may be a slow rise in systolic and diastolic blood pressures followed by a sharp fall when normal respiration is resumed and the retained carbon dioxide is eliminated. In most of the circumstances mentioned, respiration is abnormal and its correction is difficult.

Treatment

This depends on correction of the primary disturbance and in restoring normal respiratory exchange. In the acute type of disturbance which may follow open operation on the heart with cardiopulmonary bypass, so much depends on correction and control of the acidosis that repeated measurement of base excess and pH is essential.

Metabolic Alkalosis

In metabolic alkalosis the reduction in hydrogen ion concentration may be due either to the loss of hydrogen ions from the body (and thence a reduction in extracellular carbonic acid concentration) or to an absolute increase in the quantity and concentration of extracellular bicarbonate. In surgical patients this type of disturbance is commonest when in pyloric stenosis the loss of acid by the repeated vomiting of gastric secretions is accentuated by the excessive consumption of sodium bicarbonate; other antacids such as magnesium carbonate or trisilicate, bismuth carbonate or aluminium hydroxide also produce alkalosis. The chloride lost in the vomitus is replaced by retained bicarbonate, but it is important to remember that there are large losses also of potassium.

Whereas the sodium and chloride contents of gastric juice decline when vomiting persists for a long time, the concentration of potassium is undiminished and in achlorhydia is increased because of the large amount of mucus with a high potassium content in the gastric juice. The combination of this continuing loss of potassium in the vomitus, with a daily loss in the urine which is increased by intracellular dehydration, and partial starvation due to the vomiting, results after several weeks in the loss of very large quantities of potassium. Sodium is conserved efficiently by the kidneys, less is lost in the vomitus as the body content is reduced and reduction in extracellular fluid volume is now fairly readily recognised and treated by the rapid infusion of 0·9 per cent saline. The insidious loss of potassium without replacement may lead to reductions of 1000 mEq or more, a third of the original body content. This is accompanied by severe extracellular alkalosis, but because two-thirds of the potassium lost from the cells is replaced by sodium ions and one-third by hydrogen ions there is an intracellular acidosis. These changes in intracellular composition cannot be directly demonstrated in the patient in bed, whereas the extracellular alkalosis can be readily measured. For this reason in the past the therapeutic emphasis has been placed mainly on replacement of sodium chloride and water and the correction of extracellular alkalosis. A small proportion of patients with prolonged vomiting due to pyloric stenosis and very severe extracellular alkalosis do not do well when treated in this way; they improve only when their large losses of potassium are assumed and are replaced. The only way in which the loss of potassium can be measured is by estimating the total potassium content of the body, which is seldom feasible. Potassium depletion should be suspected whenever there is severe alkalosis and is almost always accompanied by magnesium deficiency.

Alkalosis with potassium deficiency may be found also in some types of Cushing's disease, with some adrenal cortical neoplasms, and after the prolonged administration of cortisone, ACTH or desoxycorticosterone acetate or the prolonged intravenous infusion of saline.

To compensate for alkalosis there is a reduction in respiratory exchange, due to inhibition of the respiratory centre by the raised pH, leading to accumulation of carbon dioxide and thus of carbonic acid and a tendency to lowering of the pH. There is also an increase in the excretion of bicarbonate in the urine, which may be accompanied by an increase also in sodium excretion unless large amounts of sodium have been lost in the vomitus, and a reduction in the output of hydrogen ions, mainly by lowering of the ammonium and dihydrogen phosphate excretion.

Clinical Features

The close association of severe alkalosis with other disturbances, especially potassium and magnesium deficiency, makes it difficult to separate the typical features of the component factors of the combined disturbance. Mild degrees of alkalosis do not cause any particular clinical feature and can be recognised only by the raised plasma bicarbonate concentration. The most striking feature of severe alkalosis is the phasic respiration. A period of apnoea, varying in duration from 5 to 30 seconds or more, is followed by the onset of respiration which is at first shallow and then increases in depth until the excursion is normal; after two or three respirations of normal range the excursion again declines to apnoea. The number of breaths in each cycle varies from 5 to 10 or more and, with the variation in depth and the duration of the apnoeic periods, seems to be related to the severity of the chemical disturbance. The blood urea nitrogen concentration is often, but not invariably, increased.

Tetany may occur in severe alkalosis, but probably only during periods of altered pH of which tetany may thus be an indication. Tetany is due to an increased irritability of the skeletal muscles, irritability of muscle being inversely related to the concentration of free calcium ions in the extracellular fluid. The proportion of free calcium ions depends on the pH, and as pH rises calcium ions tend to combine with phosphate. Hyperventilation may result in tetany, and it has been suggested that the cramp experienced by swimmers may be due to the hyperventilation induced by cold water. Tetany may also result from the administration of alkaline solutions of phosphate. Latent tetany, in which the serum calcium concentration remains just above the level necessary for tetanic contraction to appear, may be more common than has previously been suspected. It can best be detected by compression by inflating a sphygmomanometer cuff round the arm; the hand then assumes a characteristic position of flexion at the metacarpophalangeal joints and wrists and extension of the interphalangeal joints (Main d'accoucheur, Trousseau's sign). In animals, tetany indistinguishable from that due to calcium deficiency may be produced by feeding diets deficient in magnesium; the possibility that magnesium deficiency may be associated with severe alkalosis should not be overlooked.

Treatment

In severe alkalosis due to vomiting in pyloric obstruction there are large losses of hydrogen, sodium and chloride ions and water; the losses of potassium and magnesium depend on the duration of the disturbance and the degree of starvation. While the first consideration is always to ensure survival by maintaining an adequate volume of blood in active circulation by restoring extracellular fluid volume, the effects of large deficits of potassium and magnesium on cellular function should not be ignored. Ammonium chloride has been advocated for the correction of alkalosis because this salt provides chloride with a cation, ammonium, which can be converted to urea in normal renal tubules and excreted; it has been said that ammonium chloride thus provides a specific means of correcting an alkalosis caused by the loss of chloride. This recommendation is completely wrong since it ignores the loss of cations, especially of potassium, which is an important feature of alkalosis due to repeated vomiting, and the use of ammonium chloride does not provide the means of reversing the sodium transfer into cells or replace the loss of potassium from the body. Ammonium chloride should not be used when alkalosis is associated with potassium deficiency. The intravenous infusion of a solution of potassium chloride is necessary only in the initial stages and as soon as possible the oral administration should be started. To replace 1000 mEq potassium very large quantities, such as supplements of 12 to 18 grams per day for three weeks or more, are needed in addition to an abundant intake of a good mixed diet; the daily administration of a few ounces of fruit juice of unknown quality and potassium content is of little use in a problem of this magnitude.

Respiratory Alkalosis

In this type of alkalosis because of hyperventilation the tensions of carbon dioxide in the alveolar air and hence in the plasma are reduced and the extracellular carbonic acid concentration falls, the bicarbonate-carbonic acid relationship is disturbed and the pH rises. This probably occurs most commonly in surgical patients during anaesthesia because of excessive manual pulmonary ventilation in association with the use of muscle-relaxing agents. It may also occur in hyperventilation due to hysteria, at high altitudes, in men working in very hot dry atmospheres, in high fever and in salicylate or carbon monoxide poisoning. Compensation depends on the increased renal excretion of bicarbonate and is usually inadequate. During anaesthesia alkalosis is accompanied by pallor and a falling blood pressure. In both acidosis and alkalosis of respiratory origin there is some risk of respiratory arrest when the disturbance is severe, but this is much more common in alkalosis than in acidosis, possibly because overventilation is more common than too little ventilation which also produces cyanosis. Such alkalotic respiratory arrest can be corrected by the insufflation of carbon dioxide.

CIRCADIAN RHYTHMS

The small volume of urine which is produced during the 8 hours sleep which is enjoyed by most normal subjects has long been recognised and has been explained in various ways. Some have thought that it was simply due to a low intake of fluid but this is not entirely true, nor is it always related to sleep since disturbance of the normal sleeping habits for a short time may not alter the usual nocturnal reduction in urine volume. There is a close relationship with the alternation of light and darkness which appears to be a more important factor than alleged alterations in the output of antidiuretic hormone. There are also rhythmic changes in the urinary excretion of sodium, potassium and chloride. The urinary outputs of all three elements are smaller at night and increase in the morning, rising to a peak about midday or early afternoon. In addition the urine produced at night is usually acid and that produced about midday is alkaline. Variations in this pattern are common as the result of alterations in the food intake or exercise and during some kinds of infection. There are also similar rhythmic changes in the excretion of magnesium, calcium, lead and mercury but these are more readily disturbed than those of sodium and potassium. The output of phosphate, perhaps the most important renal buffer substance, falls after waking and the fall may even begin during the last part of sleep, but the phosphate excretory pattern is disturbed by changes in the habits of the subject.

Since these changes in the composition of the urine appear to be due to the effect on the kidney of extraneous influences detailed studies of circadian rhythms in patients with a transplanted denervated kidney may provide valuable information about how much influence nervous control may have. There are no satisfactory explanations based on chemical factors since the rhythmic changes in the output of sodium and potassium in the urine are unrelated to changes in the plasma concentrations of sodium and potassium or to glomerular filtration rate. In spite of their important effects on sodium amd potassium excretion neither cortisol nor aldosterone can be firmly implicated in the rhythmic changes in output of these two substances. There are also very large changes in the blood pressure, pulse rate and blood flow in the peripheral parts of the body resulting in or being related to changes in body temperature. These changes are particularly closely related to sleeping and waking. There are also circadian variations in the number of circulating leucocytes, eosinophils, red cells, haemoglobin concentration, and in blood clotting mechanisms.

The normal cycle of rhythms in the human subject is about 24·4 hours (circa dia, circadian) and variations from this depend on stimuli from the environment which have been called Zeitgebers, of which light is the most dominant in many species of animal and possibly also in man. People living for long periods in darkness or in perpetual daylight in Arctic regions tend to have less marked variations in their circadian rhythms but these are not abolished. Similarly, those peoples who go to high latitudes from say Britain maintain their circadian rhythms almost unchanged in amplitude of variation though there may be some disturbance of their periodicity. In this respect it is of interest that blind persons maintain their circadian variations but at lower amplitude than sighted people. Much more marked disturbances in the rhythms may occur when there are abnormal time routines, particularly due to the rapid movement across a number of time zones in air travel.

Whatever endogenous mechanism there may be governing the time sequence of various circadian rhythms, and however this may be disturbed by alterations in habit or time zones in rapid air travel, another conflicting factor is the alteration in environmental factors as the result of the change in daily habits; in addition some rhythms particularly for sodium and potassium are more affected by some factors than by others. It has been shown experimentally in the human subject that when a 12 hour cycle of sleep, activity and meals is adopted the original endogenous rhythm of excretion of sodium, potassium and chloride, of urine flow and pH and of variation in the eosinophil count is undisturbed, but changes in alveolar carbon dioxide tension and renal excretion of phosphate follow the new induced habits.

Circadian rhythms have numerous possible clinical applications. There is a well known tendency for epileptics to have their seizures at particular times during the day and these are commonest between midnight and 7 a.m. Intraocular pressure is higher during the day than at night. The normal renal excretory rhythms in diabetics should be maintained rather than disturbed by uncertainty of meals and changes of working shifts. A great deal of evidence has now been accumulated on the effects of rapid time shifts on circadian rhythms particularly in airline pilots. After a time change of 5 or 6 hours adaptation may take 4 or 5 days depending to some extent on the age of the individual, and this effect is exaggerated when the time of arrival is during the normal sleeping time. It is uncertain how much effect these disturbances may have in patients who shortly after such a time shift are subjected to a major surgical operation but judging by their disturbing effect on concentration, on sleep and on renal function this whole subject deserves considerably more study than it has received so far.

CHAPTER SIX

Disturbances Due to Loss of Gastrointestinal Secretions

The loss of gastrointestinal secretions is the commonest cause of disturbance of equilibrium in the body fluids. The effects of the loss of fluid from the alimentary tract depend chiefly on the rate and total volume of fluid lost. These secretions are derived in the first place from the plasma and so from extracellular fluid, and large depletions of the extracellular fluid may result from copious vomiting, repeated diarrhoea or fluid loss from an intestinal fistula. To a limited extent such losses can be compensated by the transfer of fluid from the cells to the extracellular fluid, but this process takes time. When the loss of secretion is large or continuous, the transference of cell fluid makes little impression on the rapid depletion of extracellular fluid volume and does not prevent the onset of oligaemic circulatory failure due to the reduction in volume of plasma and extracellular fluid. When the loss of secretion is less rapid but more prolonged, the effects of the primary loss of secretion combined with the compensatory changes in intracellular fluid and the administration of solutions of various kinds may result in marked distortion of the composition of the body fluids.

The fluid lost seldom consists solely of one type of sceretion, but is usually a mixture of secretions from more than one region of the alimentary tract. In addition, the composition of the intestinal secretions varies widely from one individual to another and from time to time in the same person. In general it can be said that repeated vomiting leads particularly to the loss of hydrogen ion as hydrochloric acid and so to a metabolic alkalosis, but the associated loss of sodium and water also causes reduction in extracellular fluid volume; whereas the loss of secretion from the small and large intestines by diarrhoea or discharge from a fistula leads to loss of sodium and water, and to metabolic acidosis. The sodium content of the bile, pancreatic juice and small intestinal secretions is usually high (see Table IX). The concentration of potassium in all alimentary fluids is normally as high or higher than it is in the plasma. Chloride is usually present in high concentration in gastric juice and in a lower concentration in pancreatic juice. Rapid losses of large quantities of fluid from any level in the alimentary tract lead to depletion of sodium and water. Repeated losses over a long period, especially if replaced by infusions of saline, glucose solution or other fluids containing little or no potassium or magnesium lead ultimately to depletion of potassium as well as of sodium and water. Such losses of potassium are commonly accompanied by proportionate losses of magnesium.

OESOPHAGEAL OBSTRUCTION

In both benign and malignant disease of the oesophagus progressive obstruction leads to increasing difficulty in swallowing food and fluids. This undernutrition causes a reduction in lean tissue mass and fat (McMurrey *et al.*, 1955). In the wasted adult as in the child the total body content of water per kg body weight is increased and its distribution is altered, much more being in the extracellular space than in the wasted cells. The total body solids representing all kinds of cells when expressed as the difference between total weight and total body water may be much less than half the normal quantity. It must be remembered that such huge losses are borne much more by some tissues, such as skeletal muscle, than others more essential to mere survival such as heart, brain and liver. These undernourished patients have a poor tolerance for intravenous infusions and for rapid and repeated transfusions of blood or plasma; cardiac irregularity or failure due to overloading is readily produced by even small volumes of fluid.

In complete obstruction of the oesophagus, in addition to starvation for food and water, the patient has to expectorate up to 1500 ml of saliva per day. Because of their poor tolerance to intravenous infusions, the general state of these patients can best be improved before operation by feeding them through a jejunostomy (see p. 242). The intestines are empty and contracted, and for the first two or three days only small feeds of 60 ml should be given every hour. In partial obstruction of the oesophagus the stricture may be dilated and the patient fed orally with a liquid diet, usually some form of milk mixture.

Patients with oesophageal obstruction suffer primarily from

starvation and so lose potassium and magnesium proportionately with nitrogen, as the result of the catabolism of tissue protein. There is usually no particular need to replace potassium and magnesium in excess of protein. Marked improvement in the general state of the patient often follows when a delay of 2 or 3 weeks before operation is employed in feeding a high energy, high protein mixture with supplements of vitamins.

The repeated slow transfusion of 500 ml of fresh whole blood is another valuable adjunct in the preparation of these wasted people for operative treatment.

Ileus is common after resection of the oesophagus and is generally attributed to reduced intestinal motility following division of the vagal nerves. When the stomach is drawn up into the chest and anastomosed to the stump of the oesophagus, delayed gastric emptying is common and the accumulated secretions in the stomach must be aspirated through an indwelling tube passed across the anastomosis. Rarely, aspiration of the stomach must be continued for more than a week; there is then additional delay in starting to eat, continued loss of body fluids and prolonged dependence on intravenous infusions for the supply of water and calories. The institution of a jejunostomy, before or at the end of the operation on the oesophagus, permits feeding with a milk mixture to be started immediately after operation, and has the additional advantage that fluid aspirated from the stomach can be run into the jejunostomy. The use of a jejunostomy before operation on the oesophagus has been opposed on the grounds that it interferes with the choice of a loop of jejunum for anastomosis with the oesophagus, but this can be avoided by making the jejunostomy a few feet lower in the intestine than is usual.

LOSS OF GASTRIC SECRETION

Gastric juice as aspirated from the stomach is a mixture of the highly acid secretion of the oxyntic cells and the more alkaline secretions of the other cells of the gastric mucosa. The proportions of these constituents are very variable, and in particular cases it is undoubtedly wiser to measure the volume of the vomitus or aspirated fluid and the content of potassium, sodium and chloride before judging the quantities of fluid and electrolyte which should be administered. Vomiting in pyloric stenosis results in the loss of large quantities of gastric juice containing varying proportions of hydrochloric acid and sodium and potassium chlorides. The loss of sodium and potassium leads to a reduction in total body water and extracellular fluid volume, and the loss of hydrochloric acid is followed by a compensatory rise in bicarbonate concentration in the extracellular fluid. If this were all that happens to these patients it would be easy to understand the cause of their physical disturbance, to measure approximately their depletions and to provide fairly specific treatment with a ıeasonable expectation of success in most cases.

But the loss of sodium in the gastric juice is soon followed by conservation of sodium by the kidneys with the almost complete disappearance of sodium from the urine, especially if vomiting continues. The urine becomes and remains acid so long as sodium conservation continues. This persistence of an acid urine in association with a low concentration of chloride and a high concentration of bicarbonate in the plasma, was produced experimentally in dogs by Gamble and Ross in 1925, and Hartmann and Smyth (1926) studied it in patients. Even earlier, however, in 1923, Haden and Orr had shown that this acidity of the urine could not be satisfactorily treated by the administration of sodium bicarbonate, because of the increased severity of the alkalosis which followed such therapy. It was originally thought that the acidity of the urine was simply an expression of the need to retain bicarbonate to compensate for the loss of chloride by vomiting. Gamble and Ross also pointed out that the sodium content of vomited fluid in pyloric stenosis is usually higher than that of normal gastric juice because of an increase in the production of gastric mucus with a high sodium content. Both Gamble and Ross, and Hartmann and Smyth showed that in spite of the acid urine the alkalosis could be successfully treated by the intravenous administration of isotonic saline, and at the same time the pH of the urine tended to rise. The urine always contains free carbonic acid in a concentration almost the same as that in the plasma, and when the sodium is being completely conserved there is a tendency for urinary pH to fall. Only when sodium again appears in the urine does urinary pH rise.

It is unusual for a patient with pyloric stenosis to be able to maintain a normal water content during bouts of vomiting. Extracellular fluid volume is depleted by the loss of gastric juice and can be restored only to a very limited extent, and at the cost of a fall in sodium concentration, by the transfer of water out of cells. The best that can be achieved by this transfer is usually only the maintenance of the depleted extracellular fluid volume, until it is further reduced by the next vomit. Since the water requirements of patients who vomit repeatedly cannot be adequately satisfied by drinking, water is transferred from the intracellular fluid. This intracellular dehydration causes severe thirst.

Potassium is lost in the urine as the result of tissue catabolism, secondary to starvation and an inadequate calorie intake, and probably also in association with the mobilisation of cell water for such purposes as insensible loss and urine formation. The severity of the potassium depletion depends on the number and duration of the bouts of vomiting, on the completeness of the starvation and on the extent of the intracellular dehydration. The urinary excretion of potassium is also increased by intravenous administration of isotonic saline and of 5 per cent glucose solution.

In the early stages of pyloric obstruction there may be little alteration in the composition of the plasma and extracellular fluid. The first indications of the large changes which are occurring in body composition are often an increase in the plasma bicarbonate and a decrease in chloride concentration. Sodium concentration is maintained by renal conservation and possibly by the mobilisation of sodium from bone. Potassium and magnesium concentrations are maintained by mobilisation from the cells, even when food intake is very small, and fall only when depletion is severe. This is presumably the result of the continued transfer of potassium and magnesium from the cells because of partial starvation and intracellular dehydration. Even though renal excretion of potassium remains high the reduction of extracellular fluid volume by loss of sodium and water may be associated with an extracellular potassium concentration which is in the upper part of the normal range although a large amount of potassium has been lost from the body. The recognition of these possibilities is important because the frequent finding of a high extracellular potassium concentration has probably caused many clinicians to minimise the importance or deny the existence of severe potassium depletion after prolonged vomiting due to pyloric stenosis. Often when isotonic saline is administered by intravenous infusion the ensuing rapid increase of extracellular fluid volume is accompanied by a marked reduction in the extracellular potassium concentration, but not necessarily by any other clinical signs of potassium depletion.

When large quantities of gastric secretions are repeatedly lost in a few days, extracellular fluid volume is acutely reduced and the clinical signs of sodium and water depletion appear (see p. 42). This type of acute disturbance is usually successfully treated by the rapid intravenous infusion of isotonic saline. It is important, however, to recognise that the administration of isotonic saline merely increases the volume of the extracellular fluid by providing sodium and water. It does not correct the loss of potassium and water from the cells or repair the ravages of starvation. In gastric juice the concentrations of sodium (50 mEq/litre), potassium (10 mEq/litre) and chloride (80 mEq/litre) are unlike those in extracellular fluid (see Table IX). After the loss of one litre of such gastric fluid the replacement of the sodium can be achieved with 3 g of sodium chloride (55·5 mEq), but replacement of the chloride will require 5 g of sodium chloride (85 mEq) and of the potassium 1g of potassium chloride (13·4 mEq). The intravenous infusion of a litre of isotonic saline thus provides an excess of sodium but no potassium, and is an inaccurate means of replacing the lost fluid. The reappearance of chloride in the urine is not an indication of the complete replacement of chloride, because, as Van Slyke and Evans (1947) showed, the urinary chloride concentration may increase soon after the infusion of saline is started, and may approach the plasma chloride concentration before the chloride deficit is fully replaced.

It is only in the later stages of pyloric obstruction, after loss of vomitus has been repeatedly replaced by infusions of isotonic saline, that the effects of repeated losses of potassium and magnesium become clinically evident with muscular weakness, lethargy, and a high carbon dioxide combining power.

Treatment

Treatment of severe alkalosis which is based on attempts to lower the high plasma bicarbonate does not always succeed. Indeed, the administration of saline and of ammonium chloride sometimes makes the patients worse rather than better. In alkalosis associated with potassium deficiency the correction of the potassium disturbance is of primary importance. The administration of potassium salts is known to produce marked improvement in the clinical state of patients with this combined disturbance, even when no attempt is made to correct the alkalosis by administering chloride. Perhaps this is due to the restoration of the intracellular content of potassium, which in turn displaces sodium and hydrogen ions from the cells.

The intracellular acidosis is thereby reduced and the transfer of hydrogen ion to extracellular fluid diminishes the extracellular alkalosis.

It is essential to appreciate the importance of an accurate and detailed history of how long the patient has been vomiting and how severe has been the interference with food intake. Prolonged illness is nearly always associated with potassium and magnesium depletion as well as alkalosis but this is rare with obstruction of short duration. Thus as Roberts *et al.* (1954) showed acute alkalosis is readily corrected by the infusion of saline but the chronic alkalosis developing slowly over several weeks cannot be corrected without the administration of potassium salts.

Whenever vomiting has continued for more than a week or ten days, potassium deficiency as well as alkalosis should be suspected. Some indication of potassium deficit may be obtained from change in the general state of the patient, especially recent loss of appetite and energy. The serum concentrations of sodium, potassium, chloride and bicarbonate, pH and base excess should be measured and an electrocardiographic tracing made. There is close association between potassium and magnesium and whenever there is depletion of potassium it is reasonable to assume that there is also an equally severe depletion of magnesium. Whenever potassium replacement seems necessary magnesium should also be given.

The pre-operative treatment of such a patient is designed to replace the deficits of potassium and magnesium as well as that of chloride and the smaller loss of sodium. The ideal method is by the oral consumption of as full a diet as can be eaten, combined with the emptying and washing out of the stomach at night; a supplement of up to 12 g of potassium chloride and 3 g of magnesium per day should be added to the diet. In spite of reducing the daily loss of gastric secretions and increasing the intake of food, fluid, potassium and magnesium by these means, there may be a further reduction in the serum concentrations. This is probably caused by an expansion of extracellular fluid volume, which may in part be due to the transfer of sodium from cells to extracellular fluid. It is reasonable to continue with this method of replacement if the general condition of the patient improves and the volume of gastric residue diminishes; if not, other methods of replacement must be employed. The institution of a jejunostomy allows of the provision of a full daily intake of calories and protein, together with ample potassium and magnesium chlorides. Alternatively, and in any case if there is coma, extreme drowsiness or persistent vomiting in spite of gastric lavage, the lost water and electrolyte should be replaced by intravenous infusions. Before a solution containing a potassium salt is injected, a urine output at the rate of at least 500 ml per day or 20 ml per hour should be ensured, if necessary by the infusion of a 5 per cent glucose solution. Up to 2 g (26·8 mEq) of potassium chloride in a 5 per cent glucose solution may be administered over a period of 4 to 5 hours, and up to 12 g (160·8 mEq) may be given during the first 24 hours. Because of the dangers of intravenous administration of potassium, it is wise to change to the oral route as soon as possible.

Occasionally, when prolonged pyloric obstruction has been treated by pyloroplasty, partial gastrectomy or gastrojejunostomy, the return of gastrointestinal motility is delayed for more than 48 hours. Accumulation of fluid in the stomach and upper jejunum then requires gastric aspiration and the restriction of oral fluid intake. Unsually this state lasts for at most a few days, but rarely it may persist for a week or more and it then becomes a very serious complication. The cause of this impaired motility is uncertain; but it now seems likely that the intravenous administration of excessive quantities of saline, and potassium and magnesium depletion, are possible causal factors. When, because of fear of an organic obstruction, the abdomen is reopened, the stomach and jejunum are usually seen to be immobile and stiff with oedema fluid, the stoma is widely open and across it fluid contents swill to and fro with each respiratory excursion. Restriction of the oral fluid intake is not always followed by reduction in the volume of the gastric aspirations. The stomach tube should always be withdrawn as soon as the fluid smells clean and is not thickly turbid. Intravenous saline administration should be strictly limited to a daily quantity sufficient to replace the sodium lost in the aspirated fluid, and the effect of the intramuscular injection of potassium and magnesium chlorides should be tried. It is doubtful whether any additional anastomosis should be carried out in the absence of organic obstruction; indeed, reopening of the abdomen and the inspection of the stomach and jejunum alone are often followed by early resumption of normal peristalsis.

LOSS OF INTESTINAL SECRETIONS

HIGH INTESTINAL FISTULA

Gastric, duodenal, biliary or pancreatic fistulas are rare but highly dangerous complications of operations on the stomach, duodenum, pancreas or biliary tract. The daily volume of fluid lost from these fistulas is proportional to the extracellular fluid volume, and is thus directly affected by the degree to which intravenous replacement succeeds in correcting earlier losses of fluid. Some of these fistulas dry up and close after draining for as short a time as 7 to 10 days without particular difficulty being experienced in their management. Others unfortunately persist for much longer periods and cause great anxiety and difficulty in treatment, and from a few so much fluid is lost within a short time that treatment may be unavailing.

Duodenal Fistula

The fluid which is lost from a duodenal fistula consists of a mixture of bile, pancreatic juice and duodenal secretion. It is alkaline and contains moderate quantities of chloride, but large quantities of sodium; its loss leads to reduction of extracellular fluid and plasma volume, haemoconcentration and acidosis. Duodenal fistulas most often follow leakage from the duodenal stump after partial gastrectomy and when there is any distal obstruction the fistula persists.

Up to 2 litres or more of fluid, containing as much sodium as extracellular fluid, may be lost daily. The replacement of these losses with isotonic saline may restore the sodium and water, but provides an excess of chloride. As the extracellular fluid is depleted by the loss of fluid from the fistula the volume of the loss declines, but the rate of loss increases soon after the extracellular fluid volume is restored by intravenous infusion. The oral consumption of food and fluids is soon followed by gushes of bile-stained fluid and undigested food from the fistula. Digestion of the skin round the fistula causes severe pain, but can be prevented by smearing the skin with an alumina paste, barrier cream or Karya gum.

Much of the anxiety and difficulty of treating such a fistula can be avoided by the prompt establishment of a jejunostomy. The greatest advantage of the jejunostomy is that it allows the collected discharges from the fistula to be run into the jejunum. This prevents the loss from the body of a fluid of complicated composition and there is little if any need for intravenous infusion. In addition, because the full calorie, protein, water and vitamin requirements can be readily supplied by jejunostomy feeding, all oral intake can be stopped and the loss from the fistula thereby greatly reduced.

The early establishment of the jejunostomy is essential if secondary fluid disturbances due to inaccurate intravenous replacement are to be avoided and malnutrition with impairment of wound healing prevented. Jejunostomy is of limited value when there is an intestinal fistula lower in the small intestine.

Biliary Fistula

A complete biliary fistula will produce severe disturbances in body-fluid equilibrium if it lasts long enough, the mineral composition of liver bile being very similar to that of extracellular fluid. The illness which may follow prolonged external drainage of all the bile with weakness, apathy, lack of appetite, mental confusion and often sudden circulatory collapse, is well recognised, and after deliberate surgical drainage of the common bile duct it is usually avoided by clamping the drainage tube. Fistula of the common bile duct occasionally follows inadvertent damage to the duct during dissection of the duodenum. This type of fistula usually begins to discharge within a week of the operation, but may cause biliary peritonitis and jaundice before discharging at the laparotomy wound. Specific operative treatment of the fistula is seldom required because most fistulas close spontaneously. Gradual depletion of the extracellular fluid volume may lead to sudden circulatory failure which can be corrected by the rapid intravenous infusion of isotonic saline in a volume equivalent to the total quantity of bile which has been lost by external drainage. The oral intake of potassium should be increased by the consumption of 2 to 4 g of potassium chloride per day for as long as the fistulous discharge exceeds 250 ml per day.

Pancreatic Fistula

Pancreatic juice may be lost from a fistula of an accessory duct or very rarely of the main duct, as the result of injury during operation. An opalescent fluid begins to discharge from the drainage sinus about 48 hours after operation. Pancreatic juice contains sodium, potassium and chloride in concentrations which resemble closely those in extracellular fluid; in the absence of infection the fluid from a pancreatic fistula may contain more sodium than plasma, a difference which appears to be related to the very low protein content of the pancreatic juice. The bicarbonate content varies directly with the secretory activity of the gland and is high after meals. The daily output from a pancreatic fistula may vary from less than 100 ml to nearly 2 litres. The pancreatic secretion is unique amongst body fluids in its high bicarbonate content averaging about 80 mEq per litre; the bicarbonate and chloride concentrations vary reciprocally and together equal that of the total plasma anions (154 mEq per litre). In a 47-year-old man with a pancreatic fistula Sinclair (1956) found the average daily output to be 880 ml, the greatest loss on any day being 1740 ml, a figure which is similar to that recorded from several other patients. Large acute losses of fluid from a pancreatic fistula may require replacement by intravenous infusion, when a solution containing a mixture of sodium chloride and sodium acetate should be used and potassium citrate should be administered orally. Early recognition of leakage depends very much on the presence of a drain inserted into the neighbourhood of the duodenal stump at the end of the operation.

ACUTE INTESTINAL OBSTRUCTION

Acute Primary Obstruction or Strangulation

Shields (1965) showed that soon after obstruction of the small intestine the bowel immediately above the obstruction loses its power to absorb sodium, potassium and water which therefore accumulate in the bowel because their secretion in normal quantities is unaffected. Later after 24 hours the fluid and electrolytes enter the lumen at a faster rate than normal. The bowel higher up may continue to absorb the fluid which has been secreted lower down near the obstruction. The fluid which accummulates has a composition similar to that of the extracellular fluid so that there will be no disturbance of the serum chemistry until the obstruction has been present for some time, if indeed there is any alteration at all. At all levels there is also a loss of fluid into the intestinal wall and the peritoneal cavity. The higher the obstruction is in the intestine, the more copious is the production of secretion and the loss of fluid, a reflection of the predominantly secretory activity of the jejunum and of the changing emphasis from secretory to absorptive activity down the small intestine and into the colon.

In obstruction high in the intestine, fluid is lost principally by vomiting, and in lower obstructions by simply accumulating in the lumen of the bowel. Several litres of fluid may be lost by vomiting within 24 hours of the upper jejunum being occluded, whereas the lower colon may be obstructed for 2 or 3 weeks without much loss of fluid, even into the lumen of the large bowel. The addition of a closed loop increases the urgency of surgical relief as well as the loss of fluid. In strangulation there is a loss of whole blood into the mesentery and the wall as well as into the lumen of the bowel, and when an extensive piece of bowel is involved, this loss of blood is sufficient to cause a large fall in circulating blood volume.

Patients who are admitted in emergency with acute intestinal obstruction do not present straightforward problems in fluid replacement. The urgency of surgical relief of the obstruction often allows of only a short delay for replacement of previous loss of body fluids and while it is essential to make the patient as safe as possible for operation, nothing should be done which will make the operation more difficult or hazardous. The lost fluid closely resembles extracellular fluid in its water and sodium content. If it is replaced by the rapid intravenous infusion of isotonic saline the infused saline is rapidly distributed throughout the extracellular fluid and much of it is lost into the wall and lumen of the obstructed bowel. This leakage is due to the increased vascular permeability in the obstructed segment of bowel. This increase in bowel content hampers manipulation of the bowel during operative relief of the obstruction and increases the risk of leakage after intestinal anastomosis. If the reduction in extracellular fluid volume is large, it causes sufficient reduction in plasma volume to lower peripheral blood pressure and to cause haemoconcentration with elevation of the packed cell volume and plasma protein concentration, but there is seldom any other characteristic change in blood composition.

The clinical state of the patient depends on the volume of fluid which has been lost by vomiting and into the lumen of the bowel, and on the duration of the obstruction; the general appearance usually gives an excellent idea of the severity of the depletion of the extracellular fluid. Reduction in blood pressure, poorly filled veins and sluggish peripheral capillary circulation indicate the need for restoration of blood volume before operation. This can be achieved by the rapid infusion of 0·9 per cent saline or of a plasma substitute such as a high molecular weight preparation of dextran; blood should also be used if an extensive strangulation is suspected. Although it appears to be theoretically desirable to replace completely the fluid which has been lost by vomiting or into the lumen of the bowel, in practice it is sufficient to restore blood volume and then to proceed without further delay to relieve the obstruction.

In general, if intravenous therapy has not been required before operation, it is seldom necessary afterwards unless blood volume falls during or soon after operation; in such an event the rapid infusion of 500 to 1000 ml of dextran or blood usually restores and maintains blood volume, but sometimes larger volumes may be necessary, and the volume required by each individual should be judged by the response to treatment. When it has been necessary to restore blood volume before operation it is always wise to continue the intravenous infusion at a slow rate during and for up to 12 hours after operation until stability is certain. Further circulatory impairment is treated by the rapid infusion of dextran or blood. Postoperative saline infusion is of value when large volumes of fluid have been lost before operation. Great care must be exercised in judging the volume of saline to be infused, because after operation, especially in a patient depleted by large losses of intestinal fluid, renal conservation leads to the almost complete retention of infused sodium and water. Unfortunately there is no reliable way of estimating or calculating the quantities of sodium and water which should be administered to a particular patient, and it is necessary to judge when to stop by the changes in the appearance of the patient. Restoration of extracellular fluid volume is indicated by a healthy, reddish colour in the skin, which is warm, dry and feels thicker when picked up instead of being pale muddy grey, cold, clammy and shrivelled. The eyes are no longer sunken and dark-ringed, the tongue is moister and not hard, the pulse is slower, full and firm and the blood pressure is within normal limits. As soon as possible the patient should start to drink again and should be fed as soon as he can take food.

Postoperative Obstruction

After abdominal operations there are three important types of obstruction, or delayed emptying of the bowel, which cause loss of intestinal fluid: first, peritonitis; secondly kinking or binding down of the bowel by fresh fibrinous adhesions; and thirdly, adynamic or idiopathic ileus in which the bowel appears to have lost temporarily the ability to contract.

In *peritonitis*, the intestines which are involved in the intraperitoneal inflammatory process are inflamed and stiff with inflammatory oedema. This interferes with peristalsis, and intestinal secretions accumulate in the inflamed bowel and in the intestine above. When large quantities of saline are administered to patients with peritonitis the bulk of the inflammatory exudate is increased, and interference with intestinal function is more severe and is prolonged by the formation of this excessive exudate.

When extensive or generalised peritonitis is encountered, even although the blood volume and peripheral circulation appear to be satisfactory, it has been found of value to transfuse the patient with 500 to 1000 ml of whole blood. Following the transfusion, the needle is withdrawn and the oral consumption of fluid is restricted. If the patient vomits, drinking is stopped, and if vomiting is repeated the stomach is aspirated every hour. Only very rarely is it necessary to administer fluid by intravenous infusion, and the subsidence of the inflammatory ileus and the reappearance of peristalsis appear to be earlier when the fluid intake is restricted in this way than when large volumes of saline or glucose solution are infused.

In a few patients there appears to be some impairment of vasomotor control associated with advanced peritonitis, and even the lavish transfusion of whole blood, plasma or plasma substitutes and free administration of saline do not make much impression on the circulatory failure, which is the common cause of death. In acute haemorrhagic pancreatitis and in biliary peritonitis there is often very severe circulatory disturbance, and the peritoneal reaction is due more to chemical than to bacterial irritation. Blood volume may be much reduced, but a poor response often follows the administration of blood, plasma or dextran in these two conditions. Sometimes the infusion of 500 ml of low molecular weight dextran may be followed by a marked improvement in the state of the peripheral circulation, because the dextran has washed out the aggregated red cells from the stagnant capillary circulation. The use of vasodilator or vasoconstrictor drugs is seldom of much use.

The modern habit of protecting patients from infective complications during the first week or so after operation by the prophylactic administration of antibiotics has resulted in a change in the clinical picture of post operative peritonitis following intestinal operations. The insidious onset leads almost imperceptibly into a state of severe but indefinite illness; often for several days no more can be said than that the patient does not look well. A sudden fall in peripheral blood pressure may be preceded by some increase in pulse rate. Before exploration or drainage of the peritoneal cavity can be safely undertaken it is usually necessary to prepare such patients by transfusion of blood or dextran.

Adhesions and ileus. When abdominal distension is progressive after an intraperitoneal operation, it is of the greatest importance to know whether the accumulation of gas or fluid is due to an organic obstruction, such as a fibrinous adhesion producing kinking or twisting, or to an inability of the bowel to empty itself of contents. Organic obstruction demands urgent release as soon as possible after it has been diagnosed. For true ileus or inability to empty there is no satisfactory or certain relief, and the less such bowel is interfered with the better. Because it occurs in a bowel which is active, organic obstruction causes colicky pain, which is the most important diagnostic feature of this type of obstruction. Patients with organic obstruction may have been subjected to gastric aspiration for several days before the diagnosis is made; they may not have complained of pain, or their complaints may have been minimised, ignored or misinterpreted and a copious vomit may be the first sign of intestinal obstruction. Before the obstruction is relieved by operation it is advisable to start an intravenous infusion so that if circulatory failure develops during laparotomy, blood volume can be rapidly increased. In some cases it may be wise to start the infusion of dextran before anaesthesia is induced.

At operation, after relief of the obstruction, the dilated intestine should be emptied of gas and of as much fluid as possible by suction after local puncture with a needle. The emptied loops are then better able to pass on any contents which remain in the rest of the involved intestine and the abdominal wound is more easily and rapidly closed. After operation a careful watch must be kept for signs of impending circulatory failure; gastric aspiration should be continued, but drinking should not be permitted as long as aspiration is continued. As soon as the aspirations become clean-smelling and dark green in colour, the tube should be withdrawn and should be replaced only if there is vomiting. During the period of aspiration, the intravenous infusion may be continued. Not more than one litre of 5 per cent glucose solution should be given each 24 hours. If signs of extracellular fluid depletion appear, the rapid infusion of a litre or more of isotonic saline may be required, but potassium salts should not be administered until at least 48 hours have elapsed since operation. If the blood pressure falls below normal limits, 500 to 1000 ml of high molecular weight dextran should be infused rapidly, followed by 1000 to 1500 ml of saline.

Sometimes peristaltic sounds are not heard for 2 or 3 days after operative relief of obstruction, and during this anxious period of waiting for the restoration of peristalsis, restraint must be exercised. No good purpose is served by allowing the patient to drink even small quantities of water; thirst is better relieved by frequent mouth washes of ice cold water. Urinary output will be low and it is unwise to attempt to increase its volume by administering large volumes of glucose solution. The use of enemata to stimulate the bowel to contract, or of the various drugs which have had temporary vogues in the past produces inconsistent and uncertain results and does more harm than good. Gerber *et al.* (1958) showed that after operation on a wide range of abdominal lesions there was as rapid recovery and only half as much morbidity in patients who did not have nasogastric suction as in those who did and the mortality was not increased; respiratory complications in particular were much reduced.

Altered motility and muscular inco-ordination of the intestinal musculature may result from severe depletion of potassium or sodium. Ileus which follows operation on a gastric or intestinal lesion that has resulted in prior depletion of potassium, may be due, in part at least, to depressed intestinal motility secondary to potassium deficiency. The reduced gastrointestinal motility after prolonged gastric aspiration may have a similar basis. In such cases the intravenous administration of potassium salts should be tried, success being usually indicated by an early increase in bowel sounds and by the passage of flatus. It should not be forgotten that calcium and magnesium are both liable to be depleted by the same circumstances which lead to the loss of potassium, and that the activity of calcium in extracellular fluid is diminished in alkalosis. Sometimes the intravenous administration of 20 ml of calcium gluconate has produced a striking if temporary response by initiating peristalsis in patients with ileus. When a patient fails to improve in spite of the restoration of extracellular fluid and blood volumes and the administration of potassium and calcium, magnesium depletion should be suspected. Magnesium chloride 0·5 mEq per kg body weight should be administered slowly by intravenous infusion in a suitable volume of 5 per cent glucose solution.

As soon as peristalsis is once more well established, the patient should be encouraged to drink and eat as full a diet as possible. Sometimes troublesome diarrhoea follows the relief of an obstruction or ileus, and the loss of secretions leads to an unexpected extracellular fluid depletion and to circulatory failure.

Extensive resection of the small intestine

The effects of resection of much of the intestine depend not only on the total length which remains but also on which part it is and on the age of the patient. The newly born baby is the least capable of tolerating the removal of most of its small intestine because of the large requirements for growth, in addition to the daily needs for maintenance of metabolism, although the removal of the whole of the colon is compatible with survival and good nutrition (Wilkinson *et al.*, 1963; Wilkinson and McCance, 1973). Retention of the ileum is more important than of the jejunum because of its absorptive capacity and it seems likely that the minimum length of small intestine which a neonate needs for survival is about 25 cm. Yet in older children and adolescents only 15 cm of small intestine may be sufficient for a tolerable, if sometimes precarious existence (Meyer, 1962; Anderson, 1965; Winawer *et al.*, 1966). There should not be great difficulty in keeping alive a neonate with 60 cm of small intestine providing the diet is suitably modified. There has been much emphasis on the value of the ileocaecal valve in delaying the transit of contents from the small intestine to the large and on the importance of the retention of the terminal ileum for the absorption of vitamin B_{12}, but both these claims may have been exaggerated.

The intestine which remains grows only as much as it would normally grow and there is no disproportionate increase in length in spite of claims which have sometimes been made that this happens. In the absence of intestinal obstruction the remaining bowel does not usually hypertrophy or dilate and there are insignificant changes in the mucous membrane in the absence of infection.

When a large part of the small intestine has been resected the digestion as well as the absorption of food is considerably disturbed. In the normal state of affairs the digestion of a mixed meal proceeds in such a way that the food is broken down and the products of digestion are absorbed in a well defined order down the intestine. For example, Bergstrom *et al.* (1957) showed that when a normal adult is fed a meal composed of glucose, lactose, corn oil and milk protein, absorption is complete in the duodenum and upper 100 cm of jejunum. Lactose is normally absorbed most rapidly in the duodenum and proximal jejunum, maltose in the jejunum and proximal ileum and sucrose in the distal jejunum and ileum. Normally starch is completely hydrolysed and absorbed in the small intestine.

At least half the calories consumed by a normal adult are in the form of carbohydrate, of which 300 g or more is eaten every day, mostly as starch and sucrose and some as lactose. The weaned child also eats large amounts of carbohydrate. Before they can be absorbed by the small intestine these carbohydrates must be hydrolysed to their constituent monosaccharides. This is achieved partly by salivary and pancreatic amylases but the final stage depends on the disaccharides of the brush border of the intestinal mucosa which is also responsible for the absorption of the monosaccharides produced. When the action of the disaccharides is defective little if any disaccharide is absorbed in the small intestine and the unabsorbed disaccharide and the water which it attracts and holds pass into the colon and increase its contents and cause diarrhoea. In addition these disaccharides are broken down by bacteria in the colon with the production of gas and lactic acid. The faeces become watery and acid, the pH being less than 5·5, and are passed often and noisily with much gas and cause a characteristic irritation and excoriation of the buttocks.

Disaccharide intolerance causes much more acute and severe disturbance in the young infant and neonate than in the older child or adult because the load of sugar as monosaccharide or disaccharide in each milk feed is proportionately larger. The diagnosis must be based on a knowledge of the composition of the milk feeds. This kind of diarrhoea is particularly likely to start soon after a change has been made in the feeds, such as especially the addition of a carbohydrate supplement.

To establish a diagnosis of disccharide intolerance the pH of the stool must be measured with a test paper and must be less than 5·5. Reducing sugars in the faeces can be shown by Clinitest and this should be done on a fresh stool at the bedside. Chromatographic examination will identify the individual sugars in the stool and for this test a stool must be collected freshly in a plastic bag and deep frozen immediately otherwise fermentation will continue. It is seldom necessary and in very ill children always undesirable and even dangerous to carry out a loading test with the suspected sugar. Temporary disaccharide intolerance is a common complication of the treatment of oesophageal, duodenal and small intestinal atresias, of Hirschsprung's disease and after intestinal resections for other reasons soon after birth. It seems to be much commoner in such surgical patients than in medical patients of the same age and, while it may cause a very severe acute disturbance, it lasts for only a few months and disaccharides can then be gradually reintroduced into the diet.

The digestion and absorption of dietary fat depends on hydrolysis mainly by pancreatic lipase which is potentiated by the emulsifying action of bile salts. Lipolysis is seldom affected by the operations which are inflicted on neonates and infants unless so much bowel has been removed that the contents pass through the small intestine too rapidly for the fat to be hydrolysed and absorbed.

Although some digestion and absorption of fat can occur in the absence of bile both are much more efficient when the normal daily cycle or turnover of bile acids and bile salts between the liver and small intestine is maintained. Normally most of the bile salts are deconjugated and absorbed in the distal ileum and only small amounts of bile salts are lost in the faeces. Deconjugation and absorption may be reduced when there is alteration in the bacterial flora of the ileum, or after the extensive resection of bowel so that more bile salts reach the colon where absorption is poorer than in the ileum. In addition the oncotic effect of these unabsorbed bile salts in the colon may cause diarrhoea by interfering with the absorption of water and sodium by the colon If the loss of bile salt is sufficiently severe it may disturb the normal enterohepatic cycling of bile salts, and this may so reduce the bile salt content of the jejunum that fat digestion and absorption is impaired. In the blind loop syndrome there is an abnormal growth of coliform organisms in the loop and other parts of the small bowel. Some of these bacteria can split and dehydroxylate bile salts and this causes a high concentration of bile acids in the bowel. The absorption of these acids reduces the concentration of bile acids in the lumen of the intestine and so disturbs fat absorption that steatorrheoa results.

The classical concept that protein is broken down completely to amino acids in the lumen of the small intestine by various enzymes, mainly those in the pancreatic juice, and the amino acids are then absorbed across the mucous membrane must now be revised. In newly born but probably not in older mammals, including man, whole proteins from milk, including maternal antibodies, may be absorbed intact by pinocytosis, the formation of vesicles by the invagination of the mucosal cell wall. It is now accepted that part of the ingested protein is hydrolysed to amino acids which are then absorbed, but another fraction is taken up by the mucosal cells as oligopeptides which are than hydrolysed by the peptidases in the mucosal cells. There is an obvious similarity here to the hydrolysis and absorption of carbohydrate and fat.

The digestion and absorption of dietary protein is usually very efficient. The equivalent of only 10 per cent of the nitrogen intake normally appears in the stools and some of this is endogenous. In each 24 hours in an adult up to 20 or 30 g of protein is secreted into the bowel in mucus and digestive enzymes, another 30 g is cast off in desquamated epithelium and up to 2 g of plasma protein per 24 hours normally enters the lumen of the gut. Thus in an adult nearly as much protein is secreted or lost into the gut as is taken in a good mixed diet and the same is presumably true in childhood. Interference with this intestinal cycle of endogenous protein can obviously cause the loss of large amounts of body protein and is another and important cause of protein depletion in severe and prolonged diarrhoea.

The simple idea that complete digestion and absorption of the meal depend on the food being in contact with the appropriate digestive enzyme and the intestinal mucosa for a sufficient length of time is still broadly true in health. In abnormal conditions new knowledge of other factors is having an increasing effect on our management of the patient. Steatorrhoea causes protein malabsorption which to some extent can be corrected by the administration of hydrolysed instead of whole protein. It is, however, uncertain whether this is because one stage of digestion has been cut out or because the peptides can be taken up directly by the mucosal cells in the form in which they are administered. There may be an analogy with the fact that sucrose is a better carbohydrate supplement than glucose because when sucrose is hydrolysed in the brush border the resulting glucose is in a more favourable relationship with an intracellular carrier than glucose which comes from the lumen direct. In the human adult most of the products of protein digestion are normally absorbed in the upper two-thirds of the small intestine but the lower ileum is well able to absorb these products. Resection of small intestine must be very extensive to interfere with protein digestion or absorption.

When most of the small intestine is removed absorption of water and carbohydrate usually recover first followed by that of protein. Starchy and fatty foods both reach the colon before hydrolysis is complete enough for absorption. Decomposition of starch in the colon causes the formation of much odourless gas but protein gives rise to foul smelling flatus. When fat is hurried through the shortened small intestine to the colon, the production of fatty acids irritates the colonic mucosa and causes severe diarrhoea. One way of trying to increase absorption from the short bowel is to increase the total intake of food. When Weckesser *et al.* (1949) doubled the total carbohydrate intake the percentage which was absorbed of the total calories which were consumed rose from 66 per cent to 90 per cent. When the fat intake was doubled the loss of fat and protein was so much increased that only 25 per cent of the added fat was absorbed, and the percentage absorbed of the total calorie intake fell from 66 per cent to 53 per cent.

When much of the intestine has been resected the food is in contact with the digestive juices and absorptive mucous membrane for a much shorter time than normal, even when transit time is not reduced by diarrhoea. The feed should therefore be so modified before consumption that as much of it as possible is ready for absorption. It should be based on skimmed milk, which is almost free of animal fat. The excluded fat should be replaced by medium-chain triglyceride in equicaloric quantities (Anderson, 1966), fortified with glucose, thickened with arrowroot (a simple and readily absorbed carbohydrate powder) and predigested with pork or beef pancreatic extract. An amino acid preparation can also be added. The feeds should be small and thick. Large volumes of dilute feeds only stimulate secretion of intestinal juices and increase the loss of fluid and minerals in the stools.

Steatorrhoea reduces the absorption of fat soluble vitamins A, D and K and it is essential to give adequate quantities of a complete vitamin preparation to cover all requirements. The absorption of folic acid and iron may be affected when the whole of the jejunum and some of the ileum are resected, but it is remarkable how well the lower ileum can compensate. It is generally believed that resection of the terminal ileum and ileocaecal valve results in poor absorption of vitamin B_{12} but from our experience with children with extensive resections of the intestine it seems likely that almost the whole of the ileum and right half of the colon must be resected before vitamin B_{12} absorption is much impaired. Similarly, the patient should not be given by mouth 0·9 per cent saline or 6 per cent glucose solutions because they pass so rapidly through the intestine. Sometimes it has been recommended in the past that sodium lactate should be given to counteract the tendency to metabolic acidosis, but because of the adverse effect sodium lactate has on magnesium absorption from the bowel it is better to use sodium bicarbonate.

There is now abundant evidence that for a limited time the total requirements for the maintenance of daily metabolic requirements and for growth can be provided by the intravenous infusion of various suitable combinations of amino acids or hydrolysates of beef fibrin or cow's milk casein, combined with non-protein calories derived from soya bean oil emulsions, glucose, ethanol, fructose or other carbohydrates with adequate supplies of vitamins and trace elements. Such parenteral feeding can be continued only so long as there are veins available for infusion and in the absence of infection. In the end, long-term survival and growth both depend on the ability of the patient to ingest and digest enough food taken by mouth to provide for all the requirements of daily maintenance, and growth.

There are usually three stages of recovery after an extensive resection of intestine. At first until feeding is started the bowel is inactive and little if anything comes from it. When feeding begins and even when the food is modified as described the stools are loose and frequent. For two or three weeks there may be rather profuse diarrhoea with perianal irritation and excoriation during which an adult may lose 10 or 12 litres of fluid from the bowel in a day. Sometimes the time taken by the food to pass from mouth to anus may be only 10 minutes, and not only the food but also the secretions which the intestine produces in response to it are almost completely lost.

Once the diarrhoeal stage subsides with treatment and modification of the food intake large losses of much of the ingested food may continue, the state of retention remains poor and lost weight is not regained and in the infant growth is much retarded. Gradually bowel function settles down with careful modification of the feeds and attention to the detail of the dietary modifications until in older children and in adults a considerable degree of dietary freedom is achieved.

Malabsorption may also occur when only a short length of bowel has been removed, because of the formation of a blind loop, associated with the use of a lateral anastomosis between the two segments of intestine. This method of anastomosis has now been almost entirely abandoned but occasionally patients are seen who have been operated on many years ago with this sort of anastomosis. Sometimes a similar effect results from the closure of a Bishop Koop (1957) type of enterostomy in which the piece of distal bowel which was brought to the surface is closed over and is not resected. This has resulted in a clinical disturbance similar to that found with the blind segment due to lateral anastomosis and also similar to what has been found sometimes in patients with short dilated segments of intestine (Nade and Dickson, 1972).

Some of these patients have a characteristic clinical disturbance.

They are poor eaters yet they say before a meal that they are hungry and they are looking forward to their food. They take a mouthful and chew it and perhaps swallow it but soon, after one or two mouthfuls, they lose their appetite for food and sit and just chew the same food without taking any more and never get through a proper meal. When the dilated segment or the blind end has been resected normal appetite returns. This disturbance has been reproduced in young pigs from whom at the age of about 7 to 10 days a large part of the small bowel was resected and who developed a dilated segment of bowel as the result of dense adhesions following the operation. The pig was hungry for food but when it was offered took only a few mouthfuls and then just stood with its lower jaw in the feed and slopped it about but did not swallow any more. When at a second operation the adhesions were divided and the dilated segment of intestine was freed and the delay in emptying was avoided the pig began to feed normally again. Subsequently the adhesions recurred, the dilated segment developed once more and the pig failed to eat again and when sacrificed was found to have redeveloped the saccular piece of intestine which had been present at the time of the second operation.

Such a localised dilatation is not uncommon in young patients with Crohn's disease where scarring gives rise to stenosis and proximal dilatation. The disturbance in appetite is also related to the growth of bacteria in the dilated segment because temporary improvement follows the oral or intramuscular administration of a suitable antibiotic such as one of the penicillins. It can also be relieved by a short circuit operation which diverts the stream of bowel contents from the dilated segment. An alternative method is to feed the patient orally on a mixture of synthetic amino acids and glucose which is absorbed almost completely in the upper small intestine. This changes the bacterial flora of the affected segment of bowel.

Large sudden losses of fluid in repeated liquid stools may so reduce the extracellular fluid volume that the rapid intravenous infusion of 0·9 per cent saline or a balanced electrolyte solution may be necessary; both potassium and magnesium deficiency may follow repeated disturbances of this kind and it is probably best to anticipate excessive losses of these minerals by adding supplements of them to the food as potassium chloride and magnesium acetate or sulphate.

Both the rate of transit of intestinal contents and the absorption of products of digestion can be improved by the reversal of a short segment of distal intestine (Hammer *et al.*, 1955, 1959). This procedure has not been much used but recently Venables *et al.* (1966) have reported favourably on its use in a man aged 58 years in whom only 120 cm of jejunum remained and was anastomosed to the mid-transverse colon. This procedure is limited by the difficulty of judging how long a segment should be reversed; 10 cm was effective in the patient mentioned above. If too much is reversed the resulting delay in transit causes a low grade obstruction with dilatation of the bowel above and malabsorption, which may be exaggerated by infection.

Ulcerative Colitis

The repeated bouts of diarrhoea which are a feature of the acute phases of this disease cause the loss of mucus, purulent discharge, blood and intestinal secretions, as well as interfering with the absorption of the products of digestion of food. In addition to malnutrition and the wasting of the body there are losses of water, sodium and potassium in the loose faeces, and severe secondary anaemia. During bouts of diarrhoea it is often necessary to maintain the circulating volume of blood by transfusion of whole blood, and in some cases dextran may be necessary in emergencies to keep the patient alive until blood is cross-matched. The rapid depletion of the extracellular fluid which follows bouts of diarrhoea can be treated successfully by the intravenous infusion of balanced electrolyte solution and the transfusion of blood only in the early stages. Later the progressive loss of potassium requires that potassium salts be added to the diet or to the infusion fluids. Since diarrhoea causes acidosis, Darrow's solution is of more value than saline, and potassium citrate and sodium bicarbonate should be administered orally to supplement the sodium and potassium of the diet.

Villous Adenoma of the Colon

This tumour gives rise to the production of a copious secretion of clear watery mucus which may be passed from the bowel up to 20 times a day. The mucus secretion is the result of the stimulation of the mucosa by the constant presence of the tumour in the bowel. The most important of the chronic effects of this tumour is the large cumulative loss of potassium in the mucus which is usually associated with depression of the serum concentrations of sodium as well as of potassium. Babior (1966) reviewed 22 patients with this disturbance. The concentration of potassium in the colonic mucus varied from 15 to 120 mEq per litre and of sodium from 70 to 160 mEq per litre and up to 3 litres per day might be lost. Although the blood urea concentration is usually raised in these patients this is due to the extrarenal loss of fluid rather than to primary renal impairment and responds completely to rehydration of the patient; for this up to 4 litres of saline per day may be needed with large supplements of potassium chloride.

Ileostomy

During the first 24 or 48 hours after an ileostomy has been established there is usually not much loss of intestinal fluid from the ileum. Subsequently, however, there may be repeated gushes of large quantities of thin fluid which often amount to a litre or more and sometimes to 3 or 4 litres per day (Kanaghinis *et al.*, 1963). The sodium content of this fluid varies a good deal but averages 126 mEq per litre. Losses of 40 to 100 mEq per day are usual and may be as high as 200 to 400 mEq. Potassium losses range from 1 to 20 mEq per day and magnesium depletion is common. The loss of sodium is disproportionately large compared with that of chloride and leads to acidosis, and the replacement of the lost sodium by sodium chloride results in an excess of chloride. Even when the ileostomy is well established large amounts of fluid may still be lost from it because of minor intestinal upsets or infections. Although the losses of water and sodium from an ileostomy are nearly always larger than from the normal bowel, patients with well established ileostomies may be able to drink large quantities of various fluids without disturbance so efficient is absorption in the unirritated small intestine.

Clarke *et al.* (1967) found that in a group of 21 patients with well established ileostomies there was an average reduction of 11 per cent in total body water and of 7 per cent in total exchangeable sodium. The urinary outputs of sodium and water were also significantly reduced by amounts which were similar to the losses of sodium and water in the fluid lost from the ileostomy, in spite of an increased daily intake of salt.

Moderate losses of sodium and potassium may have to be replaced by the intravenous infusion of saline, or saline and acetate with added potassium chloride (0·2 g per 100 ml, 27 mEq potassium per litre) but sodium chloride and sodium citrate can also be given by mouth. Provided renal function is good and the water intake is adequate, most patients can make satisfactory adjustments for the excessive administration of chloride. When signs of sodium and water depletion appear treatment must be thorough and rapid and its accuracy is improved if all the fluid lost from the ileostomy, as well as all urine are collected and the volume and sodium and potassium contents are measured. The serum concentration of sodium is not usually of much help in estimating how much sodium should be administered, and it is unfortunately still true, that the close and careful observation of the effect of treatment on the patient is probably the best means of judging success. If in addition a low-grade intestinal obstruction develops (Counsell and Goligher, 1952) even greater care is needed in the employment of intravenous replacement of lost fluid. It may sometimes be necessary to use dextran or blood to restore circulating blood volume, especially in the presence of intestinal obstruction, but usually the rapid infusion of enough isotonic saline is all that is necessary.

BIOCHEMICAL DISTURBANCES AFTER TRANSPLANTATION OF THE URETERS

It has been known for many years that, following the transplantation of both ureters into the colon, acidosis might follow the continuous discharge of all the urine into the lower bowel. Dilatation of the upper urinary tract, with or without secondary infection, is commonly followed by impairment of renal function. Acidosis may be accompanied by other biochemical changes and the clinical and chemical state of these patients is subject to wide individual variation.

The typical biochemical disturbance is an elevation of the plasma chloride concentration, with which is associated a lowered bicarbonate and sometimes a raised sodium concentration, and rarely potassium depletion. This disturbance is found most often in continent patients after complete diversion of all their urine to the colon; it may appear at any time after operation, but becomes more common the longer the patient survives and especially when renal function is impaired. It may also occur when the ureters have been transplanted to an isolated segment of ileum or colon when the isolated segment is too long or the urine does not drain freely from it to the surface. Patients affected in this way are usually easily tired, feel weak and have poor appetites; there may be nausea and vomiting, severe thirst and the discharge of large volumes of more watery rectal fluid than is customary. The disturbance is often precipitated in a severe form by illnesses such as influenza or by other acute infectious disease. Anuria is rare and is usually associated with progressive potassium depletion; the latter may cause flaccid paralysis, severe drowsiness and occasionally coma.

These disturbances are due to the combination of selective absorption and secretion in the colon with impairment of renal tubular function resulting from pyelonephritis. Although reflux of bowel contents with infection occurs in 50 per cent of cases after direct anastomosis (Nesbit), but in only 10 per cent of cases after indirect anastomosis (Coffey or Stiles type) there is little difference in the incidence of acidosis after either of these types of anastomosis (Jacobs and Stirling, 1952). The accumulation of urine for four or five hours or more in the colon above a continent anal sphincter, or in an isolated segment of bowel, seems to be the most important factor common to all cases, and improvement follows continuous drainage of the urine from the bowel by an indwelling tube.

The absorption of chloride from the colon depends on the relative concentrations of chloride in the bowel fluid and in the plasma. The presence in the lower colon of urine with a high chloride content makes absorption likely, and the longer the urine is allowed to remain in the colon the greater is the quantity of chloride which may be absorbed. Absorption of chloride in this way interferes with the renal regulation of chloride content of the body even when, as Mitchell and Valk (1953) have shown, renal function is better than the normal minimum. Parsons *et al.* (1952) have confirmed the old observation that when only one ureter was transplanted into an isolated pouch of colon and rectum, the urine from the bladder was strongly acid, whereas that from the pouch of colon was consistently alkaline. By adding radioactive chlorine (^{38}Cl) to urine in this pouch they showed that ^{38}Cl concentration rapidly rose in peripheral venous blood and was disproportionately high in the bladder urine. They also showed that ^{38}Cl was absorbed more rapidly than ^{24}Na from urine in the colon. When 0·9 per cent saline is instilled into the isolated colon more chloride than sodium is absorbed by the colonic mucosa, which in addition secretes potassium into the lumen to a concentration of 15 to 20 mEq per litre and bicarbonate to a concentration of 50 to 70 mmol per litre (d'Agostino *et al.*, 1962). In spite of absorption of sodium from the urine in the bowel, elevation of serum sodium concentration is not common after transplantation of the ureters.

The presence of urine in the colon stimulates the secretion of colonic mucus, which is therefore lost in large quantities when the bowel is emptied. The potassium concentration of the mixture of urine and colonic secretion discharged from the rectum is higher than that of the urine alone, and over a period of time significant quantities of potassium are lost from the body. Under normal circumstances, the loss of potassium is replaced by the potassium in the food; when, however, food intake is restricted by illness or loss of appetite, or if potassium excretion is increased by injury or infection, signs of potassium depletion may appear; attention was first drawn to this in 1951 by Diefenbach *et al.* Thirst is a common symptom in patients whose ureters have been transplanted and suggests that a low-grade chronic intracellular dehydration is fairly common. This probably accounts for the inability of these patients to tolerate restriction of their normally high fluid intakes. The chief importance of potassium depletion in association with acidosis is the greater mortality and morbidity with which it is associated.

In most patients symptoms are rapidly relieved by continuous drainage of the rectum or isolated segment of bowel with an indwelling tube, combined with the consumption of a normal diet. If rectal drainage is maintained for four or five days, the disordered blood chemistry usually returns to normal. Intravenous therapy is seldom required except when potassium depletion is severe and there is coma. The disturbance can be prevented by regular emptying of the collected urine from the rectum, at intervals of two or three hours by day, and once or twice during the night. The consumption of up to five or six pints of water per day should be encouraged. The intake of sodium chloride should be limited to that used in cooking or preparing the food, but it does not seem to be necessary to insist on the provision of a salt-free diet. To counteract the tendency to potassium depletion and enhance the effects of restriction of chloride intake, potassium citrate should be administered according to a simple plan, for example a stock mixture (20 mg in 30 ml) should be taken three times a day for three weeks out of every four and throughout any illness or infection (Wilkinson, 1954).

There is now a tendency to transplant the ureters to an isolated segment of ileum or colon, the main advantage of which is to reduce the risk of ascending infection. Such segments are designed simply as conduits for urine from the ureters to the surface and not as substitutes for the reservoir action of the bladder. The segment must be short and have a wide enough opening on the anterior abdominal wall to allow free escape of urine without delay into a suitable bag. Biochemical disturbances may still occur when the piece of bowel is too long and the urine is not rapidly discharged from it.

CHAPTER SEVEN

The Influence of Associated Disease

Patients with severe disturbances of cardiac, hepatic and renal function are commonly submitted to major surgical procedures. Success largely depends on the accuracy with which these associated disturbances are recognised and assessed before operative treatment is undertaken. This is particularly true in patients who have to be submitted to emergency operation, in whom preoperative assessment must necessarily be limited. When it is possible to investigate the patient more fully before operation the limits of freedom in treatment can be more accurately defined and greater latitude for postoperative treatment may be secured by suitable preoperative preparation.

CARDIAC DISEASE

In congestive cardiac disease restriction of the intake of sodium is usually beneficial because administered sodium is not readily excreted. Provided the sodium intake is controlled, the consumption or intake of water can be maintained at a fairly high daily rate and some patients respond well to an increased intake of water. In congestive failure renal blood flow is reduced, but an increased resistance in the efferent glomerular blood vessels tends to maintain the volume of glomerular filtrate. Nevertheless there may be a reduction in the quantity of sodium filtered by the glomerulus, and in addition increased tubular absorption of filtered sodium may also increase sodium retention. When thiazide diuretics are used to reduce or remove oedema in cardiac disease the urinary excretion of potassium is increased and negative potassium balance and a fall in the plasma potassium concentration are liable to occur. Such patients should be encouraged to take as liberal a diet as is possible consistent with control of their sodium intake. Most potassium supplements have an unpleasant taste and enteric coated tablets may cause ulceration and stenosis or perforation of the intestine.

Moore and his associates (Wilson *et al.*, 1954) have shown how water and sodium retention may increase the morbidity of patients submitted to mitral valvuloplasty. Before operation on non-oedematous patients there were only small increases in the total body content of sodium and water and total potassium was reduced; these changes are in conformity with the wasted state of most of their patients. After operation the usual features of the general metabolic response were seen, but in spite of sodium restriction water retention readily occurred. When the sodium intake was not restricted, marked sodium retention resulted and body weight increased. This tendency in cardiac patients to exaggeration of the normal post operative conservation of sodium increases the risk of generalised oedema and its many complications. Although these observations were made on patients submitted to mitral valvuloplasty, they apply equally to other operations on patients with severe cardiac disease.

The use of local analgesia may reduce some of the hazards of operation on a strangulated hernia or obstruction of the large bowel in patients with cardiac disease but is unlikely to affect the post-traumatic renal functional changes. The inevitability of these changes and their greater significance in the circumstances of these patients should lead to especial caution in the administration of sodium, and, to a lesser degree, of water, by any routes during the first week after operation.

McMurrey *et al.* (1955) found that in chronic cardiac invalids with cachexia the blood volume was larger than in health, total exchangeable sodium, the extracellular water and plasma volumes being increased as well as the total red cell volume. In such patients particular care is necessary in the use of both transfusion and infusion Patients with chronic cardiac disease or in failure do not tolerate well a hot environment and their tolerance is further reduced when the humidity also is increased. At any age chronic pulmonary disease may be associated with polycythaemia and a chronic increase in blood volume as well as with chronic respiratory acidosis.

LIVER DISEASE

Acute or chronic liver disease may lead to severe disturbances of water and sodium content and equilibrium. The precise way in which these disturbances are brought about remains obscure, but it seems fairly certain that the kidneys are closely concerned. Oliguria or suppression of urine and the delayed onset of a diuresis after the consumption of a large volume of water are well-known features of acute liver disease; and it has long been known that the onset of a diuresis is perhaps the earliest sign of improvement in liver disease of several types. In acute liver disease there is retention of both sodium and water by the kidneys perhaps because of impaired inactivation and conjugation of aldosterone; a diuresis may follow the administration of an osmotic diuretic such as mannitol.

In cirrhosis of the liver, with or without ascites, there is usually a marked reduction in lean tissue mass and the total body weight is well below the ideal weight. Yet at the same time the total body content of sodium is increased and the distribution of body water is altered, the extracellular fraction being unusually high. Protein depletion is usually marked, and with the loss of protein tissue, total body potassium falls. The total quantity of plasma protein in circulation is reduced, but the albumin falls to a greater degree than globulin. The reduction in circulating albumin is another factor leading to distortion of body fluid equilibrium. Too little emphasis seems to have been laid on the generalised nature of the protein depletion in severe liver disease.

The factors which lead to the production of ascites are puzzling. The fluid in the peritoneal cavity is in dynamic equilibrium with the rest of the extracellular fluid in the body, and there are large and continuing exchanges to and fro across the peritoneum. Ascites may appear after an operation, bleeding from oesophageal varices or during an acute infective illness; in these circumstances it seems to be related not so much to further impairment of liver function by infection, anaesthesia or anoxia as to the renal conservation of sodium and associated retention of water which are part of the general response to operation, haemorrhage or infection. In addition, bleeding from varices is usually followed by a marked reduction in plasma albumin concentration. In patients with chronic liver disease the daily renal output of sodium remains low in spite of wide variation in the daily sodium intake. Whatever the primary factor in this may be, renal conservation continues with surprisingly little elasticity. Over a prolonged period of time it may be possible to strike a balance between sodium intake and output and so to prevent the reaccumulation of ascitic fluid; this balance is precarious and can be upest by slight variations of intake or output, for example, small increases in sodium consumption or minor operations or infections.

Much attention has been given to the depressed plasma albumin concentration which is such a common feature of severe liver disease of all kinds. In severe liver disease protein depletion is generalised and the plasma albumin concentration cannot be lastingly increased by the infusion of plasma protein alone, but only by improving the state of protein nutrition in the body as a whole. Patients with advanced liver disease often do not tolerate high protein diets; the consumption of a large quantity of carbohydrate to ensure the provision of sufficient calories is of at least as much importance. It is unfortunate that reducing the sodium content of food so greatly reduces its palatability. When albumin is administered to an ascitic patient by intravenous infusion, a large part of it is lost into the ascitic fluid, in which the concentration of albumin may increase until it equals that in the plasma. Moreover when albumin is injected into the peritoneal cavity some of it may rapidly pass into the plasma. In ascites when tritium is injected into the peritoneal cavity 40 to 80 per cent of the dose has left the ascitic fluid within an hour (Prentice *et al.*, 1952) and when deuterium oxide is injected into the peritoneal cavity soon after a laparotomy equilibrium is reached in an hour (Bujant *et al.*, 1957). The surface area of the peritoneum on the bowel and its mesenteries and the abdominal wall is believed to be about equal to that of the skin and such rapid equilibration is not surprising. It must be remembered, however, that this implies an equally or even more rapid transfer in the reverse or in both directions of constituents of extracellular fluid when an inflammatory state involves the peritoneum and the organs which it covers, and as large and as rapid exchanges to and from the peritoneal fluid as occur in inflammatory exudates anywhere else in the body.

In advanced liver disease coma associated with a raised concentration of ammonia in the blood is a common and severe complication. The accumulation of ammonia may be due to exogenous or endogenous factors. It may be exogenous owing to the digestion of blood in the alimentary tract after bleeding from oesophageal varices in portal hypertension, or to an excessive intake of protein in the diet after surgical decompression of portal hypertension especially soon after operation. In these types of ammonia intoxication ammonia absorption can be reduced by the use of suitable antibiotics to diminish the breakdown of protein in the bowel, but at the risk of enterocolitis. Cation exchange resins also may be useful in exogenous intoxication. Zuidema *et al.* (1964) have recommended that the blood ammonia concentration should exceed 150 micrograms per 100 ml. before resin treatment is considered. A potassium cycle resin should be used to avoid an undesirable increase in body sodium content, as well as depletion of potassium content which is commonly low in advanced liver disease. Potassium supplements should always be provided when sodium cycle resins are used. Colonic lavage may be used to wash out blood shed into the bowel, but saline should be avoided.

Just as in severe cardiac or renal disease, many patients with advanced or severe hepatic disease are living near the margin of compensation. What is sufficient for a quiet life without injury or infection may be too little after operation. Then the chances of survival in all these conditions, like the previous maintenance of equilibrium, depend on moderation in all ways. The intravenous administration of glucose solution or saline is particularly hazardous when the normal postoperative renal conservation of sodium is distorted by loss of adaptability and the already sodium-loaded state of the body.

DIABETES MELLITUS

Diabetes affects between 1 and 2 per cent of the population and may not be recognised until it is found as a complication of a surgical illness. Even in known diabetics an acute exacerbation may result from severe infection or other surgical conditions because the requirements for insulin are increased. There may then be a gradual loss of control of the diabetic state with increasing polyuria, thirst, dehydration and even circulatory failure, drowsiness, stupor and coma. Intracellular dehydration results in the transfer of potassium from the cells to the extracellular fluid and because of the polyuria, large quantities of sodium and potassium are lost in the urine. If the blood pressure falls, renal function may be impaired, with a rise in the concentration of urea in the plasma and blood, and there may be anuria. Severe abdominal pain, with vomiting, may simulate an acute obstruction of the appendix.

It is essential to administer enough insulin to control the deterioration in the diabetic state, enough suitable fluid to correct the losses of water and sodium in the urine and by vomiting, and to control the infection when this is the precipitating cause. The initial dose of insulin should be given immediately by intramuscular injection and when an intravenous infusion is established, further insulin can be given by this route. During the first 24 hours of treatment, very large quantities of insulin may be needed because of the antagonistic action of ketone bodies on insulin.

When there is oliguria or anuria, the dose of insulin must be controlled by frequent estimation of the blood sugar concentration but if the urinary output is maintained, estimation of the urinary glucose may provide a satisfactory indication of the requirements of insulin. It is probably best to use a balanced electrolyte solution to restore and maintain the extracellular fluid volume, with the addition of sodium bicarbonate as indicated by analysis of the serum. The initially high serum potassium concentration will fall by dilution as the extracellular fluid volume is increased by intravenous infusion, and also as the result of the transfer of potassium to the cells as glucose uptake improves following the administration of insulin. As much as 100 mEq of potassium per 24 hours may be needed once treatment is established and is effective. The administration of glucose is required if ketosis persists in spite of the reduction of the blood sugar concentration towards the normal range.

Hypoglycaemia may occur in insulin-sensitive diabetics when the intake of glucose is restricted, especially when a long-acting insulin is used. In some patients there may be mental disturbance alone or in association with anxiety, palpitation, pallor and sweating; in others, the sudden loss of consciousness is the first sign. It is important to distinguish, if possible, the coma associated with ketosis from that due to hypoglycaemia. In ketotic coma there is usually peripheral circulatory failure, which does not occur in the early stages of hypoglycaemia. If there is any doubt in diabetic coma, glucose should be administered first, because if insulin is given in hypoglycaemic coma it may cause irreversible cerebral damage and death. The urinary glucose concentration is not a good guide, but a rough indication may be obtained from the use of clinistix test paper with a drop of peripheral blood from a needle puncture.

Diabetic nephropathy is a frequent complication of poorly controlled juvenile diabetics and deserves to be remembered because of the risk of renal failure.

Diabetics who are well controlled without insulin do not usually develop ketosis during deliberate operative treatment. Those who need an oral supplement may develop hypoglycaemia, and the supplement should be stopped while they are starving, and be restarted when their intake of calories is resumed. Insulin-sensitive diabetics should be maintained on soluble insulin for several days before and after operation, and glucose should be administered by intravenous infusion for 12 hours before operation, during the operation, and thereafter until the oral intake is adequate. Glucose solution should never be given orally within 12 hours of operation because it may be retained in the stomach and vomited, especially during the induction of anaesthesia. Insulin should be administered every 4 hours before, during and after operation and the dose should be controlled by equally frequent and suitably timed estimations of the blood glucose concentration.

RENAL DISEASE

The important part which the kidneys take in the regulation of the volume and composition of the body fluids has already been indicated. So great is the reserve functional capacity of the normal kidney that only in severe or advanced renal disease are the body fluids liable to distortion. The large normal reserve allows of great adaptability in function and the main effect of disease is to reduce this elasticity or adaptability. Although an individual with diseased kidneys may be able to live satisfactorily a quiet life, he no longer possesses the means of reacting to the large disturbances of metabolism resulting from a freely chosen diet, violent exercise or severe injury. Because of the impairment of concentration and reduced specificity in absorption and tubular secretion, the formation of an increased volume of urine is necessary for adequate excretion of solutes. Yet the reduced absorptive and concentrating capacity of the diseased kidneys hinders the normal conservation of constituents of the glomerular filtrate, and the unlimited consumption of water, by causing diuresis, may induce additional losses. When in chronic renal disease urinary volume is injudiciously increased, the conservation of sodium may be so far impaired as to lead to reduction of extracellular fluid volume. The combination of such sodium loss with the retention of sulphate and phosphate may cause severe acidosis.

The patient with advanced renal disease is a poor subject for a major surgical operation, and his survival may depend largely on whether his remaining renal function is sufficient to deal with the extra excretory burdens imposed by the inevitable postoperative metabolic disturbance. The impaired ability to produce a concentrated urine then demands an increased water intake, but there is also a reduction in the capacity to respond rapidly and completely by diuresis to a sudden large intake of water. If excessive water retention is to be avoided after operation, its administration must be carefully controlled. Especially in elderly patients with impaired renal function, the water intake should not be suddenly increased by intravenous infusion of glucose solution, and the administration of isotonic saline or sodium sulphate solution in an attempt to compel a diuresis is dangerous and ineffective.

Some indication of the severity of the degree of renal functional impairment may be obtained before operation from the examination of the volume and osmolality of the urine, even in the absence of elevation of the blood urea concentration. For this type of examination to be of any value it is, however, essential that the urine be collected over short periods of time, not exceeding four hours during the day, but the whole of the night urine may be collected in one sample from 10 p.m. to 6 a.m. The volume of urine passed in the night specimen is normally only about one-quarter of the total and its osmolality is high; in severe renal disease the nocturnal urine may equal in volume that passed during the remainder of the 24 hour period and be of equally low specific gravity. A large volume of urine may also be passed during the night when a large quantitiy of fluid is drunk late in the evening, or when there is urinary tract infection, prostatic enlargement, uncontrolled diabetes or adrenal insufficiency. The response to the ingestion of 500 ml of water also gives a valuable indication of the functional state of the kidneys; in a normal subject there is a prompt diuresis and the osmolality of the urine falls sharply, but with impaired function there is little change in the volume or osmolality of the urine.

When chronic obstruction is relieved there may be polyuria which lasts only a few hours depending on the state of tubular function and the accumulated osmotic load, largely of urea. It generally subsides uneventfully but rarely it may persist long enough to cause severe dehydration and sodium loss. It is important to measure accurately the output of urine when obstruction is relieved and the sodium and potassium concentration in the urine whenever polyuria is prolonged.

Uraemia

The term uraemia indicates an elevation of the concentration of urea in the blood. It is commonly used to indicate the retention in the body of urea produced by metabolism, which is a feature of many disturbances of water and electrolyte balance. Urea is an end-product of protein metabolism and is not a toxic substance; elevation of its concentration in the blood does not cause harm or give rise to symptoms, but may be a useful though unspecific index of alteration in several body functions. A high plasma urea concentration may be an index of impairment of renal function by disease, it may also be due simply to reduced or incomplete excretion; the latter may be the result of osmotic limitation when water for urine formation is insufficient to dissolve all the urea awaiting excretion or because urea formation is increased by tissue catabolism.

The normal daily output of urea by an adult is about 30 g, and its excretion in the urine results from the selective absorption of glomerular filtrate without urea, the concentration of urea in the urine (2 to 3 g per 100 ml) being about 100 times that in plasma and glomerular filtrate. Failure to maintain the excretion of urea may thus be due to reduction in glomerular filtration rate. Disturbances of tubular function affect the ability of the kidneys to concentrate the urine; unless the glomerular filtration rate is reduced, however, the quantity of urea which is excreted may not be affected, although its concentration in the urine may fall. Elevation of the blood urea concentration may indicate altered glomerular function, but is not a direct index of tubular function. The urinary urea concentration is a measure of tubular function, since it reveals the concentration in the urine at which the kidneys can excrete urea. The urea clearance test, on the other hand, is an index of glomerular function, since it measures how much of the urea in the plasma at a particular concentration can be filtered and excreted in the urine in a specific period of time, regardless of the concentration at which the urea is present in the urine. Retention of urea is related to impairment of glomerular filtration. Peters and Van Slyke (1931) concluded that urea clearance must be reduced to less than 20 per cent of normal before patients with impaired renal function exhibit a raised blood urea nitrogen concentration. The blood urea nitrogen concentration can be interpreted correctly, however, only when the rate of urea formation is known.

Many patients with renal disease can maintain their blood urea nitrogen concentration within normal limits provided the intake of calories is maintained but that of protein is sufficiently reduced; about 1 g of urea is produced from 3 g of protein. In normal subjects excretion of urea usually keeps pace with its formation even after severe injury. Patients with even moderate impairment of renal function may show elevation of the blood urea nitrogen concentration after relatively small increases in urea production but large rises may occur, if for example after burns the protein intake is much increased but urine volume does not rise enough.

Because of an antagonism to insulin many uraemic patients cannot metabolise glucose or galactose efficiently (Cohen, 1962) but can utilise fructose and xylitol normally (Luke *et al.*, 1964) since their transport into muscle occurs independently of insulin. Both fructose and xylitol are useful alternative sources of calories to glucose, and xylitol can be used instead of glucose in dialysis fluid.

The clinical state of uraemia is usually considered to be of two types, 'renal' or 'extrarenal', according to the nature of the underlying disturbance.

RENAL URAEMIA. The 'renal' type of uraemia is encountered in organic renal disease such as nephritis, or secondary to arteriosclerosis. Its importance in surgical patients is related to the degree of functional impairment which exists and to the consequent loss of elasticity of renal function. The reduced ability of the kidneys to respond to the large metabolic disturbances due to injury and inflammation of all kinds leads to slower and less delicate regulation of the composition of the internal environment.

'EXTRARENAL' URAEMIA is due rather to primary disturbances unconnected with the kidneys but which have an effect on renal function. Reduction in glomerular filtration rate may be due to a reduced flow of blood through the kidneys, or to a lowered blood pressure which reduces glomerular filtration pressure. Renal blood flow may be reduced by direct loss of blood or plasma, or by reduction in extracellular fluid volume by vomiting, diarrhoea, fistulous discharges or excessive sweating. Cardiac disease, especially with cardiac failure, may reduce renal blood flow and is particularly important in elderly patients whose reserve of renal function is low, and in the presence of arteriosclerosis. After bleeding into the upper gastrointestinal tract the blood urea concentration may be raised and then has usually been ascribed to the absorption of products of digestion of the blood in the bowel; in the absence of bleeding, however, the presence of blood in the bowel is not associated with elevation of the blood urea concentration, and it seems likely that alterations in blood urea concentration may be due to effects of blood loss other than digestion and absorption of the shed blood, for example, impaired renal excretion caused by reduction in glomerular filtration rate following severe bleeding (Johnson, 1941)

Anuria

The term anuria is usually employed when the output of urine from the kidneys has ceased. Oliguria is usually used to describe reduction in urine volume below 500 ml per day. It is probably wise to distinguish clearly between the use of these terms in patients who have lost large volumes of body fluid, because the treatment of anuria due to renal failure is usually incompatible with the replacement of large losses of body fluids.

Anuria due to acute renal failure may be caused by:

1. Primary renal disease such as acute nephritis or pyelonephritis.

2. Mechanical obstruction in calculous disease of the renal pelvis or ureter, in sulphonamide crystalluria or inadvertent bilateral ligation of the ureters.

3. Damage by specific poisons, such as mercury, carbon monoxide or diethylene gylcol.

4. Various disturbances such as mismatched blood transfusion, abortion, concealed accidental haemorrhage and other forms of prolonged renal ischaemia.

Oliver *et al.* (1951) described two types of pathological lesion in the kidneys. One type which was found only after poisoning caused necrosis of the cells lining all the proximal tubules, with preservation of the basement membrane, so that regeneration and return of function were possible. The other type of lesion affected the whole of the nephron and was patchily distributed through the kidneys; the lining cells and the basement membrane might be disrupted, but not all nephrons were affected, except in a small proportion of cases of massive necrosis. Bull *et al.* (1950) found a uniform pattern of disturbance of renal function in these conditions, characterised by evidence of gross tubular dysfunction and extreme reduction in renal blood flow, and in the fatal cases by a typical patholgical picture; they applied the term 'acute tubular necrosis' to the whole group instead of that of 'lower nephron nephrosis' proposed by Lucké (1946).

The clinical course can be divided into four stages (Bull *et al.*, 1950):

(1) *Stage of onset.* A period of severe and prolonged shock or diminution in blood flow, or a period during which a toxin such as mercury is acting.

(2) *Stage of anuria or oliguria.* During this stage, lasting up to three weeks, the renal blood flow falls from the normal of 1200 ml per minute to as little as 10 to 30 ml per minute and less than 300 ml of urine per day is secreted; complete anuria is not common except in cases of massive renal cortical necrosis. Up to half the total deaths used to occur in this stage, most often from cardiac arrest due to the accumulation in the extracellular fluid of potassium released from the cells. The plasma potassium concentration should be estimated at least once every 24 hours, since it provides a more reliable indication of progress of the biochemical changes than do electrocardiographic tracings.

The accumulation of acid resulting from the catabolism of protein causes a reduction in plasma bicarbonate, leading to a fall in plasma pH, stimulation of the respiratory centre and the characteristic deep respiration of acidosis. The plasma sodium and chloride concentrations fall, either because of a shift of these ions into cells as a compensation for the outward transfer of potassium or because of dilution by retained water.

(3) *Early diuretic stage.* This follows in patients who recover with a gradual or occasionally a sudden increase in daily urine output, the volume soon reaching a litre or more, but there is at first no evidence of tubular function. The duration of this stage is usually about as long as that of oliguria. The urine has a low specific gravity of about 1010 (400 mosmol) and is an almost unmodified ultrafiltrate of plasma. Loss of large quantities of this fluid leads to reduction in extracellular fluid volume. It is usually recommended that an amount of fluid equivalent to the urine volume should be added to the daily intake of water. Swan and Merrill (1953) have warned against the administration of excessive volumes of fluid during this stage, since they believe that this frequently leads to overloading the body with fluid and thus to prolongation of the diuresis.

(4) *The late diuretic stage.* It is said that this stage is present when there is evidence of tubular function.

When renal blood flow is diminished in the stage of onset, it affects equally glomerular as well as tubular function. When blood flow is restored, glomerular filtration is gradually resumed, but tubular function is more slowly regained. It is not known how long anoxia must last to produce tubular changes, but undoubtedly the prompt correction of hypotensive states will greatly reduce the incidence of renal disturbances and is the most important way of preventing tubular necrosis. Circulatory disturbances secondary to renal disease may result from excessive loss of sodium and water in the urine or by vomiting, and ultimately give rise to anuria. In all cases of anuria, obstruction of the renal tract must be excluded or treated.

When oliguria occurs at a time when it is not unexpected, for example after an operation or accidental injury, diagnosis of tubular necrosis is often delayed. Only when a low urinary output has persisted for several days and does not rise, or perhaps falls further, is renal functional impairment suspected. In the absence of artificially high intakes of water after operations, oliguria is normal, but the urine is highly concentrated with a specific gravity of 1026 to 1036 (1000 to 1250 mosmol). Renal failure is not invariably accompanied by oliguria and the persistent passage of pale urine of low specific gravity (1010, 400 mosmol) may also be an indication of severe renal functional damage. Once suspicion has been aroused, close observation at the bedside and repeated estimation of blood chemical changes are required. Excessive accumulation of water is shown by haemodilution with a falling packed cell volume or haemoglobin concentration and a drop in plasma sodium concentration. The accumulation of metabolic end-products is indicated by the rising blood urea and plasma potassium concentration. The provision of 100 g of glucose to an otherwise starving person will reduce the catabolism of protein to a minimum of about 40 g per day (Gamble, 1947), but the supply of 2000 calories per day and a litre of water may have other effects on metabolism. In the anuric patient the ready availability of abundant carbohydrate may lead to glycogen synthesis and to the removal of some of the excess potassium from the extracellular fluid. The consumption of protein tissue by unavoidable or 'continuing' protein metabolism can be reduced to the minimum of about 40 g per day with the liberation of 6 to 7 g nitrogen per day only in normal subjects. In patients who have suffered severe injuries, or who have had an abortion with subsequent infection, or whose uterus is undergoing postpartum involution, such reduction in protein metabolism is obscured by the much larger protein catabolism due to injury or infection.

It is usually impossible to predict by how much the blood urea concentration will rise each day, but in such patients the figure will be at least 20 mg per 100 ml, and may be much higher. After severe injury mean daily rises in blood urea concentration of 50 mg per 100 ml have been reported (Teschan *et al.*, 1955; Taylor, 1957). The catabolism of tissue protein may result in the release of nitrogen ranging in quantity from the minimum of 6 g to 20 or 30 g per 24 hours in the first week after injury. Since 2 to 3 mEq potassium may be released with each 1 g of tissue protein nitrogen, from 12 to 60 mEq potassium may reach the extracellular fluid every day (Tables XVI and XVII). The serum potassium concentration may rise 0·6 to 0·7 mEq per litre per day after severe injury.

Impaired tubular function in the second and third stages is shown by inability of the kidneys to concentrate urea and creatinine, to conserve sodium and chloride, to extract para-aminohippuric acid from the blood or to reabsorb glucose at a normal rate. There is a rapid initial loss of tubular function, but a very slow return beginning only after several days and becoming complete only after many weeks or months. During the anuric stage there is retention of potassium with the possibility of a toxic concentration being reached, and later, during the diuretic stage, a risk of a large and prolonged loss of sodium and chloride in addition to a continuing loss of potassium.

Acute renal failure carries a mortality rate of about 50 per cent at any time of life but the causes may vary a good deal at different ages. In elderly people without pre-existing renal disease Kumar *et al.* (1973) found that ischaemic renal damage was the cause in three-quarters of their patients, in more than half a poor fluid intake was an important predisposing factor and a third had recently been subjected to a major operation. The chronic and excessive use of diuretics and laxatives predisposes to potassium depletion which is not always adequately corrected by supplements. A quarter of the patients were treated by dialysis mostly peritoneal, and as many had suffered from some kind of severe infection.

Treatment

In acute renal failure the aim of treatment is to keep the patient alive until tubular epithelium regenerates. Any circulatory disturbance causing renal ischaemia must be corrected as rapidly as possible. Until glomerular filtration is re-established in the early diuretic stage, water, minerals and other substances cannot be excreted by the kidneys, and if administered in excess of the quantities lost by insensible loss and in the sweat, faeces or vomitus, will accumulate in the body. Diuretics which act by osmotic effect or on the tubules are useless and may be harmful in the anuric stage, which is also unaffected by spinal or splanchnic block, or by decapsulation of the kidneys.

TABLE XVI

Effects of tissue catabolism

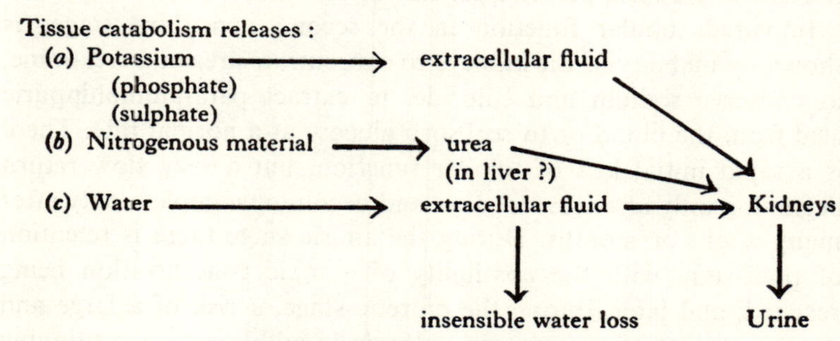

During the anuric stage water intake must be limited to 1000 ml per day to supply sufficient water for extrarenal losses. Only in this way can water intoxication and extensive oedema be avoided. Similarly, since apart from excretion in the urine the only ways in which sodium and potassium can be lost is by vomiting, in the faeces, or by sweating, there must be restriction of the intake of these elements until diuresis starts. Acidosis and alkalosis cannot readily be corrected during the anuric stage except by dialysis. As Borst (1948) pointed out, uraemic patients seldom eat unless forced to do so, and therefore seldom satisfy their calorie requirements. Any protein which they consume will therefore be deaminated and the residues used for energy, while the potassium, non-protein nitrogen and phosphate which are also released by protein catabolism increase the severity of the bodily disturbance due to failure of renal function.

DIET. Catabolism of tissue protein can be reduced without much increase in the sodium and potassium content of the body by feeding a suitable mixture of fat and carbohydrate; Folin (1905) used 400 g starch and 300 ml cream per 24 hours and reduced the urinary nitrogen excretion to 4 g per 24 hours within 7 days. Borst (1948), by feeding a protein-free diet to patients with oliguria or anuria, delayed the otherwise invariable increase in blood urea concentration associated with the consumption of protein with inadequate calories. He obtained the best results with a gruel consisting of 100 g custard powder, 100 g butter, 150 g sugar in 1·5 litres of water, which provides 1750 calories. The addition of even small quantities of protein greatly improves the palatability of this mixture, which does not always have to be administered by tube. In a normal man the use of this mixture reduced the daily urinary excretion of nitrogen to 6 g in 3 days and to 4 g in 14 days and of potassium to 30 mEq in 3 days and 10 mEq in 14 days.

Bull, G. M., *et al.* (1949) modified Borst's diet by mixing 400 g glucose with 100 g peanut oil emulsified with acacia in one litre of water. This provides 2300 calories per day free of protein and minerals and can be administered by stomach tube. Unfortunately some patients find this procedure nauseating; if vomiting or diarrhoea is persistent, intragastric feeding must usually be abandoned. Young and Scrimshaw (1968) found that when healthy volunteers lived on a protein-free diet for 16 days the daily urinary nitrogen output fell to 37 mg N per kg body weight from the ninth to the sixteenth day and very similar results have been reported by Calloway and Margen (1971). After prolonged protein depletion or malnutrition even lower outputs have been recorded, especially if the intake of calories also has been inadequate.

A solution which contains the essential L-amino acids in suitable proportions can be administered with hypertonic glucose in a volume of 1000 ml water to provide 1500 to 2500 calories per 24 hours, depending on the amount of glucose which is used. Such a solution will improve uraemia and encephalopathy but must be administered into a central vein. (see p. 261).

When uraemic patients are maintained on a nitrogen-free diet they can reuse urea nitrogen for protein synthesis provided they are also supplied with enough essential amino acids by mouth (Giordano, 1963). When the eight essential amino acids were provided by intravenous infusion in addition to a protein poor diet (2·7 g N/24 hours) (Fürst *et al.*, 1969) or an almost protein-free diet (0·2 g N/24 hours) (Bergström *et al.*, 1970) and histidine was added the nitrogen balance was more positive than when the essential amino acids were administered alone. The addition of a non-essential amino acid, arginine, further improved nitrogen retention but only by the amount of nitrogen in the arginine.

In spite of a high caloric intake, accumulation of potassium sometimes occurs, or may result from the mistaken or ill-advised administration of potassium salts. Some improvement may temporarily follow the administration of 50 units of insulin and 50 g of glucose (Bywaters and Joekes, 1948), which causes deposition of potassium in glycogen.

RESINS. A variety of cation exchange resins given by mouth or as an enema have been used to extract potassium from the body. The exchange of sodium and potassium ions from the gastrointestinal secretions for the ammonium or hydrogen ion of the resin depends on several factors such as the pH of the medium or fluid in the intestine, the amount of resin employed and its binding capacity, the total quantities and the proportions of sodium and potassium as well as other cations such as calcium and magnesium in the medium and the time the resin remains in the bowel. The theoretical binding capacity of a resin is seldom fully satisfied and is modified by other factors such as the presence of antibiotics. Perhaps the greatest disadvantage is the lack of specificity in removing any available cation. Some resins may give up ammonium or sodium in exchange and are thus unsuitable in renal failure. Berlyne *et al.* (1966) recommended the use of a calcium cycle resin as being safer and as efficient as other resins. To be most effective the resin should remain in contact with colonic mucosa as long as possible and anything which is liable to cause diarrhoea such as sorbitol should be avoided. Resins are usually administered in doses of 15 g in water or mixed with syrup, three or four times a day or 30 g daily by enema. In addition a fat glucose emulsion should be administered by mouth or 20 per cent fructose solution by intravenous infusion. When the resin is given by mouth some patients become nauseated and lose their appetite or vomit while others may become constipated which increases the extraction; others have diarrhoea which reduces the amount of potassium which is extracted. When extraction is successful 25 to 75 mEq of potassium may be removed each day which is more than is being released except in the first two or three days after injury.

DIALYSIS. When in spite of or for the lack of treatment the products of metabolism accumulate in the body to a dangerous degree they can be removed by dialysis. This process depends on the principle of equilibration between two fluids of dissimilar composition which are separated by a semipermeable membrane. There are two methods by which this can be achieved—haemodialysis and peritoneal dialysis. In haemodialysis with a so-called artificial kidney the patient's blood circulates on one side of a membrane of cellophane or other material while on the other there is a fluid, the composition of which is varied according to whether it is desired to remove or add materials to the body. In this way water can be extracted or added and excess urea and potassium can be removed. In peritoneal dialysis the peritoneum is used as the dialysing membrane, a suitable fluid is injected into the peritoneal cavity and then is removed after an interval of 20 minutes for equilibration.

Because peritoneal dialysis avoids the use of vascular cannulas it is the method of choice for babies and small children, but at any age its value is limited soon after abdominal operations or peritonitis. When it is feasible it is cheaper than haemodialysis since the equipment is simple, but it is of limited value for repeated use and when renal failure is due to very severe injury or infection. Peritonitis may occur when the catheters are left too long in the peritoneal cavity and after repeated dialysis peritoneal adhesions may form; it is not always possible to remove all the fluid which is injected and this may cause overloading of the body with the solution used. Peritoneal dialysis has the advantage however that it seldom reduces the blood urea concentration so rapidly as to cause cerebral oedema which may occur with rapid haemodialysis (Kennedy *et al.*, 1962).

Various types of apparatus have been developed for haemodialysis with disposable membranes and tubing. For repeated dialysis in chronic renal failure some types of apparatus are sufficiently automatic in action that the patients can be taught to connect themselves to the apparatus with little assistance and can be dialysed at night while they sleep and at home. Haemodialysis can be used after any kind of operation but the patient must be heparinised. These methods are still not without their complications and risks and several dialysis centres have reported outbreaks of serum hepatitis amongst both patients and staff, some of whom have died. In both types of dialysis close supervision of the biochemical changes and control of water and mineral contents and exchanges are essential. The expansion of the treatment of both acute and chronic renal failure by dialysis depends on the skill, calibre and interest of the various types of person who work in the units, and shortage of suitable staff is and will remain the most important limiting factor. This sort of treatment cannot and should not be undertaken without sufficient ancillary assistance, in particular, an entirely reliable 24 hour biochemical service.

Haemodialysis is indispensable for the maintenance of homeostasis in patients who are waiting for renal transplantation both in preparation for operation and while a suitable donor is found. It should never be used in patients with urinary obstruction in preference to a relatively simple surgical drainage operation.

Chronic haemodialysis may be associated with severe emotional disturbance in the patient and closely involved relatives. These are related partly to the dependence on the apparatus for survival and the new kinds of discipline which must be imposed on the patient and the household whether the dialysis is carried out at home or in hospital. These emotional strains are aggravated by suspense in patients who are waiting for a renal transplant.

Most patients with anuria will be receiving injections of an antibiotic and may have been given a sulphonamide drug. Sulphonamides must be stopped and the dose of penicillin reduced. Streptomycin and chloramphenicol will cause toxic effects if their administration is continued, and a single dose will be sufficient to maintain an adequate concentration during the anuric stage.

It is usually recommended that during the diuretic phase sufficient water to equal urinary volume is added to the basal 1000 ml of water intake. If this advice is followed an artificial and entirely undesirable diuresis may be induced, a diuresis which often becomes larger day by day, and which in association with some persisting impairment of renal tubular function may cause large unnecessary losses of sodium and potassium. For this reason it is better and safer to maintain a mild state of dehydration or water lack until renal function recovers more completely. Because of the rapid loss of potassium in the urine, potassium should be supplied in the form of fruit and fruit drinks, and if the serum concentration falls, as potassium chloride by mouth up to 6 g per day. The body content of sodium and chloride is similarly maintained by supplementary intake of sodium chloride, as indicated by daily measurement of the serum sodium and chloride concentration, and if possible by measurement of the urinary output of sodium and chloride.

Acute reversible renal failure is less common than it was, possibly because its clinical features as well as the factors which cause it are now so well-known that prophylactic treatment is more often successful than in the past. It is also difficult to judge how much of the improved results are due to the careful restriction of the administration of water and minerals by infusion and the much wider appreciation of the need to provide sufficient calories to prevent starvation.

CRUSH SYNDROME (ISCHAEMIC MUSCLE NECROSIS)

In this syndrome prolonged crushing injury of a limb with pressure necrosis of muscle is followed, after release from compression, by anuria and renal failure. Originally described by Frankenthal (1916) this condition affected between 1 and 5 per cent of British air-raid casualties admitted to hospital in World War II (Bywaters, 1944). It is rare in peacetime, the commonest cause then probably being compression by roof falls in mining accidents or in some road accidents. It may also occur when damage to the main artery of a limb causes ischaemia of muscles without crushing, the development of a collateral circulation to the affected muscles leading to the absorption of products of muscle damage. The typical pathological features of the true crush syndrome, ischaemic muscle necrosis and myohaemoglobinuria, have been found after other types of injury, such as lesions of main vessels or fractures, in which mismatched transfusion or sulphonamides could be excluded as important factors in the associated anuria.

Clinical Features and Pathology

Release from compression may take many hours, and by the time the patient arrives in hospital there may be a zone of erythema at the margin of the compressed area, or this may appear only after warming or resuscitation. Blistering may later appear in the normal skin adjacent to the compressed area, which remains pale grey and opaque like a deep burn. Within an hour or two of release the general state deteriorates as the result of plasma loss into the damaged crushed tissue, which swells. For a time, as in burns, the blood-pressure levels are maintained by vasoconstriction, but as plasma loss continues a point is reached when this fails to maintain an adequate circulation and there is a sudden drop in blood pressure, with a systolic pressure of only 60 to 80 mmHg or less; there is marked haemoconcentration with a haemoglobin concentration of 20·6 to 23·6 g per 100 ml unless this is masked by bleeding from other injuries. These changes are probably due to the loss of plasma into the damaged tissues which continues, as after burning, for 24 hours or more after release from compression.

The affected limb becomes swollen and hard with a shiny tense skin; the distal pulses may disappear. On incision of the swollen limb, serous fluid oozes from the oedematous subcutaneous tissues; when the muscle fascia is opened, friable, wet, greyish, swollen muscle bulges outwards.

The first urine passed after injury may be normal, having been secreted before the injury, but thereafter it is acid (pH 5) and contains albumin, muscle pigment and casts, and is smoky or dark brown in colour. As renal failure comes on, both the volume and osmolality of the urine fall and acid haematin is found in the dark deposit. After a day or two pigment excretion ceases and casts become more numerous. Urinary output may be low only for 24 to 48 hours and then increase, and the blood urea concentration may be raised only for a short time. With more severe renal damage, urinary output is reduced for up to a week before a diuresis occurs and the blood urea may rise to a very high level. Renal function recovers slowly, and clearance may not return to normal limits for several months. In the past more than half the patients died about the end of the first week after injury of cardiac arrest due to a high extracellular potassium concentration. At least some of these deaths should now be avoided by better general management of the renal failure and by dialysis.

This syndrome consists of two components: first, the loss of plasma into the crushed tissue after release of compression with the subsequent development of a form of shock due to plasma loss; and secondly, the excretion of oxymyohaemoglobin or metamyohaemoglobin in an acid urine. It appears that the combination of reduced renal blood flow, acidosis and pigment excretion is necessary for the production of the fully developed state.

Treatment

Treatment is primarily prophylactic. If possible before release the victim should be given tea to drink, and alkali as sodium bicarbonate may be given dissolved in water (a dessertspoonful to the pint). After release, the administration of water and alkali should be carefully controlled and restricted if a diuresis does not occur within an hour or two. Patients with severe crush injuries should receive dextran prophylactically before the blood pressure falls. The effect of low molecular weight dextran in improving flow through the capillaries and in dispersing aggregated red cells is of particular value in crush injury, quite apart from the effect of large molecular weight dextran on plasma volume. Up to 500 ml of dextran 40 should be given on admission of the patient and this dose may be repeated during the second 24 hour period after injury. The injured limb should be kept cool by being exposed without coverings. Oliguria or renal failure should be treated as indicated earlier.

DIABETES INSIPIDUS

Diabetes insipidus is due to a deficiency of pitressin and at all ages it is most commonly due to a space occupying lesion of the brain, of which the most frequent is a craniopharyngioma. The cause cannot always be found, but it also occurs after injury, almost any operation on the brain, or may be due to idiopathic causes as well as to leukaemic deposits, metastases from a carcinoma of the breast or after many communicable diseases such as encephalitis and vaccinia. It is usually of abrupt onset with an unusual urine output and a sudden increase in thirst.

The diagnosis depends on the discovery of a hypotonic urine and a hypertonic plasma, both of which can be corrected by the administration of pitressin. The water deprivation test of Talbot *et al.* (1952) is usually diagnostic. No water is given overnight and then 500 ml of water per m^2 per hour is given until the patient is well hydrated, has a stable body weight and a free urine flow. During the next 6 hours water is withheld and the hourly output of urine, the hourly changes in weight and the serum and urine osmolality before, at the start of the water restriction, and at the end, are measured .The osmolality of the urine is persistently less than 150 mosmol per kg of urine water, or the specific gravity is less than 1005. The osmolality of the serum is more than 290 mosmol per litre of serum water and the sodium concentration in the serum is more than 150 mEq per litre. It is very important to watch carefully for the development of acute severe dehydration during the test.

Another diagnostic procedure is the hypertonic saline test of Hickey and Hare (1944), in which a solution containing 2·5 per cent glucose is administered at a rate of 20 mg of glucose per kg body weight for one hour, followed by 2·5 per cent sodium chloride solution at the rate of 0·25 ml per kg per minute for 45 minutes. The urine is collected at 15 minute intervals after this injection is started. In normal subjects there is an antidiuresis within 30 minutes of the start of the test, but in patients suffering from diabetes insipidus the urine volume rises.

Water deprivation in patients suffering from diabetes insipidus results in severe dehydration if pitressin is not administered, and there is loss of body weight and a rise in concentration of sodium in the plasma after 4 to 6 hours. This does not occur in psychogenic polydipsia in which the pitressin output by the pituitary is normal.

Diabetes insipidus should be treated by the intramuscular injection 5 to 10 international units per 70 kg of pitressin tannate in oil. Following this the hourly urine output should fall within 24 hours and at the same time the specific gravity of the urine should rise to more than 1015. It may sometimes also be necessary to give hypertonic saline intravenously in order to raise the osmolality of the urine and the blood. When pitressin tannate is given prophylactically before operation on a craniopharyngioma it is impossible to know whether the operation has caused diabetes insipidus or not, unless the fluid intake is maintained at a low level and the serum concentration of sodium remains within the range of 135 to 145 mEq per litre for 10 days after operation. When prophylactic pitressin is not given it is obvious within 48 to 72 hours after operation whether diabetes insipidus has resulted from the operation. The use of pituitrin snuff, 40 mg of the dry posterior pituitrin extract as a powder every 6 to 10 hours, is of less effect than the injection of pitressin tannate in oil since absorption varies and occasionally cumulative effects may develop. Some patients with diabetes insipidus are completely resistant to treatment. Nephrogenic diabetes insipidus must be distinguished from that of pituitary origin, since the nephrogenic type is due to a congenital inability of the renal tubules to absorb water, quite independent of the influence of the pituitary gland.

CHAPTER EIGHT

The Effects of Injury

Since ancient times wasting of the tissues and loss of body weight have been regarded as inevitable consequences of accidental or surgical injury, inflammation and fevers, and have been ascribed to such causes as toxaemia, infection or the consumption of tissue by starvation. In the natural wild state a severely injured animal, lacking its normal capacity for defence or flight, from new as well as old predators, must hide and be able to survive for several days without food or water. If the animal does not die from loss of blood or infection, survival during this period of starvation depends on the ability to provide from its own tissues not only the materials necessary for healing the injuries but also the continuing daily requirements of water and energy. Both herbivorous and carnivorous animals survive and heal at the expense of large metabolic disturbances. Man also possesses this inherent capacity to survive the combination of injury and starvation, but only a few observations seem to have been made on the biochemical basis of these post-traumatic phenomena before Cuthbertson (1930) described the well-marked alteration he had observed in the composition of the urine of patients suffering from fractures of the long bones. Since then many other investigations have shown how complex are the chemical and hormonic processes involved in the biological response to severe injury inflicted on a well nourished body. An understanding of this normal reaction and also of how it may be affected by orthodox treatment and variation in the environment is essential for the management of patients after many major operations. It should not be forgotten that the inflammatory reaction to injury and infection is as old as life and has been observed in many species and genera other than man and that many patients recover in spite of much of the treatment they receive.

FLUID SHIFTS AFTER INJURY

Immediately after injury the development of the acute inflammatory response and the formation of an inflammatory exudate cause the movement of fluid into the injured tissues and lead to a reduction in plasma and blood volume. Following this, there is a secondary shift of fluid out of normal tissues elsewhere in the body. Subsequently, as the inflammatory exudate resolves, there is a redistribution of fluid in the body (Fig. 4).

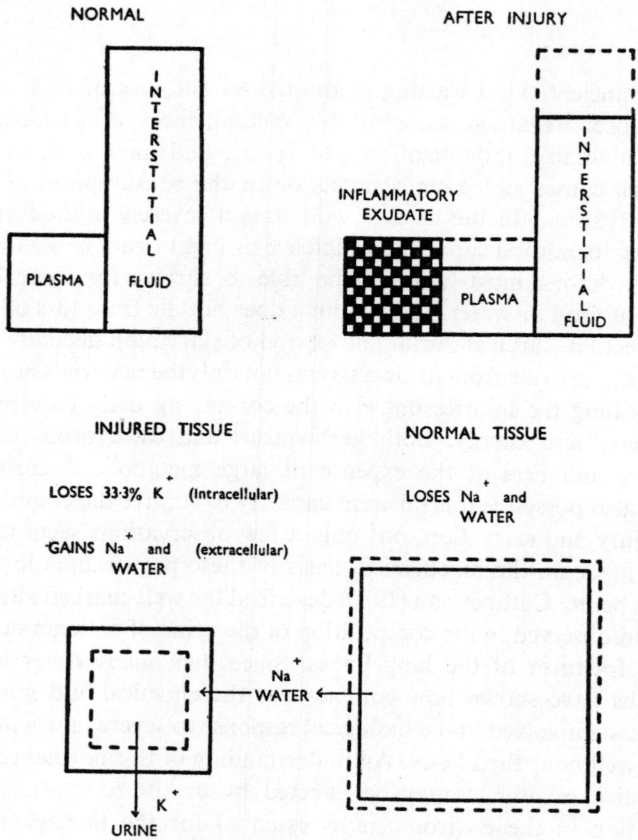

FIGURE 4. Fluid shifts after injury.

LOCAL CHANGES IN INJURED TISSUES

After all injury, even in the absence of infection, an inflammatory exudate forms amongst the injured tissues. This follows an alteration in capillary permeability which Lewis (1927) thought might be caused by substances which escaped from the damaged cells. The inflammatory exudate is rich in protein and resembles plasma, and in thermal or chemical burns is the sole cause of the swelling of the injured part. In lacerating or incised injuries there is also effusion of blood from divided blood vessels which contributes largely to the local swelling. Blalock (1931) found in dogs that handling of the intestines, crushing of a hind limb or extensive burning caused a local loss of plasma-like fluid, or of blood, equal to about 4 or 5 per cent of the body weight, or nearly half the total initial blood volume of the animal. This work has since been repeatedly confirmed and indicates that the large shift of fluid out of the blood vessels into the extravascular space in the injured tissues reduces blood volume and may lead to circulatory failure. It has also been shown by Fine and Seligman (1943) that the rate of lymph flow out of a burned limb may be increased up to eight times. At such a rapid rate of formation of lymph, albumin crosses the capillary membrane in the damaged tissues as freely as sodium (Cope and Moore, 1944), and in the injured area the intravascular osmotic effect of albumin is lost. The rapid rate of lymph formation and outflow from the injured limb shows, however, that the inflammatory exudate undergoes constant turnover; although fluid accumulates in the swollen tissues, there is a very rapid flow of that fluid through the extravascular space from damaged capillaries to the lymph vessels.

The swelling at the site of injury is due to the inflammatory exudate which is not static but is constantly changing its composition, and from this great flow of albuminous fluid through the injured tissues could be abstracted those substances which are needed for local repair. Such an exudate is a dynamic local expansion of the extracellular fluid equivalent to 4 or 5 per cent of the body weight. It is initially derived from the blood plasma to which it is nearly equal in volume, and its provision is a first charge on the available extracellular fluid, even at the expense of reducing plasma volume and circulatory efficiency. Since not all such severely injured animals or human beings die of shock caused by blood or plasma loss, even in the absence of treatment, there must be some means of compensating for the large local accumulation of fluid.

Changes in Uninjured Tissues

The amount of fluid which collected in the hind limbs of dogs crushed by a Blalock clamp was found by Ricca *et al.* (1945) to be greater than could be accounted for by the measured loss of plasma. They further showed that the water and sodium content was increased in damaged muscles but reduced in most of the uninjured parts of the body. Similar observations were made by Fox and Baer (1947) after scalding or the application of a tourniquet to the limbs of experimental animals; they also found that there was a marked loss of potassium from the cells of injured tissues. Rosenthal and Tabor (1945) found similar disturbances and calculated that after the application of a tourniquet the equivalent of all the sodium in the circulating plasma, or one-quarter of all the extracellular sodium, had accumulated in the injured area, which lost one-third of its original content of potassium. It seems clear that after injury there is a reduction in the volume of extracellular fluid (indicated by the sodium and water content) in the uninjured tissues. This is not associated with any abnormality in the capillaries of uninjured tissues, the permeability of which has been shown to be unimpaired (Fine and Seligman, 1943, 1944). In view of the compensatory shift of fluid out of undamaged tissues, the general condition and state of hydration are evidently important factors in determining the survival from severe injury.

As long as the rate of loss of fluid in the injured area exceeds that of withdrawal of fluid from intact tissues, plasma volume tends to fall, which leads to haemoconcentration in burns. By releasing pressure bandages at various times after injury, Cameron *et al.* (1945) showed that the permeability of the capillaries does not return to normal for 3 to 5 days afte1 injury, but long before this time the increased hydrostatic pressure in the swollen tissues has reduced the rate of loss of fluid from the capillaries. When normal capillary permeability is restored, most of the inflammatory exudate is usually rapidly reabsorbed.

METABOLISM DURING RESTRICTION OF THE INTAKE OF WATER AND FOOD

It is customary for the consumption of food and water by most surgical patients to be restricted for 12 hours or more before, and for up to several days after, surgical operations. The need for such restrictions varies with the site and nature of the operation, but they are commonly more lengthy and severe than is necessary. The effects of these restrictions are important and are superimposed on the disturbances in metabolism which are directly the result of injury.

The wide differences of opinion which exist between surgeons regarding the need for the provision of parenteral supplies of water, glucose, sodium or potassium during the immediate postoperative period arise partly from a lack of information or understanding of the individual and combined effects of injury and restrictions of the intake of water and food. Much of the early work on intravenous fluid therapy was done in North America, where the extremes of humidity and temperature which are inseparable from the continental type of climate may require, at certain seasons, higher intakes of sodium and water than are necessary in more temperate climates. It seems necessary therefore to examine in some detail these aspects of human metabolism. The following description of what happens in normal uninjured subjects is derived from the work of Benedict (1915), Gamble (1947) and observations on volunteers in a temperate climate (Wilkinson, 1966; Wilkinson *et al.*, 1949).

Deprivation of Water and Food

When a healthy adult is deprived of both water and food, the small carbohydrate reserve which exists as glycogen is soon exhausted, but the continuing oxidation of body protein and fat made available about 200 to 300 ml of water per day. The remaining 1300 ml of the theoretical minimal daily water requirement must be provided from water already in the body. It is obtained from both extracellular and intracellular fluid. The quantities of sodium and potassium excreted in the urine indicate the degree to which the extracellular and intracellular fluids are used to provide the continuing daily requirements of water. When the intake of both food and water is stopped, the loss of sodium and of extracellular fluid is greatest on the first day, declines during the next 3 days and is small from the fifth day onwards (Gamble, 1947).

The consumption of tissue protein is indicated by the quantity of nitrogen which is excreted in the urine; the nitrogen output usually falls on the first day of a fast, but then rises again during the next day or two before falling slowly but steadily as long as the fast continues (Benedict, 1915). On a normal diet the urinary output of potassium is related to the daily intake. When starvation begins, the urinary output of potassium usually falls to about 50 to 60 mEq per day, and then very slowly declines throughout the fast. Part of this excreted potassium comes from catabolised protein, but some may follow the movement of water and potassium out of the cells, thus allowing the endogenous provision of water for insensible water loss and the formation of urine. The volume of extracellular fluid is maintained by the renal conservation of sodium. Experiments in animals have shown that dehydration by thirsting leads to death when about 40 per cent of the initial total body water has been lost, equivalent to about 17 litres in a 70 kg man which at a steady rate of loss of 1300 ml per day would be lost in about 13 days. This estimate has received support from observations on surgical patients dying of fluid losses of various kinds (Wilkinson, 1965). In simple starvation, however, as the fast progresses there is a slow decline in metabolic rate, with a consequent reduction in the daily requirements of water for both insensible loss and urine formation, and survival is therefore possible for more than 13 days.

DEPRIVATION OF FOOD, WATER BEING SUPPLIED. When ample water is provided for the fasting subject, the loss of body water is greatly reduced. The continuing oxidation of protein and fat liberates 200 to 300 ml. of water. The renal conservation of sodium limits the loss of extracellular fluid, and the urinary output of sodium and potassium indicates that only about 500 ml of body water are lost per day. The remaining 800 ml of the minimal requirement of 1500 ml come from the water which is drunk. Gamble's subjects drank freely and in excess of their basal requirements of water; they excreted about 800 ml of urine per day, which he therefore concluded was the minimum urine volume for fasting subjects under basal conditions. Observations on surgical patients under similar conditions agree closely with this figure.

DEPRIVATION OF FOOD, WATER AND GLUCOSE BEING SUPPLIED. The consumption of 100 g glucose per day by an otherwise fasting adult prevents ketosis, which usually appears on the second day of the fast, and reduces the catabolism of body protein by about one-half (Gamble, 1947). The effect of the consumption of 500 calories and 2·5 litres of water per day on the urinary nitrogen excretion of an otherwise starving healthy volunteer is shown in Figure 5. The reduction in protein catabolism is clearly indicated and the reduced nitrogen outputs of the two controls is in marked contrast with the rise in nitrogen output which follows operation. These alterations in endogenous metabolism also halve the quantity of solutes to be excreted by the kidney and therefore the minimum daily water requirements foı urine formation. No further benefit results from the consumption of more than 100 g glucose per day, because this quantity reduces tissue protein catabolism to the minimum of about

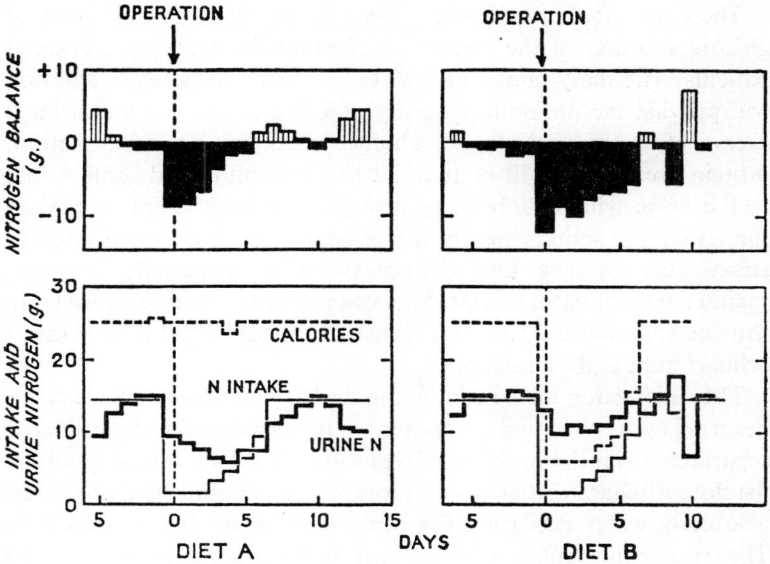

FIGURE 5. This shows the effects of restrictions of diet on urinary nitrogen in normal volunteers not submitted to operation.

In diet A the intake of nitrogen was reduced but the intake of calories was maintained at 2500 per day. The intake of nitrogen is reduced from 14·4 g (90 g protein) to 1·6 g (10 g protein) on the day of imaginary operation and the two succeeding days (this small intake was designed to make the experiment less unpleasant for the volunteers). From the fourth day the nitrogen intake was increased as nearly as possible as it increases after partial gastrectomy.

In diet B, in addition to a similar restriction of protein intake, the daily intake of calories was reduced to 500 for three days (equivalent to the calories derived from 2.6 litres of 5 per cent glucose solution) and then increased at a rate equal to that commonly achieved after partial gastrectomy.

The results in one subject are shown. The urinary excretion of nitrogen fell in both experiments but more markedly, to 5 to 6 g per day, near the minimum output possible, when the calorie intake was maintained. When the calories were reduced the nitrogen output fell only to 8 to 10 g per day. In both experiments the continued loss of nitrogen in the urine led to a negative nitrogen balance, indicating the destruction of tissue protein, but this was more severe when the intake of calories was reduced.

Reference to Figure 6 (*b*) (p. 161) will show that after an operation such as partial gastrectomy there is an increase in the urinary output of nitrogen (Wilkinson *et al.*, 1950a).

(Reproduced by kind permission of *The Lancet*.)

40 g per day. The administration of glucose also reduces the loss of sodium in the urine by about half, but the potassium loss is reduced by only about one-sixth.

These observations provide some justification for the use of glucose solution in the treatment of otherwise starving uninjured patients. The daily intake of 2 litres of 5 per cent glucose solution will provide the optimum quantity of 100 g of glucose and a large excess of water, and, in the absence of injury or inflammation, protein breakdown will be reduced to a minimum and sodium loss in the urine will be halved. If, however, in an attempt to replace the remaining sodium loss in the urine, sodium chloride is administered, the urinary loss of potassium is increased; complete maintenance of extracellular fluid volume in the fasting subject can thus be achieved only at the expense of an additional loss of intracellular fluid and potassium.

The satisfaction of the continuing daily requirements of water for insensible water loss and the formation of urine should be considered separately from the problem of replacing body fluid lost in vomitus, fistulous discharges, diarrhoeal stools or by other abnormal processes. The daily water needs are for expendable water free of minerals. The successful replacement of lost body fluids depends on the provision of solutions containing the appropriate mineral constituents.

METABOLISM AFTER INJURY

Postoperative Changes in Urinary Composition

The pattern of the alterations in the composition of the urine during the first few days after a major operation can be modified in various minor ways by the kind of treatment which is provided. It is important therefore to know what happens when surgical injury and starvation alone are inflicted on the patient. The basic biological pattern, compounded of the effects of starvation and injury, is seen when, after an operation such as partial gastrectomy, the intake of water is stopped for 48 hours and of food for 4 days, followed by the gradual resumption of water intake from 48 hours onwards and of food from the fifth day onwards (Fig. 6) (Wilkinson, 1956b, 1966). With such restrictions, which are unnecessarily rigorous for most circumstances but do not hinder recovery, the intake of calories, protein and minerals is stopped for 4 days, blood is not transfused and fluid is not administered by intravenous infusion. The volume of urine remains small for 48 hours (25 ml per hour or 600 ml per 24 hours) and then slowly increases towards the preoperative volume of about 800 to 1000 ml per 24 hours which is reached after about a week. Although there are wide variations between individuals and from day to day in the same patient, the average volumes during the first 48 hours after injury resemble the smallest volumes attainable by normal adults with good renal function (Gamble, 1954), and oliguria should be regarded as a normal response to severe injury combined with this type of starvation even when there has not been a severe loss of blood or plasma. The volumes of urine passed by patients after operation and by normal volunteers subjected to similar restrictions of their intake of water and food are much the same.

After injury the composition of the urine changes. The osmolality rises almost immediately and, especially when water intake is restricted, remains high for a week or ten days. Towards the end of the first 24 hours the quantity of nitrogen excreted in the urine increases greatly and continues to be abnormally high for six or more days, the peak being reached between the fourth and eighth days after accidental injury but rather earlier (between the second and fifth days) after various surgical operations (Cuthbertson,

TABLE XVII

Mobilisation of potassium and water from muscle

Within 6 days of operation the excretion of 120 g nitrogen, in urine in excess of normal quantity, if derived from body tissues, is equivalent to the catabolism of

(*a*) (N×6·25) 750 g protein
or (*b*) (N×30) 3600 g wet muscle
containing up to 2850 ml water and 330 mEq potassium

1936; Wilkinson *et al.*, 1950a). During the first 10 days after a severe fracture or partial gastrectomy a well-nourished adult patient may lose up to 120 g of nitrogen in the urine; if all this nitrogen is derived from skeletal muscle, it represents the catabolism of over 3·5 kg (7·7 lb) of tissue containing about 750 g of protein and nearly 3 litres of water (Table XVII). Cuthbertson found that the output of phosphorus and sulphur in the urine also increased and that the proportions of them to nitrogen suggested that the excess output might be due to the catabolism of muscle.

The urinary excretion of potassium is usually markedly increased during the first 24 hours after injury (Howard *et al.*, 1946; Blixenkrone-MØller, 1949), from less than 50 mEq per day before operation to 75 to 125 mEq per day, and this increase may last for 3 or 4 days. The urinary output then usually falls below the daily preoperative level and remains low for more than 10 days. It was noticed later (Wilkinson *et al.*, 1950b) that the excretions of potassium and phosphorus follow a parallel course and increase before those of nitrogen and sulphur. In 3 or 4 days 4 to 8 g (100 to 200 mEq) of potassium may be lost in the urine. This is equivalent to more than two or three times the total quantity of potassium in the extracellular fluid, and since the plasma potassium concentration does not appreciably change, the potassium excreted in the urine is derived from cells. The loss of 4 to 8 g of potassium represents the mobilisation of 750 to 1500 ml of water from the cells. The more rapid appearance of potassium than of nitrogen in the urine may be due to faster mobilisation of potassium, or to the slower catabolism of the nitrogenous part of the protoplasm.

Reduction in the urinary output of sodium from the preoperative daily quantity of 100 mEq or more begins soon after and sometimes even before operation, and may fall to as little as 25 mEq or less from the third to fifth postoperative days. Towards the end of the first week after operation the sodium output rises and may exceed the preoperative quantity during the second week. During this sodium conservation in the first week after operation, the pH of the urine is low. These remarkable changes in renal function are shown in Figure 6, which illustrates the large increase in urinary potassium concentration at the same time as sodium excretion is much reduced.

In the absence of infection or persistent inflammation, the urinary output of nitrogen declines during the second week after operation or injury; about this time, provided a sufficiently liberal diet is being eaten, the intake of nitrogen should exceed its output or loss from the body. When recovery is uncomplicated, it is usual for such a positive balance of nitrogen, and of potassium, sulphur and phosphorus, to be achieved after about two weeks, and to persist for a varying time until much of the tissue catabolised during the first week after injury has been replaced.

Cuthbertson (1936) showed that this post-traumatic tissue

catabolism is not simply due to immobilisation or disuse atrophy, because although when a limb is fixed in a splint there are increased urinary outputs of sulphur, nitrogen, phosphorus, and later calcium, these increases last only a short time and are not nearly as large as after injury. It has also been shown (Wilkinson *et al.*, 1950a) that while starvation undoubtedly accounts for some of the continuing urinary excretion of nitrogenous material after operation, the large increases in nitrogen, potassium, sulphur and phosphorus excretions are related mainly to the infliction of injury and their pattern of urinary excretion is different to that found during starvation.

When the intake of water by all routes is maintained at about 4 litres per 24 hours, LeQuesne and Lewis (1953) have shown that there is still invariably a period of oliguria after operations such as partial gastrectomy; this occurs even when 160 to 170 mEq of sodium or up to 200 mEq potassium per 24 hours is given in addition. In their patients the retention of water which accompanied the oliguria led to dilution of the extracellular fluid and also to a gain in weight. It is important to recognise that oliguria following deliberate or accidental injury may be just as intense in a patient who is loaded with water by intravenous infusion as it is in a patient who has been deprived of a water intake for 48 hours.

When the intake of sodium is stopped sodium is conserved by the kidneys, its absorption from tubular fluid being increased by the action of aldosterone. During starvation this sodium conservation is of gradual onset and takes several days to reach its maximum intensity. After injury its onset is rapid and it may be maximal within 36 hours of operation; moreover in some people it may begin up to 24 hours before operation. It occurs regardless of the type of postoperative treatment which is provided, and, at least in the first 48 hours, is as intense in the patient to whom large quantities of sodium are administered by intravenous infusion as it is in those who receive none at all (Wilkinson *et al.*, 1949). Subsequently, however, the effect of thus loading the body with sodium modifies to some extent, but does not entirely obliterate, the normal pattern of postoperative sodium conservation which commonly lasts for up to a week after an operation such as partial gastrectomy.

It seems likely, however, that the quantity of sodium which is excreted in the urine during the second week after operation bears a fairly close relationship to the quantity which has been administered during the first week after operation, that is to say, to the degree of sodium loading during the normal period of postoperative renal

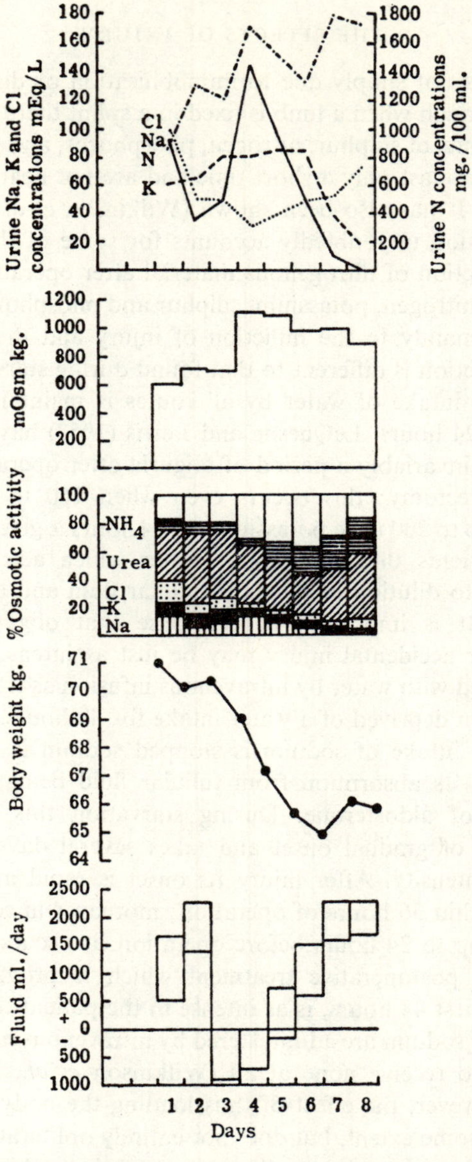

FIGURE 6. (*a*) Effects of starvation combined with restriction of water intake on composition of urine of a normal adult male. Concentrations of nitrogen, sodium, potassium and chloride are shown at the top, below this is the total osmolality of the urine; which in the third graph has been divided into the percentages which can be accounted for by the observed concentrations of nitrogenous material (calculated as urea), sodium, potassium and chloride. Weight, water intake and urine volume also are shown. (*b*) Effects of operation and starvation with restriction of water intake in an adult male plotted as in (*a*); the intake of water on the 2 days before operation has not been plotted.

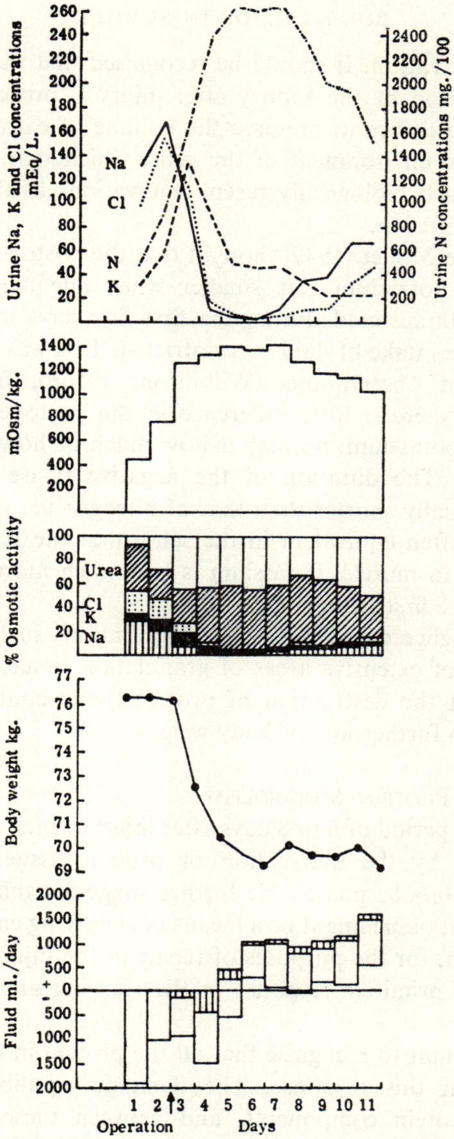

In (*a*) the output and the urinary concentration of potassium did not change much during the period of starvation whereas after operation in (*b*) there was a marked rise in urinary potassium concentration and some rise in the total output. The output of sodium rose in (*a*) during stravation but in (*b*) the urinary output and concentration of sodium both fell after operation. There was a large increase in both the concentration and the total output of nitrogen in the urine after operation in (*b*) (Wilkinson, 1966). (For method of charting see Appendix III.)

(Reproduced by kind permission of Sir Charles Illingworth.)

sodium conservation. It should be recognised that the reduction of sodium excretion by the kidney after injury is probably part of a very primitive device to preserve the volume of extracellular fluid, the immediate environment of the cells, which may not be much affected by such biologically recent innovations as the continuous intravenous infusion.

Blixenkrone-Møller (1949) thought that the postoperative urinary excretion of potassium was smaller when adequate volumes of fluid were administered during the first few days after operation than when the intake of fluid was restricted. This was not confirmed in subsequent observations (Wilkinson, 1956b), from which it appears that there is little difference in the postoperative urinary excretion of potassium, no matter how much or how little water is administered. The duration of the negative phase of potassium balance is usually shorter than that of nitrogen yet the total losses of each are often equivalent in the sense that the KN ratio is the same as that in muscle. Potassium is lost much more rapidly than nitrogen in the first two or three days.

In the presence of infection, of complications such as thrombophlebitis, or of extensive areas of granulation tissue, renal sodium retention and the destruction of protein tissue continue, and the latter leads to further loss of body weight.

Changes in Protein Metabolism

The initial period of 6 to 8 days after injury, which appeared to be characterised by the destruction of protein tissue, Cuthbertson called the 'catabolic phase'. He further suggested that this destruction of protein tissue might be a means of supplying energy or amino acids, or both, for the purposes of repair of the injury, perhaps the survival of a primitive response in the starving animal unable to obtain food.

It is important to recognise that all the protein in the body takes some part in this response. The dynamic equilibrium between individual protein components, and between these peptides and amino acids and carbohydrate and fat, first described by Schoenheimer (1942), indicates the folly of trying to consider protein economy in isolation from the other potential sources of energy and cellular components. The quantitative relationships which can be established after operation or other injury, between the urinary output of nitrogen and the decline in total circulating plasma albumin and the destruction of red blood corpuscles in the so-called 'anaemia of trauma', are further indications of the close relationships and mutual equilibria between the individual items of the total protein mass of the body. Moreover, this 'catabolic response' is not confined to man and the other mammals, but is clearly exhibited also by the shore crab *Carcinus* and earthworms (Needham, 1955, 1958). It was first described after typhoid fever by Shaffer and Coleman (1909) and Coleman and Dubois (1915), who found that the degree and duration of the metabolic response were related to the severity of the infection.

The significance of the increased output of nitrogenous material in the urine remains uncertain. In burned animals much of the nitrogen appears to come from skeletal muscle, but the weight of the liver and other very active organs may increase (Levenson *et al.*, 1967). It seems as if the integrity of organs such as the liver may be preserved at the expense of skeletal muscle. Although both anabolism and catabolism are increased, the balance between them varies in different tissues and at different times after injury. Albumin turnover may be increased after injury even when the total quantity in circulation and its concentration in the plasma are reduced (Blocker *et al.*, 1955, 1957).

Both the quantity of protein tissue catabolised and the excess nitrogen output in the urine are related to the state of protein nutrition of the body at the time it is injured and to the severtiy of the injury. Previously well-nourished patients produce a maximum catabolic response if the injury is sufficiently severe (Moore and Ball, 1952), but patients who have suffered from malnutrition and who are already deficient in protein at the time of injury produce a proportionately less marked catabolic response; when malnutrition is severe, there may be little or no increase in urinary nitrogen excretion after injury. In such wasted patients breakdown of operation wounds is more common and healing is slower. This impairment of healing in the previously malnourished subject is in sharp contrast to the normal healing, in spite of starvation after injury, which is exhibited by well-nourished patients.

After severe injury appetite is commonly lost for 3 or 4 days and the emptying of the stomach is delayed, the gastric phase of digestion is slowed and food eaten shortly before injury may be vomited unchanged 24 hours later. The futility of drinking water as a means of relieving thirst soon after major operations and the frequency with which this is followed by vomiting are also well known. Although gastric motility is greatly reduced or abolished for 24 to 48 hours after any severe injury or operation especially on the stomach the small intestine rapidly resumes its functional activity even after abdominal operations and returns to normal within 12 hours (Ross *et al.*, 1963; Wells *et al.*, 1964). Scholer and Code (1954) showed that even in normal subjects the rate of absorption of heavy water from the small intestine was 10 times as fast as from the stomach; by combining the heavy water with a barium suspension they showed that this difference was due to the rapid distribution of the water in a thin film over a large mucosal surface in the small intestine, whereas it lay in one place in a puddle in the stomach. Howard (1955) showed that the normal delay in gastric absorption of water was even greater after injury, and in later studies (Drawhorn and Howard, 1957) found that intra-abdominal injuries had a more marked effect than burns or other injuries of the chest or limbs, and that partial gastrectomy produced the most prolonged disturbance.

ENERGY REQUIREMENTS

Several explanations have been proposed for the large and rapid loss of weight sustained typically by the well-nourished adult after severe injury or a major operation. One suggestion is that in response to severe injury there is a large increase in the oxidation of fat to provide for a sudden increase in energy expenditure. Fever causes small increases in energy expenditure but does not alone explain the large increments seen in some patients. After most major surgical operations, in the absence of infection, the metabolic rate is raised for 5 to 6 days and then begins to decline. Cuthbertson (1936) found that during the first 12 days after severe fractures of the long bones or surgical operations the respiratory quotient varied from 0·76 to 0·85; thereafter it gradually rose to 1·15. He concluded that during the first 12 days his patients were deriving 50 to 80 per cent of their total calorie requirements from fat, and that later they passed into an intensely anabolic phase while fat and other tissues were being restored. For comparison it may be noted that the hibernating marmot has a repiratory quotient of 0·7 and that during the fattening of farm animals the respiratory quotient may rise as high as 1·4 (Best and Taylor, 1955).

Cuthbertson also noticed that oxygen consumption rose as the urinary nitrogen excretion rose, but fell from the fourth day onwards although the urinary nitrogen excretion remained large; about this time the consumption of food had been resumed and was again providing a proportion of the energy requirements. Cairnie *et al.*

(1957) found that in rats after fracture of the femur heat production rose sharply to a peak on the third day and then gradually diminished. The rise in heat loss and oxygen consumption was exactly parallel to that of nitrogen output in the urine. They concluded that the increase in heat production was more likely to be related to the increase in protein catabolism than to any changes in fat or carbohydrate metabolism. Cuthbertson (1957) after re-examining his earlier data concluded that, during the first week after injury, the energy liberated by the oxidation of protein could alone account for the rise in basal oxygen consumption which he had earlier observed, and that there is no indication of any post-traumatic increase in the oxidation of fat and carbohydrate. In rats, heat production does not rise after injury if the animals are not fed protein, nor does the urinary nitrogen excretion of adrenalectomised rats increase after further injury, unless they are maintained on a sufficiently large dose of cortisone.

Caldwell (1962) found that when burned rats were kept at an environmental temperature of 30°C there was no protein catabolic response to the injury. He originally suggested that this was because less heat was lost by evaporation of water at the surface of the injured skin at this higher environmental temperature. Subsequently Miksche and Caldwell (1967) have suggested that it is due rather to a smaller heat loss by radiation. Campbell and Cuthbertson (1967) and Cuthbertson *et al*, (1968) confirmed Caldwell's observations in rats and man after fracture of the femur, and it seems likely that because the higher environmental temperature reduces heat loss, and thus energy expenditure, it also reduces the need for tissue catabolism. Davies *et al.* (1969) found that when burned patients were treated in a dry environment at a temperature of 32°C the patients lost less weight, had lower basal metabolic rates, and γG globulin and albumin breakdown were reduced and albumin synthesis was increased compared with patients treated in moister air at a temperature of 22°C. It is of interest in this connection that Hey and Mount (1967) observed that when the temperature in the incubator in which a newly born baby was nursed was raised oxygen consumption and energy expenditure were reduced. A similar effect was achieved by covering the baby and protecting it from direct cooling by cold currents of air circulating in the incubator.

The intermediate products of carbohydrate metabolism are important both in the tricarboxylic cycle and in other ways in tissue economy. In the fasting mammal most of these intermediates are derived from amino acids and they cannot be obtained from fatty acids. It remains uncertain whether the increased catabolism of protein after injury in the well-nourished body is related to the requirements for carbohydrate intermediates or of protein components, at a time when too little of either may be available for the enhanced needs of a body which is responding to the need to produce an inflammatory reaction and to heal damaged tissues.

Even at the height of the catabolic period, when 20 to 30 g of nitrogen may be excreted daily in the urine, the calories derived from protein, assuming that its metabolism is complete, would amount to only 500 to 750 per day. The daily energy requirements are increased after severe injury especially when this complicated by infection, and the remaining 2000 to 2500 calories out of a total energy expenditure of 2500 to 3000 in 24 hours must be assumed to come largely if not entirely from the fat stores: this would require the oxidation of more than 200 g fat per day. Keys *et al.* (1950) found that in partial starvation without injury 5·27 kg of fat were lost in 12 weeks, an average of 63 g per day, which if completely metabolised would yield 567 calories. Kinney and his associates (Duke *et al.*, 1970) have shown that the proportion of the resting metabolic expenditure which comes from protein is only about 20 per cent and that stored fat is the only source from which the rest of the energy can come. From the examination of a very large number of published and personal metabolic studies it is evident that during the second week after injury, in the absence of secondary inflammation due to infection a daily intake of at least 1800 calories and about 11 g of nitrogen is essential before protein equilibrium (nitrogen balance) can be achieved.

The possible effects of the catabolism of body tissue after injury are shown in Table XVIII. The excretion during 24 hours of 20 g nitrogen in the urine is assumed to indicate the consumption of 600 g of whole tissue, such as muscle, with the release of 475 ml of tissue water, 55 ml water of oxidation and 500 calories; about 50 to 60 mEq (1·9 to 2·3 g) potassium also are released. If in addition 250 g fat are burned, then this provides up to 267 ml water, making a total of about 800 ml. The total daily water requirements of a 70 kg man also are shown in Table XVIII, comprising at least 1077 ml for insensible water loss and 500 ml for urine. There is a difference of at least 700 ml between the most that is likely to be provided from the tissues of the body and the basal water requirements; this water must be assumed to come from the extracellular and intracellular fluids. It is probably only this fraction of the water

TABLE XVIII

Calories and water derived from catabolism of fat and protein after operation

---

Calories

20 g urinary nitrogen = (N × 30) 600 g whole muscle
or (N × 6·25) 125 g protein
= 500 calories.

At RQ of 0·76, 80% of total calories are derived from fat.

If total calorie consumption is 2500 calories, 2000 calories are derived from fat requiring oxidation of 250 g fat.

Water derived from tissue oxidation

600 g muscle provide	475	ml tissue water
	55	ml water of oxidation
250 g fat provide	267·5	ml water oxidation
	797·5 ml	

Water requirements for consumption of 2500 *calories*

Insensible water loss dissipates 25% of total heat production
= 625 calories.

625 calories will evaporate $\frac{625}{0{\cdot}58}$ g water
= 1077 ml = insensible water loss.

Minimum urinary water = 500ml.

Therefore minimum total water requirements = 1577 ml per 24 hours, of which 797·5 can be provided by tissue catabolism.

Therefore a minimum of 700 to 800 ml water should be supplied each day.

---

requirements which can be affected by the supply of water from outside the body, since the water derived from the catabolism of body tissues will be made available regardless of the quantity of water supplied.

CHANGES IN FAT AND CARBOHYDRATE METABOLISM

Not much is known about fat metabolism after injury. Changes may be related moie to starvation and the influence on total energy requirements of environmental conditions than to injury alone. Soon after operation there is a rise in the non-esterified fatty acid content of the plasma which can be diminished by the administration of glucose (Wadstrom, 1958) but the same phenomenon may also be found in the starving newly born. There are a variety of changes in carbohydrate metabolism some of which are possibly related, if not mainly dependent, on the type of treatment which is used. Hyperglycaemia is common after severe injury and is directly related to the severity of the injury. There is need for much more information about the effects of injury on both fat and carbohydrate metabolism.

It is now evident that the protein catabolism is only one feature of a general response by the body to injury which appears to consist of two phases. In the one, retention of sodium and chloride as the result of efficient conservation by the kidneys is accompanied by the maintenance of volume and composition of the extracellular fluid. In addition, there is a transfer of extracellular fluid from the interstitial space in the uninjured tissues to the damaged tissues. In the other phase, cellular destruction results in the loss in the urine of such constituents of protoplasm as nitrogen, potassium, phosphorus and sulphur, and in the absence of intake, the water from the catabolised protoplasm is presumably available for insensible water loss and urine formation.

The so-called 'catabolic phase' lasts for 10 to 14 days after moderate injuiy but may persist for 5 or 6 weeks after very severe injury, especially when this is complicated by infection. The body then enters the 'anabolic phase', the period of reconstruction following healing of the wound when the previously catabolised normal tissues are replaced. The duration of the anabolic period depends on the severity of the injury and the intensity of the catabolic tissue destruction, and also on the provision in the diet of sufficient energy and protein to allow for the formation of new tissue in addition to the ordinary daily requirements.

Changes in Body Weight

The loss of weight which invariably follows severe injury to a well-nourished person may amount to 10 per cent or more of the initial body weight. The time of onset of this weight loss depends mainly on the way in which the patient is treated after operation. The most 'natural' response is seen in the patient who for 48 hours after operation is not given any food or fluid by mouth or parenterally, but thereafter is given small quantities of water for two days and subsequently is allowed to resume gradually the consumption of a normal diet (Wilkinson, 1956b). In such a patient weight loss begins during the operation and continues at a rapid rate for 48 to 72 hours, up to 10 per cent or even more of the initial weight being lost; this period of rapid weight loss is followed by one in which there is little change and then weight rises again (Fig. 7). When unoperated control subjects are treated in the same way, the pattern of weight change is similar, but the average weight loss is smaller in the controls than after operation, and the subsequent recovery of weight is more complete. A similar patient whose oral intake is stopped, but who receives parenteral fluid during the first three or four days after operation and then is gradually fed, loses less weight during the first four days, but the weight loss continues for a longer time and is as great after 14 days as in the patient who did not receive parenteral fluid.

The postoperative loss of weight is due to the summation of several factors. The catabolism of tissue, the insensible and urinary loss of body water and the aspiration of gastric secretions cause the rapid loss seen in the patient who does not receive any parenteral fluid. There is an increase in metabolic rate after injury or in association with infection, but Roe and Kinney (1965) found that on average this was not more than 10 per cent above the basal level in the absence of complications, although it might be up to 20 to 40 per cent in peritonitis and after burns. Such increments in metabolism would account for additional insensible losses of water, above the basal rate, of 100 to 400 ml per day.

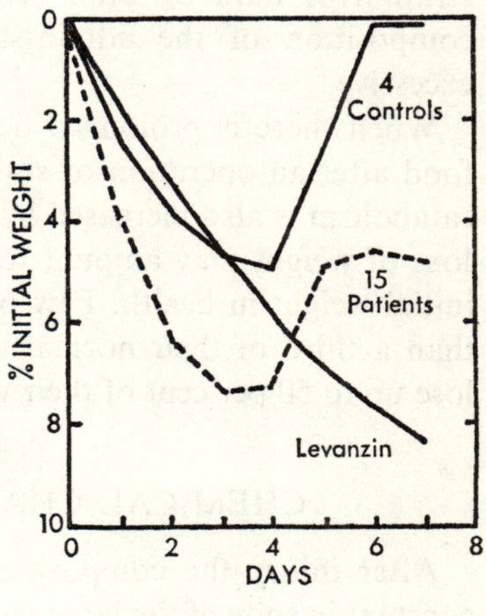

FIGURE 7. The average daily change in weight of a group of 4 adult control subjects and 15 patients submitted to partial gastrectomy. In both controls and patients the intake of food was stopped for 4 days and of water was stopped for 2 days, and on the 3rd day 720 ml and on the 4th day 1440 ml water was allowed. On the 5th day the controls resumed a normal diet and the patients began to eat a light ward diet. The weight lost by Benedict's (1915) subject Levanzin is also shown; he consumed 720 ml distilled water on the 1st day and 750 ml on each of the 2nd, 3rd and 4th days. Judging by the excretions of endogenous sodium and potassium, water was lost chiefly from the extracellular fluid in starvation alone but mainly from the intracellular fluid when starvation and operation were combined (Wilkinson, 1961).
(Reproduced by kind permission of *The Lancet*.)

When saline is administered by the rectal or intravenous route, most of the sodium it contains is retained along with water by the conserving action of the kidneys, and this offsets the normal weight reduction. Similarly, because after injury the kidneys deal less effectively with large water loads, the infusion of large quantities of glucose solution leads to temporary retention of a variable proportion of the water, which increases body weight. After about 6 days, the kidneys cease to retain sodium, and the administered sodium and water are excreted and body weight falls to its true level. It has been repeatedly observed that patients who do not receive parenteral fluids after partial gastrectomy recover their appetite more rapidly and eat more food sooner than patients who are given saline or glucose solution by rectal or intravenous infusion. When drinking is stopped completely for 48 hours after partial gastrectomy, less fluid is lost by gastric aspiration than when limited or free drinking is allowed.

It follows, too, that reduction of urinary volume does not necessarily indicate the retention of water in the body. When fluid restriction is complete for 48 hours after operation, the urine volume remains small (500 to 800 ml) for 48 to 72 hours, but there is then usually an increase to 1000 or more per 24 hours for a day or two, although the oral intake may be less than sufficient to account for this increase. This basic pattern is not much distrubed by the administration of fluid by oral, rectal or intravenous routes or by the composition of the administered fluid, unless the volumes are excessive.

When there is prolonged delay in restarting the consumption of food after an operation or severe injury, and especially when tissue catabolism is also increased by infection, before the patient dies, the loss of weight may amount to as much as 30 to 35 per cent of the initial weight in health. Few patients survive weight losses of more than a third of their normal weight although other mammals may lose up to 50 per cent of their weight in starvation and live.

CHEMICAL CHANGES IN THE BLOOD

After injury the composition of the blood remains remarkably constant in spite of the large shifts of body fluid and great catabolism and alteration of body tissues. The chemical changes in the blood which may occur depend a good deal on the quantity and type of fluid which may be administered, especially by the intravenous route, and also on renal function. When the administration of fluid is restricted, the most marked change is a rise in the packed cell volume, developing during the first 2 or 3 days, and then gradually falling over the next 5 or 6 days below the initial value, and slowly rising again towards its original level after 10 to 14 days. This change in packed cell volume is accompanied by a reduction in total plasma protein concentration due mainly to a reduction of the concentration of the albumin fraction, which usually persists for several weeks.

There is a close relationship between the urinary nitrogen output and the catabolism of albumin after various kinds of injury and also between the basal metabolic rate and the breakdown of γG globulin and plasma albumin in burned patients treated at different environmental temperatures (Davies *et al.*, 1969). These observations serve to emphasise the close relationship between all the fractions of the body protein. Davies (1970) found that 15 per cent of the nitrogen excreted in the urine probably came from albumin. The fall in plasma albumin concentration is also partly attributable to the loss of the albumin into the inflammatory exudate in the burned or otherwise injured area. For about two days after injury by burning the concentration of immunoglobulins in the plasma falls and then slowly rises towards the end of the first and through the second week and then slowly returns to normal and these changes are unaffected by the administration of plasma.

The globulin concentration may fall for only a day or two and thereafter is usually above its initial level until the albumin concentration returns to normal. The concentrations of α1 and α2 globulins, γG globulin and fibrinogen rise and that of β globulin falls. Crockson *et al.*, (1966) have found marked elevations of seromucoid, ceruloplasmin, haptoglobin and the α-acid glycoprotein of Schultze, which reach a peak about the fourth day after operation. Both the rises in β1 and α2 globulins and the fall in albumin may be enhanced by infection. Some of these changes in plasma protein fractions can be reduced but not entirely abolished by treating the patient in an ambient temperature of 30°C.

The reduction in albumin concentration may be partly due to the loss of albumin into the inflammatory exudate at the site of injury. Lynch *et al.* (1964) were able to find over 50 per cent of injected labelled albumin or globulin in the injured area in burned animals and 35 per cent in a wound of similar size. It is difficult to explain why the albumin concentration is depressed for so long; but the evidence is now against the idea that albumin synthesis in the liver is impaired, it suggests rather that the rate of turnover of albumin is increased. Weech *et al.* (1937) found that in a dog on a protein-free diet 80 per cent of the catabolised protein was derived from muscle, 18 per cent from haemoglobin and only 3 per cent from serum albumin. This catabolism of haemoglobin in starvation may also occur after injury and may be the explanation of the reduction in red cells and of the anaemia which is such a common feature about a week after severe injury, and is not lastingly corrected even by the transfusion of whole blood.

When albumin labelled with ^{131}I was injected intravenously, both controls and patients who had been subjected to operation showed a rapid initial loss in plasma activity as the injected albumin was distributed in the extravascular fluid (Sterling *et al.*, 1955). Thereafter there was a slow exponential decay of activity with a half-life of 11 days in controls, and 4·6 to 7·3 days after operation. The loss of activity was real and was not due to dilution by transfusion or intravenous infusion, and could not be accounted for by urinary excretion. Since the albumin was lost from the plasma but was not completely metabolised and excreted it is likely that the injected labelled albumin or its components were incorporated into newly formed tissues. This supports Cuthbertson's idea that the catabolism of protein after injury is related to the healing of damaged tissues and is not simply a process to provide calories during starvation.

Whipple and Elman have both shown by starvation and refeeding experiments in animals that changes in plasma albumin reflect closely changes in the total body content of protein, and have concluded that each gram of plasma albumin is in equilibrium with 30 g of tissue protein. Postoperative changes in plasma albumin concentration which are not due to dilution may therefore indicate alterations in total body protein. A reduction in plasma albumin concentration of 1 g per 100 ml, which is not uncommon during the first day or two after major operations, if not due to dilution would indicate in a patient with a plasma volume of 3 litres a reduction in circulating albumin of 30 g. This 30 g of albumin is in equilibrium with 900 g of tissue protein, which contains 140 g of nitrogen. The albumin concentration falls during the first 24 hours when the inflammatory exudate is formed, and Fischer (1947) has suggested that albumin may be the intermediary substance between fixed uninjured tissue and the inflammatory exudate and healing tissues, and the means by which protein components may be brought to the site of repair of injury.

Other changes in the blood chemistry are inconstant. When the fluid intake is restricted the serum sodium concentration like the packed cell volume usually rises for a few days. The urea concentration also often rises slowly for a day or two after operation, but there are no regular alterations in the composition of the blood except those in packed cell volume and plasma protein concentration. When fluid is administered, the subsequent changes are closely related to the composition of the fluid given, and the volume and the rate at which it is injected. The serum sodium concentration tends to be maintained by the intravenous infusion of isotonic saline, but when glucose solution is infused, there is often a subsequent decline in the serum sodium concentration.

Much attention has been given to the fall in serum sodium concentration which may follow soon after operation despite the close renal conservation of sodium, the absence of extrarenal loss of sodium, and an increasing total body sodium content, the so-called 'sodium paradox'. This reduction in serum sodium concentration is undoubtedly common in association with intravenous therapy and may be due to the retention of water, which being distributed mainly in the extracellular fluid leads to dilution of the extracellular sodium. The weight of patients who exhibit sodium dilution soon after operation seldom changes much and may increase, which also suggests that administered water is being retained in the body. When, after operation, the water intake is stopped, there is a varying degree of dehydration which affects the extracellular as well as the intracellular fluid, the packed cell volume rises and, in association with the normal postoperative renal conservation of sodium, the serum sodium concentration also increases.

HORMONAL CHANGES

For those who believe that the changes in composition of the urine after severe injury which have already been described are characteristic aspects of a normal biological response, it is natural to wonder how that response is brought about. The similarity between the metabolic disturbances after injury and in Cushing's disease led Albright (1943) to suggest that the tissue destruction, with increased output of potassium and nitrogen, and the retention of sodium and water, were in both instances due to alteration in the secretory activity of the adrenal glands.

There is now a good deal of evidence to support the idea that hormones secreted by the adrenal cortex have an important influence on the large changes in body composition and in the distribution of bodily components which follow injury; the exact way in which these changes are brought about remains unknown.

Comparisons have been made between the catabolic phase which Cuthbertson observed after injury and that which Selye (1950) described as part of the acute 'alarm reaction'. There are important differences between the acute reaction to injury as found in human patients and in animals, and the less specific type of reaction described by Selye; and the means by which these two types of reaction are produced probably differ in important respects. Although the effects vary with changes in dosage, either ACTH or cortisone will cause increases in the urinary excretion of nitrogen, potassium, calcium and phosphorus and the retention of sodium, chloride and water. Ingle *et al.* (1947) reported that such effects of cortisone diminish after about ten days, as if this substance lost its effect or the body had become refractory to it; this observation is of interest because after injury the catabolism of body tissue may be prolonged by infective complications and the change from catabolism to anabolism occurs only when infection is overcome. Campbell *et al.* (1954) found that in rats the increase in urinary nitrogen was similar after the implantation of 25 mg cortisone acetate to that produced by fracture of the shaft of the femur.

When adrenalectomised animals are maintained on saline alone they do not produce the characteristic alteration in urinary nitrogen excretion after fracture of the femur, but when they are maintained on a sufficiently large dose of cortisone the urinary nitrogen excretion rises normally after fracture of the femur. It is evident that a normal response to injury can occur in the absence of the adrenal glands provided there is an adequate quantity of adrenal extract or cortisone in the body, and an abundance of clinical experience has shown that this applies also to men and women after ablation of their adrenal or pituitary glands. When after bilateral adrenalectomy the patient is maintained with adequate doses of cortisone there are still increases in the urinary output of potassium and nitrogen and a reduction in sodium excretion in the pattern characteristic of patients with intact adrenal glands; the dose of cortisone need not be increased to enable the patient to recover from the removal of the second gland provided enough cortisone is already being given (Robson *et al.*, 1956; Wilkinson, 1956a). The production of aldosterone ceases after adrenalectomy, but provided the dose of cortisone is adequate, a normal pattern of change in renal function develops.

There is a sudden increase in the concentration of ACTH in the blood soon after injury which returns to normal within a few hours (Cooper and Nelson, 1962). The quantity of ACTH released is more than is needed to produce a maximal response by the adrenal cortex (Ganong, 1963) but a normal response to injury may be found in some individuals who show no sign of any adrenocortical response to an injection of ACTH.

It has been concluded from these observations that an increased adrenal steroid output is not essential for the production of the normal response to injury (Engel, 1951; Ingle, 1952) but that some factor other than the adrenal hormones is the primary agent after injury, although the full development of the response depends on sufficient adrenal hormones being present. Cortisone combines powerful actions, both on mineral metabolism leading to sodium retention and on protein and carbohydrate metabolism and perhaps for this reason is a more effective substitute for the adrenal glands than agents which have a poor mineral effect such as prednisone, or a mild effect on protein, but a much more intense mineral activity, such as aldosterone; neither of these substances can maintain stability after total adrenalectomy.

There has been considerable discussion of the ways in which the adrenal hormones may produce their effects after injury. Ingle (1951) suggested that the hormones 'permitted' the action of some unknown stimulus resulting from injury on a tissue or organ; this idea implies that the hormone renders a cell responsive to a stimulus and that if there is insufficient hormone circulating in the body the stimulus will not be effective. Roberts (1953) showed that the mobilisation and transfer of tissue protein, under the influence of these hormones, may in one place represent anabolism and at the same time in a different situation in the same body be catabolism. This is particularly applicable to the injured animal, in which the protein from undamaged tissues is transferred to injured structures. Fischer (1947) suggested that for such transfers the plasma albumin offered a convenient and ubiquitous vehicle, the scope of which is increased by the altered capillary permeability of acute inflammation.

If the action of a hormone is related to its concentration in extracellular fluid it might be expected that the measurement of change in blood concentration would give a better idea of the effects of injury than estimation of the urinary excretion of largely inactive conjugated residues. After abdominal operation, Steenburg *et al.* (1956) found the free serum 17-hydroxycorticoid concentration rose steeply, reached a peak within a few hours, and then declined to a normal concentration within 48 hours, but there was no relationship between serum concentration and the urinary excretion of corticoid substances. The rise in serum corticoid concentration coincided with the usual postoperative increase in urinary output of potassium and the fall in circulating eosinophils, preceded the rise in urinary nitrogen excretion, and was unrelated to the onset of sodium conservation. Samuels and his colleagues (Sandberg *et al.*, 1954; Eik-Nes *et al.*, 1955) reported similar changes in serum concentrations of corticoids and have emphasised the importance of altered liver function in determining the rate of removal of natural or infused 17-hydroxycorticoid and thus of the serum concentration.

Espiner (1966) showed that cortisol in the plasma is either free and can be excreted in the urine, or is bound to protein. Excretion of the free cortisol in the urine is the best avialable index of the activity of cortisol in the tissues and varies widely according to the severity of tissue damage. After very severe abdominal operations the plasma concentration of cortisol may increase 30 times. The increases in the production, utilisation and excretion of thyroxin just after injury resemble those of the adrenal cortical hormones but their significance is uncertain.

The concentration of aldosterone in blood and its output in the urine are very small compared with other adrenal cortical hormones. It has little effect on carbohydrate or protein metabolism (Prunty *et al.*, 1955), but has about 30 times as powerful an activity on sodium and potassium metabolism as desoxycorticosterone; both hormones are similar in causing a rapid increase in urinary potassium output and a rather slower onset of sodium conservation. After injury the urinary output of aldosterone rises promptly but there is wide individual variation both in preoperative daily output and the size of the increase after injury. It has been suggested that the postoperative increased output of aldosterone is a response to the starvation with consequent restriction of sodium intake which accompanies injury; this does not accord well with the delay in onset of sodium conservation shown by some patients or its onset 24 hours before operation in other people; moreover, the urinary output of sodium falls even when the sodium intake is maintained through the postoperative period, and in these circumstances the greater part of the administered sodium is retained in the body.

Bartter (1956) has shown that the output of aldosterone is independent of extracellular sodium concentration, or the total body content of sodium, but is related to change in the volume of extracellular fluid and especially of plasma volume. The output of aldosterone is raised in patients with oedema in hepatic cirrhosis, nephrosis or cardiac failure, in eclampsia and pregnancy and in primary aldosteronism due to tumour or to bilateral adrenal hyperplasia.

Cortisol does not reproduce exactly the effect of injury on protein metabolism, and whereas ACTH causes comprehensive adrenal secretion, a surgical operation causes the release only of cortisol and its metabolites (Johnston, 1964). It seems likely that some material which is produced in injured tissue is the most important stimulus to the total metabolic response, rather than a mainly neural process through afferent impulses from the site of injury. A normal response to injury can follow hypophysectomy in man and transection of the stalk of the pituitary in animals. A rise in the blood sugar concentration in experimental haemorrhagic shock was observed by Claude Bernard (1877). This has since been ascribed to an increased output of catecholamines causing a rise in adrenaline production which both increases glucose production by the liver and reduces the output of insulin. The clinical and experimental evidence is confusing and there is no entirely satisfactory explanation of how the hyperglycaemia which is associated with shock due to severe injury in man is produced. The inability of the mammalian organism to utilise glucose during and immediately after injury provides a possible explanation for the catabolism of protein and fat after injury, and for the apparently unavoidable destruction of body protein as an inevitable consequence of severe injury. The carbohydrate residues of the amino acids derived from endogenous protein are the main source of carbohydrate intermediates in the fasting subject and fatty acids cannot serve this purpose (Kinney 1960).

Afferent impulses arising in the injured part pass by the posterior columns to the hypothalamus (Hume and Egdahl, 1959). The adrenocortical response to a major operation does not occur when the spinal cord is divided at the fourth thoracic segment (Eisenstein *et al.*, 1962). Although after adrenalectomy a normal catabolic response occurs if the maintenance dose of cortical hormone is large enough, this dose is not nearly as large as the increase in output of these hormones after a similar injury in a normal subject. Patients who are too malnourished to produce a catabolic response show the same large increase in cortical hormone output after injury as a normal person does.

The maintenance of an adequate volume of blood in active circulation is dependent in part on the availability of adrenal steroids in adequate quantities. In adrenal failure the control of the volume of sodium and water within the vessels is lost and circulatory volume falls. It can be restored by the administration of a sufficient quantity of cortisone without the infusion of any sodium or water which alone, has only a transitory effect.

While it seems certain that survival from a severe inflammatory reaction, whether it is due to injury or infection, depends on satisfactory adrenal function or adequate substitution therapy, the precise part played by the various adrenal cortical hormones remains rather obscure. Little is known of the primary factors which initiate the hormonal response to injury or of the way in which these hormones may produce such of their effects which are known, nor indeed whether these hormonal secretory responses occur at the same intensity regardless of the environmental conditions in which the patient is treated after severe injury.

THERAPEUTIC IMPLICATIONS

It is obviously important to decide from our present knowledge of the effects of injury whether the normal response of the body can be modified beneficially in any way. The catabolism of protein tissue, the loss of potassium and nitrogen in the urine and the retention of sodium and water during the first week are determined partly by the action of adrenal cortical hormones and partly by the environmental conditions in which the patient is treated. There is good evidence that when adults who live in a so-called 'temperate climate' are injured accidentally or by the surgeon their metabolic response to such injury will be greatly modified if they are treated in the neutral thermal environment of 30° to 32°C (86° to 90°F) and that the same applies to babies and children when the temperature is varied according to their body weight (see p.272). There is less reliable evidence, however, about the effects of environmental temperature on the metabolic responses after injury in people who live in the tropics and in extremely high or low humidity (Tinckler, 1966; Badoe, 1968; Elebute, 1969). It would be surprising if there was any fundamental difference in response, but some variation is almost certain from what is known for example about racial and geographical differences in sodium intake. It is important also to remember that in the past very little attention if any was paid to the environmental temperature and humidity during metabolic studies on the human subject. The large range of humidity from 10 per cent in winter to more than 90 per cent in summer in much of the North American continent, combined with a high ambient temperature in most hospitals there, must arouse doubts about the validity of at least some of the conclusions and therapeutic applications which have been based on studies of the metabolism of the surgical patient in that part of the world.

Appetite is usually poor or absent for several days after a major operation and the patient may have little inclination to eat even if the postoperative state of his gastrointestinal tract permits the consumption of food. Delay in the absorption of water after severe injury may last for 48 hours or more even when the stomach and intestines are uninjured. The catabolism of protein tissue after injury can be somewhat reduced by the prevention or mitigation of accompanying starvation, but the degree to which this is feasible in a surgical patient depends on appetite and the ability to consume food. The maintenance of an undiminished intake of calories and protein throughout the postoperative period by the intravenous infusion of fat emulsions and solutions of amino acids is expensive and causes appreciable extra discomfort to the patient; such supplements must also provide adequate quantities of potassium, magnesium, phosphate and sulphate if protein tissue is to be spared or re-formed.

It has been recommended that potassium should be administered immediately after operation to replace the usual postoperative loss of potassium in the urine, but since the administered potassium also is excreted, this does not result in any gain in the potassium content of the body. The close renal conservation and low urinary output of sodium and chloride have been interpreted as an indication for the provision of supplements. The maintenance of a normal level of intake of sodium and chloride during the first week after injury leads, however, to the retention of large quantities of both elements. Water also is retained to maintain isotonicity in the body and results in expansion of the volume of extracellular fluid; this may be so large as to cause oedema, and the transfer of sodium into the intracellular fluid may cause disturbance of cellular function.

During the anabolic phase the consumption of an abundant and adequate diet is essential for full recovery; this is the period of

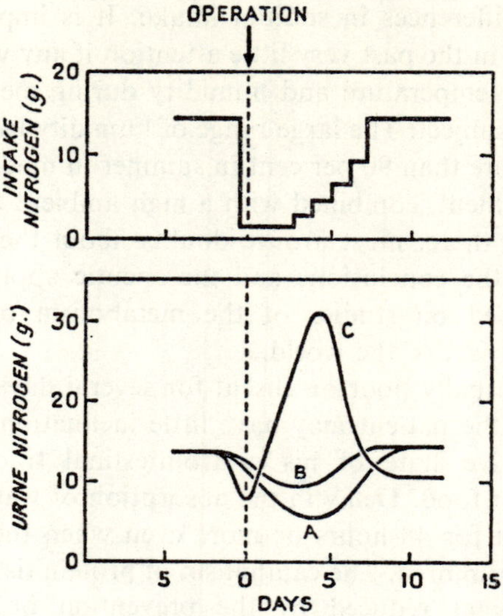

FIGURE 8. Smoothed curves of the urinary nitrogen excretions in a volunteer control subject submitted to dietary restrictions but not to operation (A and B as in Fig. 5) and in a man who was submitted to partial gastrectomy. (C) In each kind of starvation the urinary nitrogen excretion fell at a stage when after operation combined with starvation there was a marked rise. The initial fall in output after operation was related to the small volume of urine which was passed on the day of operation. It was concluded that the difference between the lower two curves was related to the amount of tissue protein spared by the maintenance of the calorie intake in diet A, while the difference between the upper two curves reflects the protein catabolism resulting from partial gastrectomy in a well nourished adult man (Wilkinson *et al.*, 1950a).

(Reproduced by kind permission of *The Lancet*.)

convalescence when there is a particular need for protein, and probably also additional potassium and some vitamins such as ascorbic acid and riboflavin. These requirements are supplied by a good mixed diet containing adequate quantities of high quality protein, fresh fruit and vegetables.

In the absence of abnormal fluid loss, such as that caused by repeated gastric aspiration, the recovery of a patient from a major operation or severe accidental injury is usually uneventful; provided that the consumption of food is resumed as soon as appetite returns, the parenteral administration of fluid, calories or protein is not required. After injury human beings, like other animals, are able to tolerate a period of starvation for water and food during which the body lives on and heals from materials derived from its own substance; if excessive bleeding or infection does not cause death, survival depends on the patient having at the time of injury sufficient bodily resources and the hormonic means of using them to live long enough to heal.

CHAPTER NINE

Shock

In the past the term 'Shock' was used mainly to cover the varied circulatory disturbances which may follow injury, and there has been much criticism of its continued use. Its value depends on the use of qualifying phrases indicating the underlying cause of the circulatory disturbance; for example, shock due to loss of plasma or shock due to bleeding. When thus qualified, the term is probably more useful and widely understood than any of the alternatives which have been suggested. The extension of the use of the term to the circulatory disturbance after myocardial infaction (cardiogenic shock), or that associated with septicaemia due to bacteria and fungi (septicaemic or septic shock), simply emphasises the importance of the use of suitably specific qualifying terms. The main problem is one of diagnosis, the recognition from the history and clinical examination of the patient of the causes of the disturbance.

CLASSIFICATION

After injury the most important factor concerned in the production of circulatory disturbances is a reduction in the volume of blood in active circulation in the body. This may be due to bleeding with the loss of whole blood from the vessels (shock due to blood loss) or of plasma from the unusually permeable capillaries in burned or scalded tissues (shock due to plasma loss). The volume of blood in active circulation may also be reduced when blood accumulates in dilated blood vessels in one part of the body as the result of a nervous mechanism (neurogenic shock). Shock was formerly classified according to the time of onset. All shock appearing within two hours of injury was called primary shock and was assumed to be due to an ill-defined nervous mechanism. All shock which appeared more than two hours after injury was called secondary shock and was thought to be due to blood or plasma loss, the action of toxins or the products of tissue breakdown, and other factors. Severe bleeding may cause shock within a few minutes of injury, and pain arising during the examination of dressings or splints may cause neurogenic shock several hours after injury. Shock should therefore be classified according to its main cause rather than to the time of it onset or diagnosis, into two main types:

(1) Neurogenic shock or vasovagal collapse.
(2) Shock due to fluid loss, either blood or plasma.

While this classification serves admirably in the younger and previously fit individual it may be less applicable to the elderly person who may already have suffered for years from debilitating or degenerative disease. In such people shock may be better or additionally classified into three types:

(1) Cardiogenic shock in which the heart is unable to produce a output large enough to maintain an adequate peripheral circulation.
(2) Shock due to reduced blood volume which leads to such a small venous return and cardiac output that the peripheral circulation is impaired.
(3) Shock due to the loss of blood into a stagnant circulation in the peripheral arterioles, capillaries and venules with consequent poor venous return and cardiac output and the absence of improvement in circulation even when the pooled blood is replaced.

Neurogenic Shock

This may follow accidental bleeding or the bleeding of transfusion donors; it may be associated with emotion, pain, the manipulation of injuries such as fractures, or with change in posture. The characteristic features are pain, a fall of systolic blood pressure to about 60 mmHg (the diastolic pressure may be too low to be recorded), slowing of the pulse rate to 40 or 50 per minute, coolness and pallor of the skin, especially on the face, hands and feet. There may be yawning, nausea, vomiting and fainting. This reaction is due to vasodilatation of the arterioles of the skeletal muscles by nervous impulses mediated through autonomic fibres in the mixed peripheral nerves (Barcroft *et al.*, 1944). Amongst blood donors the incidence and severity of the reaction are related to the quantity of blood which is removed; practically all professional donors faint after the removal of 1200 to 1400 ml blood. Recognition of this disturbance depends on observation of the very slow pulse rate combined with the low systolic pressure.

Recovery generally follows recumbency, but this may make little difference. The administration of a vasoconstrictor drug usually constricts the dilated vessels in the skeletal muscles and returns the blood from these vessels to active circulation. This disturbance may follow a surgical operation in which the blood loss has been small, but it may be associated with severe blood loss when the clinical picture may be modified by the effects of the bleeding, amd diagnosis is made more difficult.

Circulatory disturbances of the vasovagal type are common immediately after operations in which relaxant drugs have been used. Rapid recovery from a light general anaesthetic, the cessation of assisted respiration and a return to perhaps rather light spontaneous respiration, combine to increase the severity of the circulatory effects of drugs which diminish vagal tone. In addition, blood pressure may have been maintained during anaesthesia by carbon dioxide retention, caused by inadequate assisted respiration; the subsequent elimination of carbon dioxide is followed by a fall in blood pressure. In these circumstances the administration of a vasoconstrictor drug usually increases the difficulties of judging the state and progress of the patient, and increases confusion, especially if the blood pressure falls again when the effects of the drug decline.

Shock Due to Loss of Blood or Plasma

Because there is loss of blood or plasma or of both out of the vascular system into the wound or damaged tissue, there is reduction in the volume of blood in active circulation within the vessels. It is now generally agreed that this extravascular loss of blood or plasma is the most important single factor in causing the syndrome of shock, and it follows that rapid and complete replacement of this loss is the chief factor in the successful treatment of shock due to this cause.

SHOCK DUE TO BLEEDING. In shock due to bleeding, the rate of loss and the total volume lost are both important factors. The rapid loss within a few minutes of 2 pints (1·12 litre) of blood may cause severe circulatory disturbance; repeated small losses of blood spread over a longer period of time, especially during anaesthesia, may however be less well tolerated than a single rapid loss of the same total volume. Compensation for acute blood loss by the formation of red cells is slow, and restoration of volume by transfer of interstitial fluid into the vessels is partial and takes 24 hours or more to be effective. Reflex vasoconstriction increases the peripheral resistance and reduces the capacity of the veins and so redistributes the remaining available blood to maintain an adequate blood supply to those organs and tissues on which survival of the organism primarily depends. This implies intense vasoconstriction in the less essential organs or those which, because of less highly specialised function, can continue to exist at a lower rate of oxygen utilisation. When bleeding continues slowly the blood pressure is maintained by vasoconstriction and alone gives a misleading idea of the total circulatory state. Increasing pallor and coldness of the skin and diminishing bleeding in the wound are better indications of the deterioration. The general vasoconstrictor effect of blood loss may be overcome locally by a strong stimulus like heat, as in the improvement in the rate of venous flow brought about by warming the limb before transfusion or by warming the fluid to be injected.

In assessing the condition of a shocked patient and the rate and direction of change in his condition, it is still necessary to make a clinical judgement based largely on past experience. The clinical data required are a history of the accident, some indication of the amount of blood lost, the nature and extent of the injuries, the systolic and diastolic blood pressure, the pulse rate and the colour and temperature of the skin in various sites, the filling of the superficial veins, and the rate of return of skin colour after digital compression. By repeated observation of these clinical features at intervals of half an hour, or less during critical periods of rapid change, it is possible to build up a picture of the disturbance in a particular patient. No two shocked patients are ever wholly alike, and such direct observations enable a closer assessment to be made of the reaction of any individual to a particular injury than any system based on a full description of many types of reaction.

The effects of an acute loss of blood vary greatly. In a fit young man with an initial blood volume of about 8 pints (4·5 litres), up to a pint of blood may be lost without much change in the colour or temperature of the skin, pulse rate or blood pressure.

After 2 pints of blood have been lost, cutaneous vasoconstriction leads to pallor and coldness of the skin, and the pulse rate rises to about 100 per minute, but there may be little change in blood pressure. When the blood loss exceeds 3 pints, the increasing vasoconstriction causes pallor with cyanosis, which affects even the lips; the pulse rate usually rises rapidly and the systolic blood pressure falls below 80 mmHg; the diastolic pressure may be too low to be recorded, and later the pulses may become impalpable. The patient is often mentally alert, garrulous and perhaps excessively apprehensive. As his general condition deteriorates he may become restless, exhibit air hunger and even maniacal excitement. In the terminal stages, after rapid loss of very large quantities of blood, respiration becomes gasping and spasmodic, consciousness may be lost and death may seem to be imminent. Provided that this state is of only short duration, complete recovery may follow rapid replacement of the lost blood by transfusion.

The vasoconstrictor reaction may at times exceed the exact degree of intensity necessary to compensate for the particular fluid loss which has occurred; this causes what is known as the *hypertensive response or reaction.* This is more common in young subjects, especially children; pallor is usually marked, the extremities are cold, the pulse rate is increased and the blood pressure is raised above normal to 170 to 180 mmHg systolic or even higher and to 100 mmHg or more diastolic. The hypertension may be suddenly succeeded by a profound fall in blood pressure, especially if the patient is warmed. A hypertensive reaction should therefore always be an indication for caution and careful observation. Patients who have been excessively chilled are in general more difficult to resuscitate; it is often hard to predict how they will respond.

The commonest type of accidental injury giving rise to shock is a wound of the limbs, especially in association with a compound fracture. The severity of the shock is related directly to the volume of blood which is lost from the circulation, which in turn is usually related to the mass of muscle involved. Shock is therefore most severe in association with large lacerated wounds of the upper thigh and buttocks, and in compound fractures of the shaft of the femur. Grant and Reeve (1941) suggested that a quantitative estimate of the tissue damage, and so indirectly of the blood loss, might be obtained by estimating wound size in units of the size of the open hand or closed fist, which is about equal to 500 ml. In closed fractures, blood loss may also be calculated from measurements of change in the length and girth of the limb compared with those of the uninjured side. Bleeding is due chiefly to laceration of the surrounding muscle bellies by the sharp and jagged ends of the broken bone. Fractures of the femoral shaft associated with severe violence may be followed by the loss of up to 5 pints of blood; bleeding is increased by movement of the fractured bone or the affected limb and is minimised by early immobilisation with some traction in a suitable splint. In wounds of the limbs, division of main vessels is comparatively uncommon in peacetime, but extensive venous bleeding may follow superficial lacerations of the arms caused by pushing hands through windows.

Abdominal wounds are a common cause of severe blood loss during warfare, but in civilian practice their incidence varies widely in different countries and even districts. Bullets and other missiles with a high initial velocity may injure any abdominal organ and often pursue unexpected courses after penetrating the abdominal wall Because of the frequency with which mesenteric vessels are divided, severe blood loss is common, but injuries of the great vessels within the abdomen are comparatively rare. Before laparotomy, therefore, a hopeful attitude should be maintained towards all cases of intra-abdominal bleeding. Direct blunt injury to the abdominal wall and lower chest wall may cause severe laceration or rupture of the liver, kidney or spleen, with subsequent immediate, rapid and extensive bleeding, or concealed or delayed bleeding. In all these injuries the cause of shock is predominantly loss of blood, and recovery should follow timely arrest of the haemorrhage, combined with adequate replacement of the lost blood.

SHOCK DUE TO PLASMA LOSS. Shock due to plasma loss follows injury by burning or scalding. In the injured area the capillaries become unusually permeable and plasma leaves the vessels and accumulates in the interstices of the tissues; there is also a large increase in lymph flow out of the injured tissues. Evidence of plasma loss can be seen in superficial blisters and in the exudation of plasma on the raw surface when blisters have been broken; there is also a larger loss into all the damaged tissues, causing an inflammatory oedema, which is conspicuous in the face and on the back of the hands. The net result, a local increase in interstitial fluid, is due to fluid leaving the vessels more rapidly than it can return, either by re-entering capillaries directly or by returning through the lymphatic vessels. The local swelling which results is limited by rising tissue tension as well as by the limited duration of the altered permeability of the capillaries.

This inflammatory swelling is a dynamic exudate in which there is continuous exchange of the constituents between the exudate and the intravascular fluid and, at least temporarily, it is the potential destination of much of any fluid which may be injected into the body. The formation of this exudate diverts from the remainder of body a part of the extracellular fluid and some of the plasma protein and thus, by increasing the volume of distribution of the plasma in the body, decreases the proportion of the total plasma volume which at any moment will be found within the blood vessels. The normal concentration of protein in plasma falls from 6 or 7 g per 100 ml to 4 or 5 g per 100 ml or even less. The fluid in the blisters and presumably also that in the interstitial space contains up to 4 or 5 g per 100 ml of plasma protein which is mainly albumin. If this plasma loss is replaced by the transfusion of plasma, a proportion of the small plasma proteins, albumin and possibly also α and β globulins, which are thus added are liable to be lost into the exudate. The effect of plasma on the shock state is therefore not directly proportional to the volume administered. Gum saline and large molecular weight dextran are more effective than plasma in burn shock, because a smaller proportion of the administered colloid is lost into the exudate, and more remains in the blood vessels of all sizes, occupying space, suspending the red blood corpuscles and maintaining their circulation.

In deep burns, plasma loss is smaller than in superficial injuries of similar total extent since it is largely confined to the marginal areas of superficial injury; in the deeply burned tissue the vessels are coagulated by heat and blood flow ceases. Many red cells are ruptured and damaged by heat, and the plasma becomes stained with pigment. Davies and Topley (1956) found that a small proportion of red cells were destroyed within a few hours of injury apparently by the direct action of heat; between 12 and 48 hours after injury up to 30 per cent of the red cell mass might be destroyed, as had been found earlier by Wilson (unpublished observation) and even transfused cells disappeared at an increased rate. There was subsequently a slow return to a normal rate of red cell turnover, but this might be delayed by infection or extensive deep injuries.

The loss of plasma leads to increasing haemoconcentration, the degree of which initially may give some indication of the magnitude of the plasma loss and of the effects of treatment. As in shock due to loss of whole blood, the state of the peripheral circulation in the ear lobes or in the nail beds of the fingers and toes, the rate of return of colour after digital compression, and, if possible, pulse or heart rate, systolic and diastolic blood pressure should all be frequently recorded; these repeated observations provide the closest indication of the progress of a burned patient and are the best guide to treatment.

Plasma loss begins soon after injury and may continue for up to 40 hours, but the chief loss occurs during the first 12 hours, and this is also the time when shock is more severe and dangerous. At first blood pressure is usually maintained by vasoconstriction, and in children this may sometimes be excessive and lead to hypertension. As the plasma loss increases, compensation becomes less effective, the pulse rate tends to increase, and then, following a rise in diastolic pressure, there is a sharp fall in both systolic and diastolic pressures. Unless the lost plasma is rapidly and completely replaced, continued reduction in blood volume leads to progressive deterioration, and in extensive superficial injuries death may occur at any time after 12 hours.

Fluid loss into the injured tissues continues at a diminishing rate for up to 40 hours. After about 48 hours, as the exudate begins to resolve, there is obvious reduction in the size of the local swelling with wrinkling of the overlying skin, crust or eschar. The rate of removal of exudate now greatly exceeds the rate of formation, and there is a large shift of fluid from the region of the injury into the rest of the body which may cause a diuresis about 60 hours after injury. It is at this stage that the adverse effects of previous excessive infusions of fluid become most serious; the greater size of the burn exudate, caused by the injection of large volumes of isotonic saline and glucose solution during the first 48 hours, results in circulatory overloading and oedema. If large volumes of glucose solution have been employed in vain attempts to induce diuresis, there may be marked dilution of the extracellular fluid.

The systemic disturbances which may arise between 40 and 120 hours after burning have still not been satisfactorily explained. The 'acute toxaemia' which Wilson *et al.* (1938) described, and which was attributed to the effect of absorption of toxic derivatives of tannic acid, has not been observed with other coagulants such as silver nitrate, but disturbances associated with other methods of local treatment, which somewhat resemble 'acute toxaemia', have been reported. The stupor, drowsiness and other mental disturbances, vomiting, reduced urinary output, raised body temperature and increased pulse and respiration rates suggest some disturbance of body-fluid equilibrium. This may be either water retention with sodium dilution or an excess retention of both sodium and water.

The 'toxaemic' state may also be due to the flooding of the rest of the body with large quantities of materials derived from the breakdown of damaged tissue and the resolving inflammatory exudate.

The object of treatment of shock is to maintain the blood volume by replacing the lost plasma. In extensive injuries it is wise to start replacement even before the onset of signs of circulatory disturbance and so to try to prevent the onset of shock; when the blood volume is already reduced, it should be restored as rapidly as possible by the rapid injection of dextran. In large deep burns the loss of red cells by coagulation or damage in the burned area may be sufficient to require the transfusion of the whole blood in addition to dextran.

Formerly the local application of a strong solution of tannic acid (20 per cent) or silver nitrate (10 per cent) to the burned surface was believed to be an essential part of treatment in that the surface loss of plasma was reduced. Such local applications do not affect the much larger loss of plasma into the burned tissues beneath the surface, which is the cause of the swelling of the injured areas. However, when the coagulum dried the loss of water from the burned surface may have been greatly reduced. The raw surface may now be treated by exposure after cleansing and fluid is lost from it until a dry coagulum forms after about 36 hours. In some centres the raw surface may be spread up to four times a day with a cream containing para-aminomethylbenzene sulphonamide or silver sulphadiazine; both these methods involve repeated interference with the injury. The local application of 0·5 per cent silver nitrate caused metabolic alkalosis and the loss of sodium and potassium. None of these three methods reduced the loss of fluid from the burned surface or into the underlying tissues affected by the heat. It follows that the replacement of this lost fluid is an essential part of the treatment of shock; it is usually assumed that such replacement must be by intravenous infusion and consist of plasma, or a fluid similar to plasma in that it contains a colloid of suitable molecular weight.

Evans *et al.* (1952) found that the administration of plasma in volumes of 1 ml per kg body weight for each 1 per cent of the body surface which has been burned in the first 24 hours after injury, and half of this volume in the second 24 hour period gave satisfactory results. A number of other treatment plans or 'formulas' have been devised for the calculation of the fluid replacement of burned patients which differ mainly only in detail.

The need to use plasma or a solution containing colloid has been questioned by Fox (1944), Moyer *et al.* (1944) and Markley *et al.* (1950, 1959), who have all suggested that various hypotonic or isotonic saline solutions are as effective as plasma. Davies (1964) compared the effect on blood volume of the intravenous infusion of reconstituted freeze dried plasma with that of Hartmann's solution or the oral consumption of a solution containing 0·3 per cent sodium chloride and 0·15 per cent sodium bicarbonate. About half the patients who were started on the oral solution had to be given intravenous lactate saline within a few hours, either because of vomiting or because of a deterioration in their general condition. The patients had suffered from burns of varying extent and were of widely varying age; when red cell volume measurement showed low values blood was transfused. The volumes of plasma which were given were between two and three times as much as were estimated by the formula of Evans *et al.* (1952) and maintained the blood volume at between 80 and 90 per cent of the estimated normal value. The patients treated with saline received the equivalent of about 12 per cent of their body weight in the first 24 hours, and up to 25 per cent by the end of 48 hours, and their blood volumes were maintained at between 70 and 80 per cent of the normal value.

It is surprising that the use of plasma in the treatment of shock due to burns remains so popular. The value of the most useful component in plasma, albumin, with its relatively greater oncotic effect in addition to its higher concentration, is limited by the ease and rapidity with which it can traverse the unusually permeable walls of the capillaries in the area of the injury. This plasma albumin does not simply accumulate in the burned tissues but moves through them and returns through capillaries and lymphatics to the general circulation; so much of the total available plasma protein is deviated in this way that the volume of plasma in general circulation is diminished. Rhoads *et al.* (1941) reported that when large plasma transfusions were given to burned patients soon after injury the subsequent increase in plasma volume was smaller and of shorter duration than had been expected. It has been the common experience of those who have used gum acacia or large molecular weight dextran (weight average molecular weight of 150,000), or plasma that very much larger volumes of plasma than of gum saline or dextran must be used to produce comparable effects on the blood pressure. The capacity of inflamed injured tissues to accept plasma protein is large, and until this capacity is satisfied or exceeded little of the transfused plasma protein will be left over to fill the normal vessels and maintain the circulating volume. The process of 'stuffing' the 'third space' of the inflammatory exudate in this way with plasma and with saline, both of which are able to pass readily out of the damaged capillaries, is clearly only an indirect and unspecific way of increasing and maintaining the volume of blood in active circulation in the blood vessels.

Jackson and Cason (1965) found that about 70 per cent of patients with burns of up to 30 to 35 per cent of the body surface could be safely treated by the oral consumption of the saline bicarbonate solution but that vomiting occurred in a third of the children and half of the adults. The patients must be carefully watched and plasma or a plasma substitute, must be infused as soon as peripheral circulatory failure appears.

In many parts of the world facilities for intravenous therapy with plasma or a plasma substitute are very limited. The oral administration of a balanced electrolyte solution is cheap and easy, especially when large numbers of patients must be treated after a disaster. Success depends on the careful and continued observation of the patients, but this may be as difficult to achieve as a supply of plasma.

It has been repeatedly recommended that a minimum output of 30 to 40 ml of urine per hour should be regarded as an important index of the successful resuscitation of a burned patient, and that failure to achieve this output is a sign of inadequate treatment. Oliguria is a normal response to injury and Hardy *et al.* (1955) showed that it persisted after burning even when cardiac output and blood pressure were within satisfactory limits. This oliguria may be overcome only when the body is overloaded with water by the intravenous infusion of excessive volumes of glucose solution. Such attempts to compel a diuresis often lead to the administration of very large volumes of 0·9 per cent saline or glucose solution and cause excessive oedema. The free consumption of water by burnt patients often leads to vomiting and the loss of more water than is consumed. The use of mannitol to maintain the output of urine after burning has been repeatedly recommended, but its use at an early stage is not always followed by a continued or enhanced flow of urine. The risk of renal failure after burning has been exaggerated. Cason (1966) found an incidence of only 1·3 per cent in 3690 patients of all ages. The chance of survival is certainly less in patients who are grossly overloaded with water, saline and other fluids during enthusiastic attempts to force a diuresis in the first two or three days after injury. When shock due to loss of blood or plasma is treated by the rapid infusion of crystalloid solutions the circulating blood volume is temporarily restored, but more lasting restoration seems to depend on the infusion of at least three times the volume of such solutions as is necessary when blood or large molecular weight is used. In some patients the use of such large volumes of crystalloid solutions is associated with progressive respiratory inadequacy due to pulmonary oedema, the so-called 'wet-lung syndrome', and a high mortality rate.

SEPTIC SHOCK

During the last 15 years infection with Gram-negative organisms has become much more common in hospitals all over the world. This seems to be due to a combination of the effects of almost routine prophylactic administration of large doses of antibiotics with the increasing severity and sometimes duration of surgical operations on infants and elderly and infirm patients, the prevalence of strains of organisms resistant to antibiotics, at least in ordinary dosage, and the use of steroids and cytotoxic drugs, intravenous and intra-arterial infusions, catheterisation and tracheostomy. About three-quarters of these infections are acquired in hospital and septic shock associated with septicaemia is becoming increasingly common.

Altemeier *et al.* (1967) found that of 398 patients with Gram-negative septicaemia it occurred in the first, seventh and eighth decades of life in 63 per cent and had increased steadily in numbers from 1957 to 1966. More than 60 per cent of those affected in the first decade were newborn infants but only 21 per cent of these died, whereas the mortality overall was 52 per cent and over the age of 40 years it was 67 per cent. The infection entered by the urinary tract in 56·7 per cent and in half of these after the passage of an instrument. The incidence of septic shock in this series was 40 per cent. The organisms most frequently causing septic shock were *Escherichia coli*, *Aerobacter aerogenes*, *Proteus*, *Bacteroides* and *Pseudomonas aeruginosa*.

MacLean *et al.* (1967) classified patients with septic shock into two groups according to whether the central venous pressure was above or below normal limits, and these two groups were further subdivided into those who were alkalotic and those who were acidotic. In the early stages a normal or increased blood volume, high central venous pressure and respiratory alkalosis were associated with a high cardiac index, low peripheral resistance, hypotension, warm, dry, pale skin in the extremities, oliguria, hyperventilation and a raised blood concentration of lactate. Such patients usually responded well to the administration of blood and saline combined with isoproterenol in small doses (2 μg per minute), blood pressure and cardiac output rose and central venous pressure fell. Adequate surgical treatment of the infection was essential. This sort of disturbance may be associated with infection complicating septic abortion, severe accidental injuries, renal and liver disease or peritonitis.

When a high venous pressure was combined with acidosis there was usually also notable restlessness and tachycardia as well as hyperventilation and oliguria and these signs indicated that a later stage of the whole process associated with the infection had been reached. Patients in this state do not respond well to any form of treatment.

A low central venous pressure may be associated with the loss of fluid due to peritonitis or gangrene of bowel. In addition, metabolic alkalosis is combined with a low cardiac index, raised peripheral resistance, hypotension, cyanosis, oliguria and a raised blood lactate concentration. Successful treatment depends on adequate transfusion of blood or the infusion of saline, according to the packed cell volume, but the addition of isoproterenol may cause a marked rise in cardiac index, and further doses of the drug may be necessary to maintain the circulatory improvement. The association of acidosis with a low venous pressure usually again indicates that a late stage of septic shock has been reached and in this type the response to treatment is bad.

The onset of severe circulatory depression associated with peritonitis may be insidious, but the disturbance will be soonest recognised by those who observe the patient most keenly. Unusual restlessness and a rising pulse rate are earlier signs than changes in $P\text{CO}_2$ or central venous pressure and it is on early recognitions that successful treatment most often depends. The early and if necessary repeated administration of blood or saline may prevent the further development of the shock state, provided that surgical treatment of the infection is also adequate.

Both vasopressor substances (isoproterenol) and vasodilators (phenoxybenzamine) have been tried in the appropriate clinical situations but their value is very uncertain and their use is not recommended. The use of large doses of corticosteroids to improve the state of the circulation is liable to have an adverse effect on the resistance to infection. Some patients who are recovering from septic shock, and who have been adequately transfused and have warm red peripheral skin, well filled veins, and pass adequate volumes of urine, may have a systolic blood pressure of 80 mmHg or less. It is wrong to give such patients vasopressor drugs or steroids because their blood pressure will gradually rise in the course of a few days and this so-called 'benign hypotension' will pass off.

A form of circulatory collapse of sudden and unexpected onset may occur after operation on the biliary tract to relieve obstruction due to a stone in the common bile duct complicated by infection. The patient who has been making satisfactory progress for two or three days after drainage of the biliary tract may be restless for a short time or may suddenly collapse with a pale but warm skin in the extremities, bradycardia and a very low or even unrecordable blood pressure. This may be assumed to be due to a coronary occlusion but the electrocardiographic tracing is normal. It seems more likely that this form of septic shock due to the effect on the myocardium and the peripheral circulation of bacterial toxins from the organisms in the infected bilary tree. Provided coronary occlusion and acute bleeding can be excluded as causes of the hypotension, the blood volume should be increased by the rapid infusion of dextran and, if bile was taken for culture at operation, the appropriate antibiotics should be given by intravenous injection.

FACTORS PREDISPOSING TO SHOCK

Any factor which minimises or interferes with the immediate normal reaction to injury with blood or plasma loss may increase the severity of the shock. Neurogenic shock may be induced or aggravated by fear or pain. Pre-existing reduction in body water, and especially of extracellular fluid, reduces the fluid available for compensatory transfer after bleeding or plasma loss. Chronic anaemia due to repeated small blood losses, for example from a peptic ulcer or a carcinoma of the large bowel, or generalised wasting disease, also reduces the tolerance to further blood loss at operation. Exposure to cold may increase the intensity of vasoconstriction and usually makes later resuscitation more difficult. A hot environment may impair the general vasoconstrictive response to injury, and survival may be shorter; excessive heating of the shocked patient under 'shock cages' or 'cradles' by interfering with cutaneous vasoconstriction may cause a fall in blood pressure and may increase bleeding or plasma loss. Other injuries such as those of the chest wall or lung, brain or spinal cord may hinder the treatment which might otherwise be employed for shock, or may complicate operative measures or anaesthesia.

Any rough handling of injured limbs or compound fractures tends to increase bleeding and tissue damage, and to cause further nervous stimulation. The shocked patient is peculiarly sensitive to changes in posture and position and tolerates badly sudden shifts or rolling; rapid levelling of the table at the end of even a short operation may cause marked deterioration in the condition of a shocked person. Gentleness and the elimination of unnecessary manoeuvres are essential during operation on severely injured patients. The shorter the duration of the operation consistent with thoroughness and gentleness the better, but speed alone is not enough; traction on mesenteries and interference with the upper abdominal organs cause depression of blood pressure, presumably by autonomic reflexes.

Adrenocortical Factors

Occasionally after injury or operation, or during severe infections, circulatory failure is associated with extensive bleeding into both suprarenal glands. Sudden acute circulatory failure may also occur during and several days after operation on patients who have for long periods been treated with cortisone or similar adrenal hormones or when, after bilateral adrenalectomy, the maintenance dose of cortisone is inadequate. The normal outputs of ACTH, and of cortical hormones by the adrenals, are believed to be determined by chemoreceptors in the hypothalamus which are sensitive to the concentration of cortical hormones circulating in the extracellular fluid. The weight of the adrenal glands, and their sensitivity to injected ACTH, are both reduced by the prolonged administration of adrenal cortical hormones, which reduces the need for production of hormones by the adrenal glands.

In patients with Addison's disease, or those whose maintenance dose of cortisone is inadequate, circulatory collapse is usually preceded by an insidious deterioration in appearance and condition, accompanied by bad temper and irritability, poor appetite and nausea or vomiting. Although these changes are noticed, the subsequent sudden failure of the circulation, with a sharp fall in blood pressure, poorly filled veins and rising pulse rate often comes as a surprise. By withholding the maintenance dose of cortisone from adrenalectomised patients Hills *et al.* (1953) showed that this type of circulatory collapse is associated with a loss of sodium from the extracellular fluid and reduction of the volumes of extracellular fluid and plasma. They thought that sodium and its accompanying water were lost into the cells or the connective tissue gel. This type of circulatory disturbance responds rapidly to the administration of cortisone or hydrocortisone, without the administration of sodium chloride or water, and thus is probably due to an alteration in the distribution of sodium and water between the cells and their environment. A similar type of circulatory disturbance may occur during, or several days after, operations on patients to whom adrenal cortical hormones have been administered for a long time. In such patients the usual dose of steroid hormone should be maintained before and after operation. Hydrocortisone should be immediately available in the theatre and at the bedside for at least 48 hours after operation and should be administered as soon as signs of circulatory disturbance appear. It is probably not necessary to increase the dose of steroid at the time of operation. It now seems that patients who have not had steroid hormones for 3 months before operation do not need prophylactic steroids at the time of operation.

There is no convincing evidence that the administration of hydrocortisone or other adrenal cortical steroids is of any value in the treatment of shock due to reduced blood volume. Adrenal failure with a reduced level of circulatory corticosteroids occurs only in patients whose adrenal function has been suppressed by previous corticosteroid therapy.

DIAGNOSIS

In accidental injuries it is important to make a complete examination of the whole body as soon as possible. Clothing should be cut off, note being made of the quantity of blood on the garments, dressings and stretcher; when the injuries are very extensive and shock is very severe, it is usually wise to leave the patient undisturbed until blood volume has been increased by rapid transfusion. Fractures should be splinted and bleeding controlled by pressure with pads. The most important indication of the amount of blood lost is the size of the wound, for it is seldom that blood soaking of clothes or dressings indicates accurately the whole volume which has been lost. A large wound is usually a good indication for starting a transfusion as a precaution (Table XIX). It should be remembered that changes in blood pressure and in the cutaneous circulation lag behind changes in blood volume and are late indications of deterioration. Nevertheless, when combined with evidence of vasoconstruction such as pallor and coldness of the skin, and an increased pulse rate, a systolic blood pressure of 100 mmHg is an indication of moderate shock; of 80 to 100 mmHg of severe shock; and of below 80 mmHg of very severe shock. Progressive decline of the blood pressure when accompanied by evidence of vasoconstriction indicates continued bleeding or plasma loss; such deterioration can usually be arrested only by rapid transfusion and suitable surgical treatment. Restlessness, if not caused by pain, is usually a sign of progressive reduction in blood volume and should be treated by immediate transfusions. In general, it is wise to transfuse all patients whose systolic pressure falls below 80 mmHg because of blood or plasma loss.

TABLE XIX

Diagnosis of shock

Type	*Volume of loss*	*Skin*	*Blood pressure*	*Pulse rate*
Neurogenic	Varies	Warm, pale	<60/?	<80
Blood or plasma loss	<2 pints (<1 litre)	Unchanged	>100/60	80–100
	2–3 pints (1–1·5 litres)	Cool, pale	100–80/60	100–120
	3–5 pints (1·5–2·5 litres)	Cold, pale (cyanosed)	<80/?	>120
	>5 pints (>2·5 litres)	Cold, pale (cyanosed)	<60/?	>120
Hypertensive response	Varies	Cold, pale	>140/100	>100

The chief exception to these recommendations is in the case of vasovagal or neurogenic shock. The distinction between vasovagal shock and that due to blood or plasma loss can usually be made on the blood-pressure level, pulse rate and the state of the skin. In vasovagal shock the systolic blood pressure may be 60 mmHg and the diastolic pressure too low to be recorded; these changes are associated with a slow pulse rate in the region of 40 or 50 beats per minute and pale but warm skin. In shock due to loss of blood or plasma the systolic blood pressure is not often as low as 60 mmHg, the pulse rate is fast, 100 to 120, and rarely even 140 beats per minute the skin is pale and cool or cold. A vasovagal reaction may develop during or soon after surgical operations and general anaesthesia; because of blood loss, a mixed picture is produced, the blood pressure being unexpectedly low for the observed blood loss and the pulse rate faster (60 to 80 per minute) than would be expected for a pure vasovagal reaction; the administration of a large dose of atropine may also partially prevent the usual bradycardia.

The unusal combination of a normal blood pressure with severe injuries is usually an indication of a hypertensive response, and special caution is required; the pulse rate is usually raised and the skin is pale and cold. When a small wound is associated with an unexpectedly low blood pressure, the pulse rate often provides the clue to the correct diagnosis. If the pulse is very slow, a vasovagal reaction is indicated and external blood loss has probably been very small. If the pulse rate is fast, it suggests either a poor vaso-constrictive response or the impairment of this by heating. Another possibility is that severe blood loss has occurred and may have been due to injury to a large artery or vein.

TREATMENT

General Principles

Except to a very limited degree in the first two or three hours after injury, delay is not of value in the treatment of shock. When patients reach hospital very soon after injury it is usually wise to allow them a short period for stabilisation before surgical treatment of the injuries is undertaken. Apart from this reservation, the sooner the lost blood is replaced and the injuries are treated, the better is the prognosis.

The ratio between surface area and weight is high in babies and diminishes as body weight increases. The cutaneous circulation is thus more important in children than in adults; superficial injuries such as burns have a more serious effect in children than in adults and interference with compensatory vasoconstriction by excessive warming is more harmful. On the other hand, children and young adults respond more readily and completely to thorough treatment of severe shock and extensive injuries than do older patients.

Wounds in certain situations are associated with a bad prognosis because of the associated large blood loss and the difficulty involved in adequate haemostasis and treatment of the wounds. Such wounds are those of the buttock and upper thigh and the internal lacerations associated with severe and bilateral fractures of the pelvis. Injuries resulting in the pulping of large masses of muscle lower in the thigh or in the calf are associated with severe shock, which may be resistant to transfusion until the pulped muscle has been excised. Multiple limb injuries, such as compound fractures, are sometimes best treated in stages, for the additional blood loss associated with excision and suture of the wounds may render immediate manipulative reduction of the fractures unduly dangerous; it may sometimes be wiser merely to immobilise the limbs after wound treatment and to delay accurate reduction of the fractures for one or two days. Intra-abdominal injuries always carry a serious prognosis because of the risk of secondary complications such as peritonitis and ileus. Chest injuries alone usually do well and shock is not severe, but when combined with abdominal or limb injuries they impose some limitation on the freedom with which blood and other fluids may be transfused.

It seems hardly necessary to emphasise that the treatment of patients shocked by blood loss from severe or extensive injuries comprises more than just the replacement of the lost blood. It is essential to visualise at the outset the whole process which may be involved in the treatment of a particular patient. An attempt must be made to predict how much blood will probably be necessary, how long resuscitation may take, and the amount of further bleeding and injury which may be inflicted by operation. Once having made such an assessment, as treatment progresses the surgeon must be prepared to modify the original estimates and decisions according to the response of the patient, for the shocked patient is liable to rapid deterioration or improvement. The management of the severely wounded patient demands continuous close attention, repeated measurement of pulse rate and blood pressure, and observations of the cutaneous circulation and general state. The sooner operative treatment can be carried out the better, and damaged tissue should be removed as soon as possible. When a number of shocked patients are admitted at the same time, decision as to priority depends to some extent on the nature of their injuries, but the rate at which they can be resuscitated may vary and may prove the more important factor.

In ideal circumstances the surgeon should conduct the resuscitation of the patient as well as the operative and postoperative treatment. Close co-operation between surgeon and anaesthetist is essential, and if the surgeon is unable personally to supervise resuscitation, the anaesthetist is the best alternative person to do so. It is usually easy to recognise when the condition of a patient has been restored to normal by measuring pulse rate and blood pressure and by observing the other signs of circulatory improvement, and with reasonable precautions the subsequent management of such patients does not give rise to difficulty.

Unfortunately, many patients with severe injuries do not respond so completely or in a consistent fashion to transfusion, and in these circumstances difficult decisions must be made. For example, a patient with a gunshot wound of the abdomen may respond well to the rapid transfusion of three pints of blood during a period of 45 minutes, then blood begins to flow from the small wound of entry, and blood pressure, which had risen from an unrecordable level to 100/50 mmHg, once more falls. This deterioration continues in spite of an increase in the rate of transfusion. It is obvious that intra-abdominal bleeding has restarted, or has increased in rate and equals or exceeds the rate of replacement by transfusion. The only worthwhile course is to proceed at once with laparotomy in the hope of being able to control the bleeding vessels and then by rapid replacement of the lost blood by transfusion to make the remainder of the operation feasible and safe. An equally urgent decision may be required after rupture of the spleen or kidney, laceration of the liver or in severe limb injuries where there is a large quantity of mangled muscle. In the course of resuscitation of such patients a peak of condition is reached which is soon followed by deterioration; although later by increasing the rate of transfusion a further period of improvement may be achieved, the first peak of improvement is invariably the highest. The optimum time for operation is just before this peak is reached; its recognition demands calm assessment, firm decision and a willingness on the part of both surgeon and anaesthetist to accept the unusual risk.

The use of external pressure with a a G suit (Gadner and Storer, 1966) may be of much value in controlling some kinds of intra-abdominal bleeding, for example from wounds of the aorta or vena cava in the abdomen or from a ruptured aortic aneurysm.

The changes in renal and respiratory function which accompany such external pressure are usually transient and last only as long as the pressure is applied, and are a small price to pay for the much increased chance of survival and the time for more deliberate preparations for operation. Similarly, the immediate use of the aorta clamp devised by Stone (1971) may allow the control of aortic bleeding for long enough to give the surgeon a chance to make a more deliberate control of bleeding of a severity which otherwise would kill the patient within a few minutes of the abdomen being opened.

General Measures

After arrival at hospital, a short period of rest for the patient is often followed by a marked improvement in general condition. It is important that he should be made as comfortable as possible. Splints and dressings may require adjustment and the foot of the bed should be raised on 10 inch blocks. Reassurance is of the greatest importance to the patient, and he should be told something of the nature of his injuries and of his treatment. Morphine should be administered only for the relief of pain, and should always be given in moderate doses (not more than 1 mg or $\frac{1}{4}$ grain) by deep intramuscular injection. Absorption from the subcutaneous tissues is delayed in severe shock and the simultaneous absorption of repeated doses when blood flow is improved by transfusion may cause morphine poisoning. The slow intravenous injection of morphine is permissible, but is dangerous in severely shocked patients because, on account of redistribution of the circulating blood by peripheral and splanchnic vasoconstriction, an unusually large proportion of the dose may reach the central nervous system.

If possible, any wet clothing should be removed and the patient should be placed in a warmed bed or in blankets. The best way to restore the peripheral circulation in a shocked patient and to make the skin warm is to replace the lost blood or plasma by transfusion. To heat such a patient with hot-water bottles, electric blankets or 'shock cradles' causes vasodilatation and is harmful, since it impairs the vasoconstrictive redistribution of the diminished blood volume to the cardiac muscle and the higher centres of the brain on which survival may depend. Provided the patient is covered with enough blankets to retain body heat, he will become warmer as he is resuscitated by transfusion.

Thirst is best alleviated by sucking gauze moistened with cold water. Large drinks of water or tea will be greedily consumed by the severely shocked patient, but usually result in vomiting, which is particularly dangerous during the induction of anaesthesia. To avoid this danger, patients who have been allowed to drink should have their stomachs aspirated before anaesthesia is induced. Unless there has been a long delay between injury and arrival at hospital, few civilian patients in temperate climates suffer from such severe deficiency of body water, apart from that due to bleeding or plasma loss, that intravenous infusion of glucose solution or saline is required before operation. When there has been delay, the best preoperative treatment is still probably adequate blood transfusion.

In hot climates, and especially in the tropics, water loss by sweating may require replacement even before operation, but it is also important to reduce water loss as much as possible by shading the patient from the sun and by cooling him with fans. Intravenous infusions of glucose may be necessary if there is vomiting or if the nature of the wounds prevents drinking. Saline should be used with caution, because of the retention of sodium and associated water by the injured subject. Sweating during operation should be minimised by cooling the theatre, by dispensing with rubber or other impermeable sheeting and by reducing towel draping as far as possible.

Vasovagal Syndrome

The significance of this disturbance is often difficult to determine, especially when it occurs in association with severe injury or blood loss. Usually some improvement and occasionally complete recovery follows elevation of the foot of the bed. When a vasovagal disturbance is combined with severe blood loss, for example just after a major abdominal operation, it is unwise to use vasoconstrictor drugs to combat the vasovagal element on the combined disturbance. Close observation combined with adequate replacement of any accompanying blood or plasma loss is probably the wisest course to adopt. Vasoconstrictor drugs cause a temporary elevation of blood pressure and of heart rate lasting 2 or 3 hours, but if when these effects pass off the vasovagal disturbance continues, the resulting secondary fall in blood pressure may be difficult to interpret. Instead of employing a vasoconstrictor agent, the foot of the bed should be raised on blocks and a close watch kept for change in the general condition; deterioration caused by continued bleeding can usually be readily recognised. The persistence of a low blood pressure for several hours after operation does not appear to do any harm and may reduce post-operative bleeding.

Restoration of Blood Volume

Transfusion is indicated (1) in all patients with a pulse rate above 100 per minute and a systolic blood pressure below 80 mmHg, and in other patients when there is any doubt, or if spontaneous improvement does not result from simple general measures; and (2) in the presence of severe injuries with tissue damage exceeding the size of two fists in volume, even when blood pressure is within normal limits and the pulse rate is not raised.

The lost fluid should be replaced as completely and as rapidly as possible, blood with blood, and plasma with dextran. Complete replacement is usually indicated by the restoration to normal of colour and temperature of the skin, peripheral blood pressure and venous filling, and by the reappearance of bleeding in the wounds. The two factors, rate and volume, are to some extent interdependent. The slow transfusion of a very large volume of blood may be ineffective when the rapid injection of a small volume would have produced marked improvement. The sooner transfusion is begun, the more likely is the rapid administration of a small volume of fluid to be effective. Delay can be avoided by starting replacement with dextran while blood is being cross-matched; dextran may also be used instead of blood when only limited quantities of blood are available, or when only small volumes of replacement fluid are required (up to 1 litre). The importance and value of replacing lost blood completely with blood is doubted by few. Shires *et al.* (1961) have suggested, however, that the results of even such adequate replacement of blood loss will be improved by the administration in addition of saline lactate or Ringer's lactate to correct or diminish the acidosis which accompanies shock and may be increased when tissue perfusion is restored following the replacement of lost blood or plasma. There is a great deal of animal experimental work in support of this idea but the clinical evidence is somewhat confusing.

When blood transfusion is supplemented by an electrolyte solution this dilutes the blood and reduces its viscosity and thus improves blood flow and cardiac output. Although the blood has been diluted improved blood flow may increase oxygen transport and may have some advantage in severe shock. Whether dextran is as effective in clinical practice as Drucker *et al.* (1962) have claimed, both in restoring blood volume and in correcting the metabolic disturbances resulting from shock, probably depends on how soon after blood loss has been sustained replacement begins. It should be remembered that the original recommendations of Shires and his colleagues were based on their observation that during experimental shock, due to bleeding, there was a large expansion of the ^{35}S space which they took to be an indication of extracellular volume. The validity of their assumption that changes in ^{35}S dilution accurately reflect changes in extracellular fluid volume has been questioned. ^{35}S may be bound to plasma protein or may enter cells. Moreover, Shires *et al.* (1961) suggested that a balanced salt solution in volumes of 1 litre per hour should be administered after severe operations up to a maximum of only 2 to 4 litres. Some surgeons have since given very much larger volumes than this up to 10 litres or even more, sometimes with results which were far from desirable. Lowery *et al.* (1971) have questioned whether the very large volumes of electrolyte solution and blood which some have recommended are necessary or desirable in young healthy men with severe battle injuries, or are they simply well tolerated because of resilient cardiovascular, pulmonary and renal functions.

It seems not unreasonable to conclude that the most important factor in successful treatment after large blood loss is the very early, rapid and complete replacement of the blood lost, before gross secondary effects can develop as the result of poor tissue perfusion. When metabolic acidosis has developed and especially when this is accentuated after successful restoration of the blood volume by 'wash-out' from previously poorly perfused tissues, there may well be a place for the use of buffered Ringer's lactate solution or something of this kind.

In severe shock the fluid should be injected as fast as it can be made to run through the largest needle, cannula or polyethylene catheter that can be inserted into a vein. When veins are in such a tightly constricted state that they cannot be punctured readily with a large needle, to avoid delay a vein should be exposed under local anaesthesia and a polyethylene tube inserted; even in very young children, size 2 polyethylene tubing is the finest calibre which should be employed and not less than size 3 should be used in older patients. It is important to reduce resistance to flow to a minimum by making the segments of narrow calibre, such as cannulas and needles, as short as possible. In addition, turbulence in the liquid should be reduced by tapering the junctions where the calibre of the tube changes.

Disposable sets of delivery tubing and containers have been designed incorporating these improvements. Pressure may be applied to the air inlet of the standard transfusion bottle at the risk of an air embolism, whereas with a plastic container pressure can be applied externally with complete safety by wrapping the plastic container in a sphygmomanometer cuff which is then inflated. Venous spasm can be reduced by warming the limb and the blood or other fluid before administration. Especially in abdominal injuries, veins in the arms should be used in preference to those in the legs. By transfusing into two or three veins simultaneously 3 or 4 litres can be injected in thirty minutes, but such rapid replacement should not be continued after the systolic blood pressure has been raised to 100 mmHg. It is now recognised that intra-arterial transfusion into a peripheral artery is no more effective than early and determined intravenous transfusion. The total volume to be given to a particular patient depends on the quantity which has already been lost, on whether blood loss is continuing and on the response to treatment. Apart from incompatibility the greatest danger of blood transfusion arises from the risk of transmission of viral hepatitis. Grindon *et al.* (1967) estimated that out of every 1000 patients who were given one unit of blood 100 would develop hepatitis, 10 would become jaundiced and one would die of liver failure.

The treatment of severe blood loss by rapid transfusion is not invariably successful. Most failures are due to giving too little blood too slowly or too late, a combination which is rarely unavoidable. In some patients cardiac failure may appear during transfusion, while in others a deterioration in general condition is accompanied by a rising venous pressure and both these types of disturbance may be due to citrate intoxication, rather than to the rapid rate of transfusion. Disturbances in the electrocardiographic tracing during the transfusion of citrated blood were reported by Furman *et al.* (1951), who observed a progressive increase in the QT interval, an increased ST segment and a reduced amplitude of the T wave, which were abolished by the injection of calcium gluconate. The onset of citrate intoxication seems to be related to the rate of transfusion, but because citrate is excreted in the urine, or metabolised in the liver and muscles, is also more likely when there is severe disturbance of hepatic or renal function. The possibility of citrate intoxication should be considered when the response to the rapid transfusion of a large volume of blood is unexpectedly disappointing, especially in patients with poor liver function, during whole body cooling, or during exchange transfusions in erythroblastic infants.

Both in animals and in the human subject of all ages citrate intoxication has usually been associated with a very fast rate of transfusion. Nonetheless, at least in the early stages of replacement of a large loss of blood, rapid transfusion is an important factor in survival. Citrate intoxication can be treated by the intravenous injection of 10 ml of a 10 per cent solution of calcium gluconate.

Even when blood volume has been fully restored before the operation is begun, the intravenous infusion should be continued slowly during and for a time after operation, to enable the rapid replacement of any further blood loss to be made without delay. During the operation, the general progress of the patient is best judged by repeated measurement of blood pressure, pulse and respiration rates and by observation of the state of the peripheral skin circulation. The colour of the blood and the rate of bleeding in the operation wound may provide some additional information. It may be necessary at times to stop maniuplation in the upper abdomen or of a fractured limb because of the neurogenic hypotension which this may cause. Anaesthetic techniques and drugs which cause marked hypotension are dangerous and should not be used in severely injured patients. They are dangerous because replacement of lost blood may have been inadequate and the residual vasoconstriction on which circulatory efficiency depends may be abolished by these hypotensive agents. This risk is not outweighed by the possible reduction of operation blood loss at a lower blood pressure.

After operation, a slow intravenous infusion of glucose solution may be continued for 12 to 24 hours so that any further blood loss may be replaced without delay. In chest injuries, only the minimal quantity of blood should be employed and the infusion should be stopped as soon as blood loss has been replaced. In abdominal injuries involving the alimentary tract, the oral intake of fluid is usually restricted or stopped for 24 hours or more and gastric aspiration is instituted; fluid intake is generally maintained by intravenous infusion until the oral intake of fluid can be resumed.

In burns, the blood pressure should be restored by the rapid intravenous injection of dextran and thereafter the vein kept open by a very slow infusion of glucose solution; further dextran may then be administered immediately it is needed and the basal requirements of water can be satisfied by the glucose infusion. In deep burns there may be sufficient destruction of red blood corpuscles by coagulation in the burned tissues to warrant replacement by whole-blood transfusion. The former reluctance to use whole blood under any circumstances in the treatment of shock due to superficial burns has been shown to be unfounded.

PREVENTION OF SHOCK IN DELIBERATE SURGERY

General Measures

The patient should be brought to operation in the best possible condition and all unusual and violent methods of preparation, such as repeated drastic purgation, which might disturb his fluid equilibrium, should be avoided. Restriction of food and fluid intake should be reasonable and mobility maintained as long as possible. Taylor *et al.* (1945) showed that when healthy young subjects are confined to bed and kept at rest for two weeks blood volume falls by 10 per cent. The importance of mobilising patients who have been bed-fast for several weeks before submitting them to surgical operation is well recognised; a delay of 10 days or so for physical rehabilitation is well repaid by the improvement in morale as well as in circulating blood volume and pulmonary function. Blood volume should be restored and anaemia corrected by transfusion. In wasted subjects it is probably better to use packed cells than whole blood, but whichever is chosen an interval of at least three days should be allowed between the last transfusion and operation. Disturbances of water, sodium, potassium, chloride or bicarbonate equilibrium should have been corrected and an interval allowed for stabilisation before the day of operation.

Hypotensive procedures designed to limit blood loss have been used for many years. Spinal analgesia produces arterial hypotension by vasodilatation in the distribution of the spinal segments affected by the drug. The resulting diminution in bleeding in the operation wound has been of value in many operations, and the extension of this method to very high (T2) spinal block has provided bloodless fields for various operations. A similar reduction in blood pressure may be achieved by the use of the methonium compounds in suitable dosage. The advantages of these methods are: first, that blood loss being reduced, blood transfusion is less often necessary; and secondly, smaller doses of anaesthetic drugs are required to produce particular effects than in normotensive patients, and recovery from anaesthesia is usually more rapid. These methods are not without risk, and the chief disadvantages are the difficulty of precise control and judgment of the individual dose required; some patients tolerate hypotension of this type badly and there are occasional failures to recover to normal blood-pressure levels after operation. Their use is contraindicated in children, and in frail or cachectic patients in whom a diminished blood volume maintains circulatory efficiency only with the aid of vasoconstriction, and in shocked patients in whom there is compensatory vasoconstriction.

To reduce bleeding from certain cerebral tumours, blood may be withdrawn into a sterile container before the operation is started, and in addition the patient may be operated upon in the sitting position. At the end of operation the blood which was withdrawn is reinfused.

Measurement of Blood Loss

There are several ways in which an estimate may be made of the quantity of blood which is lost during an operation but none is entirely satisfactory. The swabs can be weighed on one pan of a scales and dry swabs of the same size and material can be placed on the other pan. This method always underestimates the blood loss, even on the swabs, possibly because of evaporation, and is even less accurate when the used swabs have been soaked in saline before use. Alternatively the blood in the used swabs can be soaked out and the haemoglobin converted to acid haematin and the concentration measured in a colorimeter; this method may be accurate to within 10 per cent according to who does it and the efficiency of the washing out process. It is also necessary to measure repeatedly the haemoglobin concentration of the patient's blood in order to calculate the amount of blood lost. A small domestic washing machine can be adapted for washing swabs. The blood volume of the patient can be measured directly on several occasions using labelled red cells or plasma albumin or better still both, but this is much more expensive. None of these methods except blood volume estimation measures the blood lost into tissues or body cavities. The best alternative to actual measurements is for the surgeon to learn what various volumes of blood look like when they have been spilt on to swabs, towels or the floor and to realise that in practice most estimates of blood loss are too small.

Central Venous Pressure

The central venous pressure as measured in the right atrium or superior vena cava is an indication of the capacity of the heart to accept and pump out returning venous blood, but it does not alone accurately indicate changes in blood volume. The measurement of central venous pressure with a saline manometer connected to a catheter, the central end of which lies in the right atrium, has been strongly recommended as the most direct means of following changes in circulating blood volume and their relationship to total circulatory efficiency. It is important to remember that the veins are actively contractile; and that their capacity is subject to much variation and is related to the volume of blood in the venous side of the circulation. Although a normal central venous pressure does not necessarily imply that blood volume is normal, it is often assumed that when a low venous pressure is restored by transfusion a previous deficit has been corrected, and that so long as the pressure does not rise above the normal range an excessive volume of fluid has not been administered. These assumptions are not always valid, and while they may be reasonable, in young previously healthy individuals during the early stages of treatment of their injuries, they are not necessarily so in the elderly and infirm with myocardial disease and weakness, or in the late stages of shock. However, Northfield and Smith (1970) found that in patients with acute bleeding from the gastrointestinal tract replacement transfusion until the central venous pressure was normal (5 cm water) brought the blood volume to within the normal range in 95 per cent of patients. In addition the rapid fall in venous pressure to zero in those patients who bled again was the best and earliest diagnostic indication of further bleeding. Wilson *et al.* (1971) found that neither central venous pressure nor blood volume measurements alone were consistently reliable indications of the need for fluid replacement or of the effect of its administration. In addition there was an almost complete absence of correlation between the simultaneous measurements of these two parameters. Large volumes of fluid were administered with little if any change in venous pressure and in some of these patients pulmonary oedema appeared with unchanged central venous pressures of less than 5 cm of water. The use of central venous pressure seems likely to lead to the infusion of excessive volumes of fluid, especially when the rate of administration is slow and the venous system as a whole has sufficient time to accommodate its capacity to the increased volume of blood.

During rapid infusions on the other hand a rise in venous pressure may be the earliest sign of heart failure or pulmonary congestion.

Central venous pressure can be measured by connecting a simple saline manometer to a radio-opaque catheter which is inserted through a vein in the cubital fossa to the superior vena cava. The zero level on the manometer should be fixed in line with a point 4 cm vertically below the manubriosternal joint in the recumbent patient. Measurement of venous pressure is probably most useful when it is combined with measurement of cardiac output with indocyanin green and the calculation of cardiac index, an expression of cardiac output per square metre body surface per minute, and with the arterial oxygen tension and the carbon dioxide tension of right atrial blood. These measurements depend on the availability of suitable apparatus and skilled people and are usually possible only when an organisation for the intensive study and care of very ill patients has been set up. They are probably of most value after operations on the heart and in elderly patients. It must be remembered that the incidence of complications of central venous catheterisation is high and is related to the length of time the catheter remains in the vein.

CHAPTER TEN

Plasma Substitutes

A plasma substitute is a preparation of a colloid such as gum acacia or dextran, which is designed to replace human plasma or serum in the treatment of low blood volume states, such as that in shock due to the loss of blood or plasma. The term plasma substitute is only one of a number which have been employed for these preparations. They are substitutes for plasma only in the sense that they are expected to occupy an equal space within the vascular system. Both gum acacia and dextran are carbohydrates with complicated molecular structures and neither contains any protein. The best alternative term is blood volume expander, but this also is not entirely accurate, since it is the plasma, or non-cellular fraction of the blood volume, which they are designed to increase.

Plasma substitutes are necessary, first, when the available supplies of blood and plasma are insufficient to meet the existing requirements, and secondly to provide a stored reserve in readiness for use in future large-scale emergencies. In addition, they are of value in some countries where transfusion services do not exist or where donors are scarce because of the fear of losing 'vital force' by giving blood and the maintenance of steady supplies of blood is difficult; in these circumstances plasma substitutes provide valuable alternative agents to whole blood and its derivatives. They also have the advantage that when properly prepared and used they are much less likely to cause serum hepatitis and other infections which may be due to the transfusion of blood and blood products such as plasma.

An effective plasma substitute must have certain properties. In solution its viscosity should resemble that of plasma, and it should exert an osmotic pressure similar to that of the plasma proteins. It must be stable for long periods over a wide range of temperature. It must be easily sterilised but free of pyrogens, and yet be capable of cheap manufacture in a constant form. When injected in therapeutic quantities it must not be toxic or antigenic; although being retained in the blood stream long enough and at a sufficiently great concentration to cause a lasting increase in blood volume, the material should also ultimately be completely excreted from or metabolised in the body.

The purpose of a plasma substitute is to increase in a lasting fashion the volume of fluid in active circulation within the blood vessels. The success of a particular preparation in thus occupying space within the vessels depends on how completely its molecules, with their associated molecules of water, are retained within the capillaries. This retention depends on the physical properties of the substance, and in particular on the size and shape of its molecules. Size is probably the more important factor, but at certain critical points shape may determine whether the molecules of different substances, but of the same weight, will pass through the capillary wall. It has been suggested that molecules of substances used as plasma substitutes may adhere together in loose aggregations; these aggregations may then produce unexpected physical effects on blood pressure which are not easily explained. It is also possible that some of the effects of these substances may be due to their molecules adhering to plasma protein molecules.

It has been assumed that most of the osmotic effect of plasma is due to the plasma albumin (Scatchard, 1952) and that the efficiency of plasma substitutes is similar in plasma and in solutions of albumin. The molecular weight of the plasma proteins varies from albumin 69,000, through β globulin 90,000, and γ globulin 156,000 to fibrinogen 400,000. In a discussion of the factors concerned in capillary permeability, Pappenheimer (1952) pointed out that the diameter of the pores in the capillaries is about 6 nm. The smallest dimension of the plasma protein molecules is about 3·5 to 4·0 nm, which is regarded as the smallest size of particle which can be retained within the blood vessels. Since none of the plasma protein molecules is spherical, none is concerned solely with the maintenance of plasma volume. The permeability of the capillary walls is subject to wide variation, albumin for example being largely confined within normal capillaries but leaving the unusually permeable capillaries of inflamed tissues as rapidly as water or sodium (Cope and Moore, 1944).

All the plasma substitutes in current use are colloids of large molecular weight; they are prepared by chemical synthesis or degradation and always contain a mixture of molecules of various sizes. The behaviour of a particular mixture depends on the relative numbers of molecules of different weights which it contains. The efficiency of a particular preparation of a suitable substance as a means of increasing the volume of fluid in circulation within vessels depends on whether it contains a sufficient proportion of molecules which are retained in the vessels for a worthwhile peroid of time.

Not much is known of the factors which govern the retention of colloid material within the vascular system. However, Grotte *et al.* (1951) have shown that in the case of dextran there may be rapid diffusion of injected material from the plasma into the urine, interstitial fluid, lymph and intestinal secretions. The rate and degree of loss are related to the molecular weight of the dextran molecules. Bayliss *et al.* (1933) studied the urinary excretion of protein by anaesthetised cats and rabbits and by the isolated perfused kidneys of dogs; they found that all the proteins excreted were of molecular weight less than 70,000 whereas all those retained had molecular weights in excess of 70,000. They further showed that the molecular weight, rather than the origin or nature of the molecule, was the critical factor in deciding whether the material crossed the glomerular membrane. Their conclusions regarding the critical size of molecule for renal excretion generally have been confirmed by Marshall and Deutsch (1950), and Metcalf *et al.* (1954) have stated that the kidneys probably fractionate dextran at a molecular weight of about 70,000.

Plasma substitutes contain mixtures of particles of varying molecular weight. Immediately after an injection most of the injected material will be found in the circulating blood. The smaller molecules which are able to cross the capillary membrane, rapidly leave the circulating blood stream for the surrounding interstitial space, and an unsteady equilibrium is established between plasma and interstitial fluid, about three-quarters of the smaller molecules being thus lost from the circulation. This process of equilibration throughout the extracellular fluid is disturbed, however, by the rapid coincident loss of small molecules from the renal glomeruli into the urine (Fig. 9). As this urinary excretion lowers the plasma concentration of small molecules, other molecules of similar size pass back into the plasma from the interstitial fluid to restore the disturbed equilibrium between plasma and interstitial fluid, and in due course are also excreted in the urine. It is clear, therefore, that the smaller molecules of a plasma substitute behave in a manner similar to inulin, which reaches an equilibrium between plasma and interstitial fluid within about an hour of injection, and about 95 per cent of which is excreted within 24 hours (Schachter *et al.*, 1950).

The production of a lasting increase in plasma volume evidently depends on the injection of a sufficient dose of material with a molecular weight too large to be excreted in the urine or rapidly lost into the interstitial fluid. The osmotic activity or water-holding capacity of a molecule in proportion to its weight diminishes as its size increases, but in the production of a plasma substitute it is essential that this activity is exerted within the vessels and some

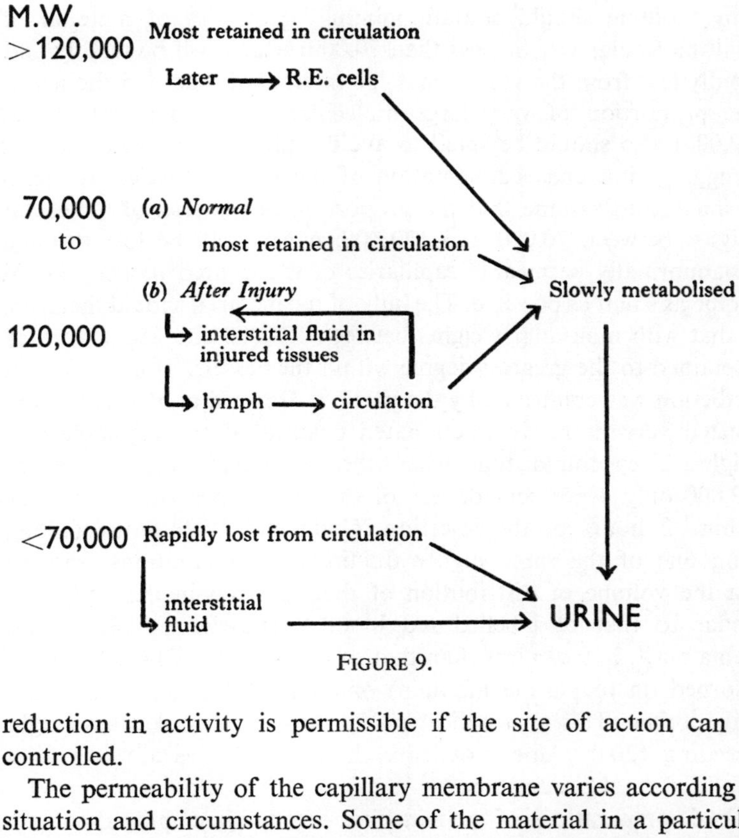

FIGURE 9.

reduction in activity is permissible if the site of action can be controlled.

The permeability of the capillary membrane varies according to situation and circumstances. Some of the material in a particular solution which exceeds the probable limit (mol. wt 70,000) for rapid urinary excretion may be lost into interstitial fluid through even normal capillaries. Capillary permeability to protein is markedly increased after injury and in other kinds of inflammation, and in such circumstances it is likely that plasma substitutes of molecular weight up to about 120,000, midway between β and γ globulin, may readily be lost. Larger molecules than this are probably largely retained within the vessels until the material is metabolised, excreted after partial breakdown, or deposited in the reticuloendothelial cells of the liver, spleen and lymph glands. It is undesirable to inject material the molecular weight of which exceeds 250,000 because of the adverse effects which are caused, in particular marked aggregation of red blood corpuscles and marked increase in blood viscosity and the erythrocyte sedimentation rate.

The ideal preparation for producing a lasting increase in circulating volume should contain minimal quantities of material of small molecular weight (less than 70,000) which will be readily and rapidly lost from the vessels into the interstitial fluid and the urine. The proportion of very large molecular weight material (above 250,000) also should be small to avoid undue increases in viscosity or aggregation and sedimentation of the red corpuscles. It seems reasonable to assume that the proportion of material of molecular weights between 70,000 and 120,000, which may be lost through the abnormally permeable capillaries of the injured tissues, should also be as small as possible. The bulk of the material should therefore be that with molecular weights between 120,000 and 250,000 which is retained to the greatest degree within the vessels. This theoretical prediction was confirmed by the work of Howard *et al.* (1956), who injected very narrowly fractionated dextran of varying molecular weight. They found that when the molecular weight exceeded 129,000 only 4 per cent or less of the dose appeared in the urine within 72 hours of the injection. Craig and Waterhouse (1955), using one of the same highly fractionated preparations, showed that the volume of distribution of their dextran in the body was similar to that of labelled red blood corpuscles or the venous haematocrit, but was less than that of the blue dye T1824 (which is adsorbed on to plasma albumin) or albumin labelled with radioactive iodine. This also indicates that dextran of molecular weight exceeding 120,000 does not leave the capillaries as albumin does even in normal circumstances.

Crude preparations of the materials commonly employed contain molecules of weights ranging from a few thousands to several millions. To reduce the crude product to a preparation suitable for injection the material must be hydrolysed and the larger and smaller molecules must be removed by fractional precipitation. The manufacture of closely fractionated preparations is wasteful in material and costly in apparatus. The more closely the ideal is approached, however, the greater is the proportion of the injected material which remains in circulation and the smaller is the dose which must be injected to produce a satisfactory response.

The mode of action of plasma substitutes is not completely understood and may vary from one preparation to another. Haemodilution is a constant effect following the infusion of plasma substitutes and may be associated with reduction in the total plasma protein concentration. The change in protein concentration has been ascribed entirely to dilution (Bull, J. P., *et al.*, 1949) or to suppression of albumin synthesis (Rosenqvist and Thorsén, 1951), but there is evidence that the total quantity of protein in circulation may be increased in spite of the reduction in concentration (Hammarsten *et al.*, 1953; Wilkinson and Storey, 1953). The state of protine nutrition of the body may be as important a factor in this type of response as it is in the alterations in total circulating protein after the infusion of saline (Shearburn, 1952). The explanation of this mobilisation of plasma protein is uncertain, but it may be related to the expansion of the extracellular fluid which follows the infusion of saline and of small molecular plasma substitutes; the consequent increase in the rate of turnover of extracellular fluid and of lymph formation may increase the rate of circulation of plasma protein. Thus part of the effect of a plasma substitute on plasma volume might be due to this mobilisation of plasma protein.

Gum Acacia

For many years before Bayliss (1916, 1919) suggested that it should be used for the treatment of shock in battle casualties, gum acacia in saline had been used for the maintenance of blood volume in laboratory animals. Gum acacia is a hydrophilic colloid derived from the natural gum of the acacia thorn. It is believed to have the property of forming aggregates of its smaller molecules, which then are retained longer in the circulating blood. The selection of raw material and the preparation of solutions are largely empirical, but satisfactory preparations of a 6 per cent solution in 0·9 per cent saline are available and give excellent clinical results. Although it is theoretically possible for the gum acacia molecule to be metabolised in the human body, there is no evidence that this occurs. It is known that it may be stored for long periods and in large quantities in the reticuloendothelial cells of the liver and elsewhere, and a similar type of storage has been observed after the infusion of other plasma substitutes. Bollman (1951) found, however, that 10 years after the administration of very large quantities of gum acacia to dogs, their liver function was not impaired in spite of large hepatic deposits of acacia, and that these deposits had not produced a tissue reaction. Patients have been followed up for more than 25 years after infusions of gum acacia and are in good health.

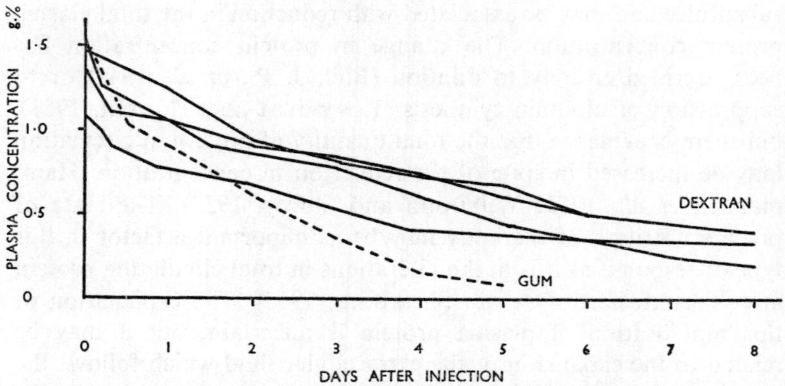

FIGURE 10. To show the rate of decline of plasma–dextran concentration after the injection of 1 litre of 6 per cent solution of dextran into four normal subjects. The curve for gum acacia has been calculated from the data quoted by Amberson (1937).

Amberson (1937) reviewed a large number of reports on the use of gum saline and concluded that retention of gum acacia in the body and in circulation was good, 61, 43 and 25 per cent of the injected dose being still in circulation 24, 48 and 72 hours respectively after injection (Fig. 10). Hartman (1951) recovered 25 per cent of the injected material from the urine in the first 24 hours after injection and 60 per cent in 7 days. Anaphylactic and urticarial reactions to gum acacia have been recorded at intervals since its introduction and have done much to discourage its use. Provided that reliable preparations are employed, it is a valuable and safe agent. The chief disadvantages arise out of the lack of knowledge of the chemistry of gum acacia, the empirical methods of production and the potentially uncertain supply of raw material. It is usually cheap to manufacture and is widely and satisfactorily used in a number of countries where exchange difficulties limit the purchase of more expensive preparations such as dextran.

Polyvinylpyrrolidone (PVP)

This is a synthetic water-soluble substance made from formaldehyde, acetylene and ammonia. It is also known as Periston, Kollidon or Polyvidone. It was developed in Germany and first used there as a plasma substitute by Hecht and Weese (1943). It is usually employed as a 3·5 per cent solution in a mixture of minerals in the same concentrations as those in which they are found in the blood; the viscosity and osmotic pressure exerted by such a solution resemble those of plasma. PVP is not metabolised in man. Such a high proportion of the injected material is excreted in the urine that its effect on blood volume is of short duration.

Dextran

Dextran is a polysaccharide composed of glucose molecules joined in a long branched chain by three types of glucosidic linkage. The pattern of the branching is related to the strain of the polymerising organism and to the substrate. It is now possible to produce dextran with a small number of branches and it has been shown that the incidence of allergic reactions is much more closely related to the number and type of linkages within the molecule than to the molecular weight of the preparation. Native dextran varies in molecular weight from a few thousands to millions and is toxic. Before crude dextran can be used clinically it must be reduced by hydrolysis to a suitable molecular weight range which is then more narrowly defined by fractionation (Fig. 11 and Table XX). The potential value of dextran as a plasma substitute was recognised both in Britain and Sweden. Grönwall and Inglelmann (1944, 1945) first developed a fractionated preparation suitable for clinical use.

When dextran is used to restore blood volume after plasma loss due to burns or scalds the duration of its effect on blood volume will largely depend on the proportion of large molecular weight material in the solution used.

Although dextran of an average molecular weight of 150,000 has been widely used in Great Britain without complications, the unfounded fear of allergic reactions and of red cell aggregation led to the general use of solutions with an average molecular weight of 110,000 or less in Europe and North America. Such a solution is less effective than dextran 150 but superior to dextran 70, both in the degree and duration of effect on blood volume.

It should be remembered that all types of preparation contain molecules of a wide range of sizes, and that there is some large molecular weight dextran even in dextran 40 and some small molecules in dextran 150. Thorsén and Hint (1950) showed that although large molecular weight dextran caused aggregation of red blood corpuscles this could be reversed or prevented by the addition of small molecular weight dextran. Gelin (1956) showed that increased aggregation of red cells due to the infusion of large molecular weight dextran could be reversed by infusion of dextran 40. After injury red cells tend to aggregate and accumulate in the capillaries and Gelin also found that this tendency was diminished by the infusion of a solution of low molecular weight dextran. It has been suggested that this effect is related to the fall in the concentration of the smaller plasma proteins, especially albumin, after injury and that dextran 40 is an effective replacement for them in the promotion of capillary flow.

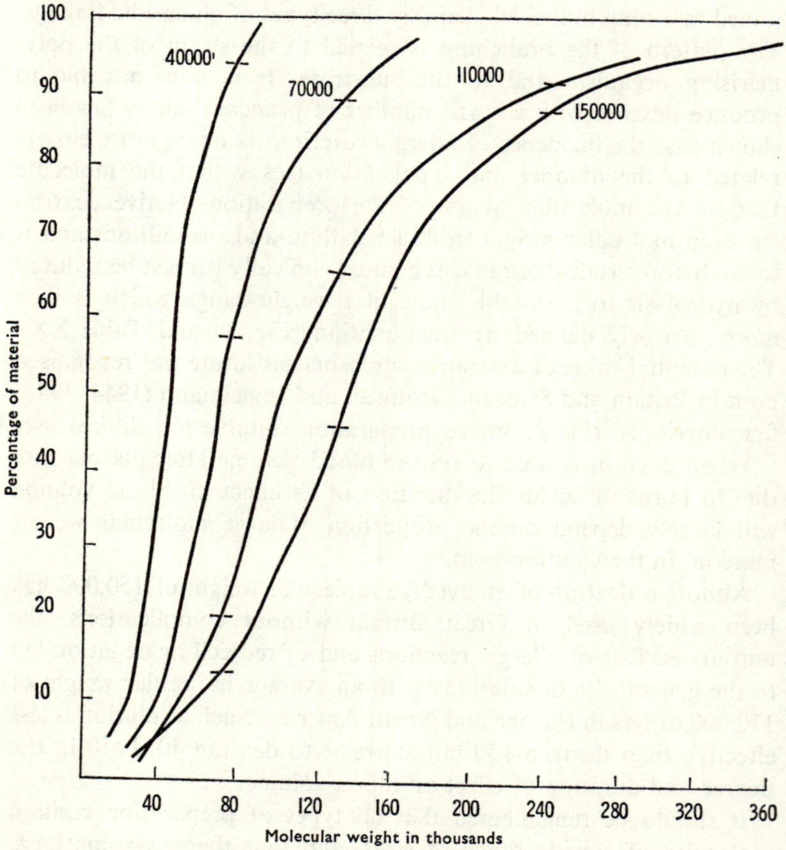

FIGURE 11. Percentage distribution of weight-average molecular weight dextran in four clinical preparations.

(The author is indebted to Messrs Fisons for this information and the permission to use it.)

For a short time after the infusion of dextran 40 there is a reduction in plasma viscosity, an increase in suspension stability of the red cells and aggregations of red cells tend to break up. After burns, dextran 40 has little more effect on blood volume than an equal volume of 0·9 per cent saline, but it has been claimed that it prevents the sequestration of red cells in the capillary circulation by improving blood flow in the capillaries. It is difficult to substantiate such a claim since measurements of plasma and blood volume are very unreliable after burns or scalds. It seems likely, however, that such solutions as dextran 110 and 150, which have an undoubted and lasting effect on blood volume, will continue to be of most value in the treatment of burns. These solutions also contain a proportion of low molecular weight dextran which appears to be enough to prevent or diminish red cell aggregation and improve capillary blood flow.

TABLE XX

Percentage distribution of various fractions in four clinical preparations of dextran

Molecular weight	%	*Type of dextran*			
		40	70	110	150
<70,000	%	95	55	20	13
70,000 to 125,000	%	5	35	45	32
>125,000	%	—	10	35	43
>240,000	%	—	—	8	12

When dextran is used to increase blood volume the duration of the increase in blood volume will depend on the proportion of larger molecules in the preparation which is used. Whatever effect the small molecules may have in bringing aggregated red cells back into free circulation will be limited in time and degree by the rapid excretion of the smaller dextran molecules by the kidneys. The value of small molecular weight dextran in the treatment of burn shock is uncertain. It has been suggested by some surgeons that the rapid excretion of low weight dextran by the kidneys improves urinary output but this is not supported by the thick syrupy urine which some burned patients pass in the first 24 hours after dextran infusions. Similar thick urine may be passed after infusions of PVP. Even the smallest dextran molecules are considerably larger than those of mannitol (molecular weight 182) which also has an uncertain effect as an osmotic diuretic in the burned patient.

Dextran 40 may be of specific value when blood flow is impaired for example in peripheral vascular disease, in gangrene, frost bite, mesenteric vascular occlusion, and for priming circulation pumps.

The serological activity of dextran varies with the type of dextran. Amspacher and Artz (1951) for example found that a dextran synthesised by the B512 strain of organism did not cause reactions even when injected into normal volunteers, and this was confirmed (Wilkinson, 1956c) even with large molecular weight dextran of this type. The strain of polymerising organism, and thus the structure of the dextran molecule, is of greater importance than the molecular weight of the dextran. Allergic reactions are extremely rare with current dextran preparations. Haynes (1965) treated a large number of burned children with dextran and did not see any antigenic reactions or unusual bleeding and this has been my own experience since I first used dextran in 1950.

Prolongation of the bleeding time has been reported after the infusion of large volumes of dextran solutions, and on a few occasions even after the infusion of less than a litre. This complication is more common after the infusion of more dextran than is necessary to restore blood volume to normal and is due mainly to the overloading of the circulation. Although some interference with blood coagulation is associated with the presence of critical concentrations of any macromolecule, no other specific effect of dextran on blood clotting has been described.

Other Plasma Substitutes

Several other plasma substitutes have been developed such as gelatin, oxypolyglucose and hydroxyethyl starch. As at present made they are all comparable in their effect on blood volume to dextran with a weight average molecular weight of about 70,000 and with the exception of hydroxyethyl starch about 65 per cent of the injected material is lost in the urine within 24 hours. Hydroxyethyl starch appears to be hyperosmolar and produces a larger increment of blood volume than the volume injected but has not yet been approved for clinical use.

EFFECT OF PLASMA SUBSTITUTES ON BLOOD GROUPING

All large molecular colloids cause some aggregation of the red blood corpuscles and false rouleaux formation, and may thus interfere with blood grouping and compatibility tests. A sample of blood should therefore always be withdrawn before any plasma substitute is injected. When this is not done, blood grouping can still be carried out but the red cells should first be washed or suspended in concentrated albumin, rather than in saline (Marston, 1954).

Mode of Use

To produce the optimum effect on blood volume, a plasma substitute such as dextran should be injected rapidly. At first only as much should be given as is necessary to raise the blood pressure to within normal limits. When in extensively burned patients the peripheral blood pressure cannot be measured the state of the peripheral circulation should be used instead, as judged by the rate of return of colour after compression of the nail bed or the pulp of the fingers or toes, and the quality of the colour changes. When the circulation is normal the colour is red and returns within three seconds of compression. Poor peripheral circulation is associated with a slower return and cyanosis or persisting pallor. More dextran should be given fast whenever there is a rise in diastolic pressure or any deterioration of the peripheral circulation. Such additional dextran should not be given slowly, especially if it is not dextran 150,000, because the small molecules may then escape from the blood stream almost as fast as they are injected, while there may be a gradual and undesirable accumulation of the largest molecules; the resulting increase in blood volume is not as great as it would be after a more rapid injection of the same volume of solution. The intravenous infusion should be kept running slowly with glucose solution until there is no longer any need for supplementary replacements.

Since the administration of large volumes of plasma substitutes causes haemodilution, it may give rise to marked anaemia, especially when there has been considerable bleeding. In addition to a plasma substitute, the administration of whole blood may thus often be desirable and, after the loss of very large quantities of blood, may be imperative. It is probably wise to administer whole blood whenever the haemoglobin concentration falls below 60 per cent of normal.

Plasma substitutes are of most value in the treatment of shock due to plasma loss after superficial burning or scalding. The blood pressure and the peripheral circulation can be restored to within normal limits and maintained there with smaller volumes of high molecular weight dextran than of plasma. In view of the comparatively poor response which often follows plasma infusion in burn shock (Rhoads *et al.*, 1941), dextran is preferable to plasma for this purpose. Consistently good results in the resuscitation of shocked burned patients have been obtained in the past with reliable preparations of gum saline, which also is superior to plasma.

Plasma substitutes are of value to supplement blood transfusion and so to reduce the requirements for whole blood. They can be employed instead of blood and are very useful for starting the resuscitation of severely shocked patients in the interval while blood compatibility test are being carried out.

It has been repeatedly recommended that in treating shock due to blood loss not more than 1 litre of dextran should be used. This limitation was proposed partly because of the fear of reactions, which are almost unknown with modern clinical dextran, and partly because of the alleged undesirable effects of large molecular weight dextran on blood clotting; bleeding after dextran infusions is usually due to giving too much and overloading the circulation. There was also the fear that adequate replacement of the lost blood with dextran would dilute the remaining blood too much and reduce its capacity to carry oxygen. When dogs were repeatedly bled and the whole blood was replaced with dextran of an average molecular weight of 75,000, haemodilution was tolerated until the haemoglobin concentration was reduced to 3 g per 100 ml, and three-quarters of the animals survived this degree of reduction of haemoglobin concentration, equivalent to the replacement of 80 per cent of the blood volume with dextran. At lower haemoglobin concentrations irreversible changes occurred in cardiac output (Takaori and Safar, 1967). Smaller molecular weight dextran (40,000) and hydroxyethyl starch solutions were both less effective and led to earlier decompensation. Ringer lactate solution without colloid was not effective. It is obvious from these experiments that it is better to use a good plasma substitute than Ringer's lactate after severe blood loss, and that with dextran oligaemia can be overcome and cardiac output and oxygen transport can be maintained. When large volumes of dextran are used there is a danger of circulatory overloading if subsequently the lost haemoglobin is replaced by the transfusion of whole blood, and packed cells are then safer.

CHAPTER ELEVEN

Diagnosis

An accurate and detailed history of the illness is the most important factor in the diagnosis of fluid and electrolyte disturbances. There must be careful inquiry into the consumption of food and fluids as well as into the losses by vomiting or diarrhoea, for on the disparity between intake and loss depends the justified suspicion of water and ionic disturbances which leads to specific investigation. The severity and duration of loss of weight, especially when combined with the best previous weight and the ideal weight for the height, sex and age of the patient, are of particular importance in judging the significance of fluid losses. The physical condition, and sometimes the mental state also, provide further evidence of the effects of fluid depletion; the effects of loss of water (p. 18), sodium (p. 36), potassium (p. 56) and magnesium (p. 69) have already been described; in obese people some of these clinical appearances may be obscured by fat. The proper partition of weight loss, and the assessment of the proportions caused by fat catabolism in partial starvation or by fluid losses and protein catabolism, is uncertain and difficult, particularly in fat people.

All patients should be weighed on admission; if an accurate stretcher type of weighing machine is available, frequent weighing provides valuable information regarding the summated effects of fluid losses and therapy. A normal adult whose intake of water and food has been stopped will lose weight at a slowly declining rate; initially in a temperate environment water loss and tissue catabolism will amount to about 1·5 kg per day. When water is freely supplied the daily weight loss diminishes to about 500 g per day. A patient who is losing large volumes of fluid by gastric aspiration or diarrhoea loses weight more rapidly than if he were only starving; conversely, when a fluid loss is replaced, its retention in the body offsets weight loss. Although a patient may thus gain weight, this does not give any indication of the location of the added fluid which, instead of reaching the interior of the cells as was hoped, may instead be accumulating as oedema fluid in the lung bases or in the buttocks. Failure to lose weight or an unexpected gain in weight is an indication to search for oedema. Although a steady loss of weight may be due to normal consumption of tissue and loss of body water in starvation, it may also be due to the failure to replace losses adequately. There cannot be fixed rules for the interpretation of changes in body weight which must be regarded rather with intelligent curiosity.

Apart from the common ground of good history-taking and clinical examination, the degree of diagnostic accuracy and refinement which is possible in any particular unit depends to some extent on the accurate collection and recording of the urinary output and fluid losses by vomiting, fistulous discharges or faeces, and in part on the biochemical facilities available for the examination of blood and other fluids. The most important factor is, however, the use which is made of the information thus obtained. The possible effects of change in bodily composition are endless. It is essential, therefore, to try to follow some simple plan by which the important and lethal disturbances receive first attention in recognition and treatment. The evidence which is obtained from the type of scheme shown in Table XXI enables some estimate to be made of the total quantity of abnormal fluid losses and of the interference with normal intake of food and water; from this a rough approximation can be reached of the potential loss of such constituents as potassium, sodium, chloride and water.

A hypothetical example of the kind of information which can be obtained by calculation when the patient's height, sex, age and the recent changes in body weight are known is shown below.

A man aged 45 years, height 5 ft 6 in (157·1 cm), who suffered from duodenal ulcer with pyloric stenosis, weighed 11 stones (154 lb; 70 kg) at the onset of a prolonged series of bouts of vomiting which lasted 9 weeks. At the time of admission he weighed 7 stones (98 lb; 44·4 kg). The best weight he had ever achieved was 12 stones (168 lb; 76·3 kg), and the ideal weight for a man of his height and age is 10 stones (140 lb; 63·4 kg). By using the formula of Allen *et al.* (1956) (p. 6), the fat content of this man at the various weights can be calculated and then the information shown in Table XXII can be obtained. The estimate of total body water based on ideal weight is a good deal higher than those based on fat free weight. From these calculations the total loss of weight 56 lb (25·6 kg) can be divided

TABLE XXI

Diagnostic plan

1. General History } of primary disease
   Clinical features }
2. Specific to fluid disturbance
   (i) History of fluid losses
      Type
      Volume
      Duration
   History of food intake
      Remote in relation to primary disease
      Recent in relation to fluid losses
   (ii) Clinical features
      Evidence of: Disturbances of water content
         sodium content
         potassium content
         magnesium content
         acid base balance
   (iii) Body weight
      Actual
      Previous best
      Ideal weight for age, sex, height
   (iv) Urine
      Volume per 24 hours
      Specific gravity
      (Chemical analysis)
   (v) Gastric aspirate, vomit, discharge, faeces
      Volume per 24 hours
      (Chemical analysis)
   (vi) Blood
      Packed cell volume or haemoglobin concentration
      Plasma concentrations of sodium, potassium, chloride, bicarbonate
         urea nitrogen

TABLE XXII

Total body weight		*Fat*	*Fat-free weight*	*Total body water*	
				60% of ideal wt	*70% fat-free wt*
lb	kg	kg	kg	litres	litres
168	76·3	24·99	51·3		35·91
154	70·0	20·71	49·29		34·5
140	63·4	16·22	47·18	38·04	33·02
98	44·4	5·19	39·21		27·44

into 34 lb (15·5 kg) of fat, 15·5 lb (7·06 litres) of water and a remainder of 6·6 lb (3·02 kg) of tissue solids.

There are several ways in which such estimates of the fractions making up lost weight can be interpreted, and the best choice depends on obtaining a sufficiently detailed history of the illness. A chronic loss in which starvation is an important factor produces a set of changes which are more likely to reflect the findings of McMurrey *et al.* (1955), with only small reductions in the extracellular fluid volume and sodium content but large reductions in the volume of intracellular fluid and the body content of potassium. These changes are also likely when the loss of weight is associated with prolonged diarrhoea as in ulcerative colitis or neglected malignant disease of the colon or rectum. The more acute the disturbance, the more likely are reductions in sodium content and the volume of the extracellular fluid and the smaller is the fraction of the total weight loss which can be safely ascribed to the catabolism of storage fat. Fortunately in acute disturbances depletion of the extracellular fluid is usually readily recognised and promptly treated. In the hypothetical case which has been described there was a loss of 7 litres of body water, and if the reduction in extracellular fluid volume is of the order of only 10 per cent (1 litre) of the original volume of 9 to 10 litres the remaining 6 litres can be attributed to intracellular water. This quantity would contain 660 to 700 mEq of potassium, and if there has been disproportionate loss of potassium from the body the potassium deficit may be even larger.

It should always be the main object of the clinician to make an accurate diagnosis from the history and physical examination of the patient, and to resort to the chemical examination of the blood only for confirmation of that diagnosis. In some patients a complete diagnosis can be made only with biochemical assistance, but if in all cases undue reliance is placed on biochemical evidence, misleading conclusions more commonly follow.

It is important to measure those constituents of the blood which will be of most value in confirming the diagnosis and in guiding treatment. Repeated measurement of the same few constituents is of more value than sporadic measurements of a large number of substances. In surgical patients most help is usually obtained by measurements of the plasma concentrations of sodium, potassium, chloride and bicarbonate; urea nitrogen is also of value when renal function may be disturbed. It is necessary also to measure on the same specimen of blood the packed cell volume (haematocrit) or haemoglobin concentration as an indication of the degree of concentration of the blood; change in extracellular fluid volume without alteration in red cell content causes haemoconcentration or haemodilution. It should be remembered that the concentration of the constituents of the plasma or serum are indications only of the concentrations of those substances in extracellular fluid. No method yet exists which will conveniently provide any indication of change in the composition of intracellular fluid, apart from the measurement of the difference between intake and output of substances, such as nitrogen and potassium, which are largely distributed in intracellular fluid. Clinical examination is also the main means of assessment of progress and of the response to treatment, although repeated chemical analysis of the blood, and sometimes also of the urine, may often be essential for the accurate control of treatment and in judging when correction of previous abnormalities is complete.

When chemical analysis of urine and collected fluids is possible, a more detailed estimate can be made of the continuing loss of sodium, potassium, chloride and water. These analyses are an indication of the present state of the body and of its secretions, as they have been modified by compensatory reactions; they are thus only indirect indices of previous losses. The greatest value of such analyses, like those of the blood constituents, is as a reference base for comparison with future analyses of the same fluids after treatment has been instituted, and thus as a means of controlling replacement of lost body components. It is important to recognise that apparently paradoxical changes may occur in the components of plasma and urine as the result of treatment.

CHAPTER TWELVE

Treatment

GENERAL PRINCIPLES

When there has been loss of body fluid, the objectives of treatment are three:

1. To ensure survival by maintaining an adequate volume of blood in active circulation.
2. To stop the loss of fluid.
3. To repair the damaged and distorted body fluid pattern by the administration of an appropriate combination of water and electrolyte, and in the long term by feeding as normal a diet as possible.

Success in treatment depends on the individual consideration and management of each patient and on gaining and keeping control of the fluid and electrolytic balance of the patient. The first step is to make an assessment of the present state of the patient, and then to try to estimate the rate and direction of progression of the disturbance and so to decide the measures which must be adopted.

The duration and severity of fluid loss can be judged from the history and clinical appearance of the patient. Signs of circulatory impairment are of first importance; those of loss of water or wasting of tissues, although notable, are not of such immediate therapeutic concern. Body weight may give an indication of the total water state of the body, and the volume and composition of the urine may show how renal mechanisms have compensated for losses of body fluid. Changes in the serum concentration of sodium, potassium, chloride and bicarbonate will show what alterations have occurred in the composition of the extracellular fluid, and may give indirect evidence of changes in intracellular fluid, but the volume, osmolality and concentrations of sodium and potassium in the urine may give even more useful indications. The haematocrit or packed cell volume indicates the presence and degree of dilution or concentration of the blood. The response to treatment also is judged by the changes in the clinical state of the patient, by repeated estimations of serum electrolyte concentrations, blood pressure, pulse rate and peripheral skin circulation, volume, specific gravity and composition of the urine, and, if possible, by repeated weighing of the patient.

The cellular environment depends primarily on the maintenance of an adequate circulating blood volume; transfusion of blood, plasma or a plasma substitute is therefore the first measure to be considered in all cases. Replacement of deficits of water and electrolyte is important, but in many surgical emergencies it is a secondary consideration, provided blood volume is maintained. In diseases for which operative relief is less urgent, attention may be given to replacement of electrolyte deficiencies, but it should be recognised that time is required for the normal distribution throughout the body of administered water and electrolyte.

In designing any required combination of fluids for complete intravenous maintenance, care must be taken that provision is made for the secondary changes of acidosis or alkalosis, and that the replacement fluids do not themselves create further biochemical disturbances. In addition, water to cover the daily insensible loss and for urine formation, and 100 g of glucose daily to prevent ketosis and reduce tissue catabolism, must be provided. The complete and accurate intravenous replacement of lost body fluids is impossible, and the best approximations to this ideal inevitably omit some of the constituents of the lost fluid; when intravenous replacement is continued for a long period, secondary disturbances, due to the inaccuracies in the replacement fluids, are almost unavoidable.

Prevention is better than cure and reduces the difficulties of compounding suitable mixtures of minerals for intravenous administration. If possible, therefore, losses should be reduced by curtailing the oral intake of food and fluid, and when direct surgical attack on the lesion causing the loss is not feasible, fluid lost by gastric aspiration or from biliary, duodenal or pancreatic fistulas should be collected and returned to the alimentary tract at a lower level through a jejunostomy. The opposite procedure may be required, for example in ulcerative colitis when the alimentary contents are diverted from the irritated colon by an ileostomy, or in the treatment by rectal drainage of acidosis following transplantation of the ureters.

Fluids injected into the blood stream are beyond the control of the administrator as soon as they leave the needle, and their fate and effects then depend on the conditions within the body. The only components of blood which will remain to any large extent within the vessels are the red blood corpuscles. Albumin is normally retained by the walls of peripheral capillaries, but freely traverses the capillary membrane in viscera such as the liver. After injury and during inflammation, in the affected areas even the peripheral capillaries are freely permeable to albumin and globulin. Crystalloid and glucose solutions rapidly leave normal capillaries until a new equilibrium is established in the extracellular fluid; in the absence of any loss by diuresis this would imply the transfer of up to 75 per cent of such solutions to the interstitial fluid within about two hours of their infusion.

PRE- AND POSTOPERATIVE TREATMENT

Most patients are in good condition when admitted to hospital and do not require any special preparation for operative treatment. A small number have lost body fluids or are suffering from malnutrition, anaemia or other disturbances which increase the risk of subsequent complications. An accurate and detailed history of their illness and a careful clinical examination usually enable this minority to be readily recognised.

In the average uncomplicated patient, it is usual to maintain a normal intake of food and fluid until about 24 hours before operation and then to provide a lighter diet for the last three meals. Even on the day of operation some fluid should be provided in the early morning, although the quantities should be strictly limited in view of the inhibitory effect of preoperative nervousness on gastric function. After all major operations there is a loss of appetite lasting in varying degree for 2 to 4 days and it is unusual for even light food to be taken for 48 hours. Thirst is usually very severe and is relieved only transiently by drinking and not at all by intravenous infusion of glucose solution or saline.

There is a welcome tendency to return to the older mode of postoperative treatment, in that apart from maintenance of blood volume by blood transfusion, fewer and shorter routine intravenous infusions are being used. After operations on the alimentary tract, gastric aspiration is being used more as a necessity when there is an accumulation of gastric secretion than as a routine measure in all cases. Although postoperative treatment varies very greatly in different clinics, the results of different kinds of treatment are so similar that it is likely that the good results are achieved in spite of much of the treatment that is provided. The sooner the patient resumes the consumption of food and is able to return to a full diet the better, and any treatment which delays this should be avoided as far as possible.

After all major operations it is desirable to record the intake and output of water. The value of such records varies directly with the interest shown in them by the medical staff; the charts must be checked and the use made of the information thus collected must be made evident to the nursing staff. Inaccurate routine fluid records are dangerously misleading and may be worse than none. Not only must the record for each 24 hour period be inspected but a cumulative total must be kept of output and intake and twice a day these totals should be carefully examined and treatment modified according to the information thus obtained. It is obvious that control of replacement will be much more accurate if it is possible for the chemical composition of urine and aspirated fluid or discharges to be measured before any decision is made about the mineral and water requirements. Measurements of this kind are of much more value than those of the serum concentrations which indicate only the temporary endpoints of extracellular concentrations after the compensatory reactions stimulated by the fluid losses have corrected the original disturbance. To reduce the burden on the nursing staff, fluid records should be maintained only for the minimum essential period. To many surgeons their main value lies in the record of urine volume which they provide. If the osmolality or the specific gravity is also measured, an excellent crude indication of renal function is provided. For several days after major operations it is normal for the urinary volume to be between 500 and 1000 ml and its specific gravity to exceed 1026 (1000 mosmol). Abnormal renal function is indicated by a low specific gravity combined with oliguria or by unusually severe or prolonged oliguria. In seeking a cause for such urinary variation, extra loss of water by vomiting, gastric aspiration, fistula or diarrhoea, inadequate intake, or renal disease or failure should be considered.

The ability of the body to recover from severe accidental or surgical injury has been underestimated for too long. It is exceptional for patients to require the intravenous or other administration of fluid after uncomplicated operations. The introduction of the continuous-drip intravenous infusion about 40 years ago gradually led to its indiscriminate use, with little regard to its adverse effects.

Only when loss of body fluid causes a significant reduction in extracellular fluid volume, with obvious changes in appearance or reduction in blood pressure, is replacement necessary for survival. Intravenous infusions should therefore seldom be necessary even after operations on the alimentary tract.

Many surgeons as a matter of routine arrange for an intravenous drip infusion to be maintained during and after all major operations. This unnatural state of fluid 'balance' does not cause ill effects so long as the volume of fluid which is administered is carefully controlled; but the procedure causes additional discomfort and anxiety for the patient and is biologically unsound.

After injury, renal function is altered but is very rarely impaired and renal damage due to severe injury is extremely uncommon. Oliguria is the natural response to injury in a well-functioning organism, and, except when the environmental conditions are suitably controlled, so is a large excretion of potassium in the first 48 hours, and of nitrogen for a week after injury; the close conservation of sodium and chloride is the equally natural obverse of the survival process. Therefore it seems important to emphasise that, after operation, before fluid losses are replaced, their volume and if possible their electrolyte components should be accurately measured and a judgement made of the possible harm the loss will do if not replaced. It may then be decided that replacement of all or some of the constituents is advisable. The volume, composition and rate of administration must be carefully controlled. The fluid should be drunk if possible. The dangers of administering excessive quantities of fluid by intravenous infusion are well and widely recognised, but it does not seem to be so well appreciated that the subcutaneous and rectal infusion of fluid is just as dangerous as intravenous infusion, and often as uncomfortable and even more distasteful. These methods also lack the certainty of intravenous infusion.

The routine use of a prophylactic intravenous infusion during operation makes the transfusion of blood or plasma substitutes too convenient. So much is done to patients nowadays that every reasonable reduction in the number of precedures should be made. Whole blood is a potentially dangerous as well as a precious fluid and should not be lightly used. The practice of routinely infusing 2·5 litres of fluid (2 litres of glucose and 500 ml 0·9 per cent saline) in each 24 hour period for 24 or 48 hours or longer after major operations such as gastrectomy, colectomy or excision of the rectum lacks precision and is an orthodox routine unrelated to the actual requirements of the patient. In the absence of severe bleeding, or large or repeated loss of intestinal secretions, such patients do not need blood transfusions or intravenous infusions, and provided they have been properly prepared for operation, are capable of surviving in good condition without a water intake until, after 24 hours, they are able to drink. Such routine postoperative infusions may not do much harm, but neither do they relieve thirst nor prevent eventual loss of weight and have not been shown to promote recovery (Wilkinson, 1956b). They increase the risk of complications such as chemical phlebitis, and of water intoxication or sodium retention if errors are made in their administration; they may delay the return of normal gastrointestinal motility and lead to undesirable restrictions of movement.

If fluid is administered by intravenous infusion, the total quantity should be limited to something near the daily requirements, of up to 1 litre for insensible water loss and 500 to 700 ml for urine formation. Not more than 2 litres of glucose solution per day should be given, and most patients do better with less than this. It is uncommon for the urine output to rise much above a litre per 24 hours in the first week after operation. The postoperative urinary loss of potassium cannot be stopped and usually lasts for only 48 to 72 hours. It will be replaced when food is again consumed, and its routine parenteral replacement is not indicated. It has been suggested that up to 80 mEq potassium (6·0 g potassium chloride) should be administered per 24 hours to patients who are receiving intravenous infusions; within 48 hours after operation the administered potassium will be excreted in the urine, and because of oliguria its administration is dangerous and unwise; after 48 hours potassium salts should be administered only if some deficiency existed before operation and if repeated gastric aspiration must be continued, or if there are other losses of body fluid.

The number of patients who need specific replacement therapy before operation is small. In these few patients sufficient time must be allowed for the administration of adequate quantities of water and appropriate ions, and for the subsequent adjustment of equilibrium within the body before the operative injury is inflicted. In emergency, when operative treatment can be delayed only for an hour or two, the restoration of deficient circulating blood volume is all that should be attempted. In patients who have been losing fluids or partially starving for several weeks, even a week or two may be too short a period over which to attempt to correct the resulting disturbances in bodily composition, some of which may be finally overcome only late in convalescence after operative treatment. In these patients, some compromise or balance must be reached between the restorative treatment of the general bodily disturbance by intravenous and other types of replacement therapy, and the operative surgical attack on the causal lesion. Time spent on improving protein and general nutrition is worth a delayed operation and the possible extension of the primary disease, if postoperative recovery is to be smoother and more certain.

The importance of improving the nutrition of surgical patients as well as the difficulty in doing so are now more widely recognised. The advantages of attacking formidable disease processes by stage operations have long been recognised and accepted; a similar stage-by-stage approach to the severe and sometimes complicated chemical disturbances in surgical patients also deserves wider application. The use of an ileostomy in ulcerative colitis as a preliminary step to colectomy has the double advantage of diverting the faeces from the colon and of reducing the irritation of the diseased colon and thus the loss of blood, purulent exudate and intestinal secretion.

Patients with intractable pyloric obstruction may lose by starvation and vomiting up to 40 per cent of their initial weight. Although part of this loss is made up of catabolised fat, the larger part consists of lean tissue, mainly skeletal muscle, with considerable associated losses of potassium, magnesium, sodium, protein and water. The sodium and part of the water losses can be made up rapidly by the intravenous infusion of saline. Part of the potassium and magnesium depletion also can be corrected fairly rapidly, though still more slowly than is the case with sodium, simply by the intravenous and oral administration of potassium and magnesium salts; the remainder is only slowly restored and depends on the reformation of previously catabolised protein tissue. Until the consumption of food and an adequate daily intake of energy are resumed, correction of potassium depletion is incomplete and there is a variable liability to recurrence or the appearance of the clinical disturbances due to potassium deficiency after operative treatment of the pyloric obstruction. In severe cases, even gastroenterostomy should be postponed until nutrition has been improved and potassium and magnesium depletion fully corrected by two or three weeks of jejunostomy feeding.

RESTORATION AND MAINTENANCE OF BLOOD VOLUME

Acute reduction of circulating blood volume by severe bleeding, due to accidental injury or surgical operation, is best corrected by the rapid transfusion of a volume of blood equal to that which has been lost. Even when such preoperative replacement is early and adequate, further transfusion may be necessary to replace continued or recurrent blood loss. Plasma loss in burns should be rapidly replaced by dextran, but because of the continued loss of plasma for up to 40 hours after injury, repeated infusions may sometimes be required after extensive injuries. Dextran may be used instead of blood for the replacement of the loss of up to a litre of blood or if there is delay in obtaining suitable blood. In extensive deep burns blood transfusion may be necessary, as well as dextran, if there has been much red cell destruction in the burned tissue. Blood volume may be acutely reduced by the rapid loss of intestinal secretions in acute intestinal obstruction. This is best treated by the rapid infusion of 0·9 per cent saline.

Chronic Blood Loss

Chronic reduction of circulating blood volume follows the repeated loss day after day, for weeks or months, of small quantities of blood, for example from a gastric or caecal carcinoma or from bleeding haemorrhoids. In severe chronic anaemia great care must be exercised during the transfusion of blood, or any other fluid, because although circulating blood volume may be only 2 litres, the blood pressure is within normal limits (McMichael *et al.*, 1943); Sharpey-Schafer (1944) showed that under these circumstances, there is, increased cardiac output which depends on an elevation of right auricular and venous pressures, a type of compensatory 'heart failure' which is liable to cause acute pulmonary oedema or auricular dilatation when the circulation is further overloaded by transfusion. This disaster can be avoided by the repeated slow transfusion of small volumes of blood or packed cells and by the close observation of the state of the neck veins of the patient. Severe anaemia should be treated by transfusion until the haemoglobin concentration reaches 10·4 g per 100 ml (70 per cent Haldane). Such transfusions should be completed several days before operation so that reactions do not occur on, or just after, the day of operation.

Although transfusion of whole blood is undoubtedly beneficial to patients who are malnourished and anaemic, the duration of some of the good effects of transfusion is limited. In a protein-deficient patient the protein of the administered red cells and plasma becomes part of the common protein 'pool' of the body, and may be used simply as a source of protein components. Correction of anaemia by transfusion of whole blood or packed cells thus has only a temporary effect, lasting as long as it takes the body to utilise about 80 per cent of the injected protein.

INTENSIVE CARE UNITS

These units were originally started because there were too few nurses in some hospitals to care adequately for very ill patients, unless they were concentrated in a small area. Such concentration does not necessarily or invariably result in the best use being made of scarce skilled nurses, but it does allow of the more convenient use of apparatus by anaesthetists and others whose help is needed.

There is an increasing tendency among some clinicians and senior nurses to demand that all patients with acute clinical and nursing problems shall be segregated to a special area of the hospital. One result of this is the reduction in the severity of the problems that remain in the ordinary wards which inevitably leads sooner or later to some decline in the stimuli to skill and interest of at least some of the medical and nursing staff of these wards. What is perhaps more serious in the long run is the inevitable physical and mental exhaustion and professional destruction of those, who chosen for their skill and excellence, are condemned for too long to the unremitting care of nothing but desperately ill patients of all kinds, of whom too few recover and survive.

Of the serious disadvantages of such units the most obvious and best recognised is infection, and for this reason alone it is not feasible to assemble in one place patients who have had operations on the heart or the intestine, those who are suffering from coronary infarction, pneumonia or extensive burns. Even when such patients are segregated into suitable groups those with infection must still be isolated and the arrangements must be duplicated. Infection thus implies duplication even when every patient is infected, because the prevention of cross infection requires some degree of isolation. Patients do not like to be moved about in hospital and to see too often too many new faces amongst the nurses and doctors who look after them. Too much emphasis on specialised skill and care, and especially on the use of complicated apparatus and investigation, detracts from the old-fashioned tradition of individual care of the patient in its most humane forms.

The effects on conscious patients of the constant activity in an intensive care unit is now more widely appreciated. No matter how well the postoperative situation may be explained to the patient beforehand, even the most stoical person will find the reality often hard to bear. The intravenous infusion, arterial and central venous cannulas, tracheostomy and perhaps a ventilator, the flashing lights of the oscilloscope, the crack of the infusion drop counter and the rhythmic cough of the positive pressure apparatus, multiplied by those of other patients in the same room; the failure of the staff perhaps to say much and especially the absence of familiar faces and voices; the sudden emergency bell or buzzer and bursts of activity for a crisis in another patient, but above all the constant disturbance for measurements and adjustments of all the apparatus and the lack of peace and sleep for perhaps 48 hours, have driven some patients into acute mental crises. Kornfeld *et al.* (1965) found that the conditions in the recovery room after open heart operations contributed to the production of psychotic reactions, which subsided when the patient was moved to a more normal environment and was allowed to sleep. Moreover, Levison (1972) has shown that postoperative delirium is two or three times as common in patients who are treated in intensive care units without windows and occurred in up to 40 per cent of patients. He suggests that this is due to the combination of sensory deprivation and prolonged sleeplessness in an ill patient after a major operation.

It is more and more widely assumed that survival may often depend on this sort of multiple monitoring and automated function, but all those concerned with the postoperative care of such patients should repeatedly stop to consider how much of it is really essential for survival. This constant critical review of practice is particularly important because the surgeon must delegate much of the highly specialised procedure to others. Teamwork is essential but the surgeon retains the final responsibility for decision, which depends on proper appreciation and understanding of the therapeutic methods which are being used and his knowledge of the needs and state of the patient.

The original idea that all patients who need special care should be segregated in one place is impracticable simply because of the complexity of modern medicine and surgery. It is evident, however, that the pioneers in these units have raised the standard of postoperative care and especially the general understanding of respiratory physiology and the use of tracheostomy and assisted respiration. They are the expensive modern substitute for the screened off beds at the proximal end of the ward in which the desperately ill or dying were formerly segregated, and in this sense they avoid disturbance of the less seriously ill majority.

THE MAINTENANCE OF NUTRITION

Tube Feeding

The feeding of unconscious patients, sometimes for weeks or months, is an increasingly important problem in patients with head injuries. Such patients do not commonly have any abnormality of their intestinal tract and nutrition can be maintained cheaply and easily through a nasogastric tube passed through the stomach. The same kind of feed can be used through a nasogastric tube and with a gastrostomy or jejunostomy. It is very important to remember that tube feeding deprives the patient of any choice in the dietary intake and removes that protection from excess of some foodstuffs that appetite and nausea confer on the conscious people. Excessive intakes of protein and carbohydrate should always be avoided and the water intake must be sufficiently large to allow of the urinary excretion of the products of metabolism. Tube feeding is very much less expensive than intravenous feeding and, provided certain precautions are observed, much less dangerous to the patient, since there is little risk of infection and an adequate intake of calories and protein can usually be achieved without difficulty. Provided hypertonic solutions are avoided and the intake is carefully controlled it is usually possible to maintain satisfactory intakes of both fluid and electrolyte.

The risks of tube feeding should be clearly recognised. The most serious of these is aspiration into the respiratory tract of feeds which have been regurgitated from the stomach, whether this has been given by a nasogastric transoesophageal tube or by gastrostomy. It is essential to make certain that a nasogastric tube is in the stomach before each feed is started and this also applies to a gastrostomy tube which should be pulled back so that its flange or shoulders are in contact with the anterior wall of the stomach and of the abdomen.

In nasogastric feeding there may be some difficulty with absorption if the patient has not been fed for a week or more and it is essential to start with small and dilute feeds. The size and strength of the feeds should be increased gradually as they are tolerated by the patient. Diarrhoea is usually the result of giving hypertonic feeds, especially when they are administered into the duodenum. Dehydration may have resulted from the use of diuretics and should be corrected independently, preferably by intravenous infusion.

The objective of tube feeding is to provide adequate protein and calories for the daily requirements of the patient and if possible additional quantities for the restoration of tissue lost by previous starvation and wasting disease. In addition to an adequate supply of protein and sufficient non-protein calories to prevent its deviation for fuel, sufficient minerals and vitamins and enough water to allow of the easy excretion of the products of continuing metabolism should also be provided. Depending on the state of the patient, an adult should probably receive 20 to 30 ml per kg body weight of water per 24 hours.

Many types of feeds have been devised, from the homogenisation of ordinary meals which are then administered by tube, to complicated preparations composed of eggs, milk, milk powder and other ingredients. A simple mixture consisting of 2 pints of fresh whole milk, 240 g lactose and 200 g of dried skimmed milk powder will provide a daily intake of 2400 calories, 120 g protein, 1·75 g (76 mEq) sodium, 4·48 g (116 mEq) potassium and 3·38 g (90 mEq) chloride. This mixture should be made in the cold by the addition of the lactose and dried skimmed milk to the whole milk; the dried milk goes more readily into solution if mixed with gradually increasing quantities of whole milk. After the mixture has been stirred, the supernatant solution is poured off and sufficient cold water is added to dissolve the sediment; the two solutions are then mixed together and kept in a refrigerator until used. To prevent intestinal spasm and the deposition of sediment in the tube, the feeds should be warmed before administration. Other feeds can be based on preparations such as Complan (Glaxo Limited) or modifications of it. Most commercial preparations contain adequate quantities of vitamins and trace mineral requirements, except iron, but when these are not included in the preparation they should be added. Iron supplements are nearly always necessary if the feeds are based on milk protein because of its content of iron is so low. There is usually adequate calcium in any milk based preparation but in patients who are recumbent for a long time the output of calcium in the urine is increased and there is then a risk of the formation of calcium stones. Some patients are intolerant to lactose which causes diarrhoea and it should then be replaced by glucose. When diarrhoea is caused by the use of solutions which are too strong or which contain too much cardohydrate the use of a carbohydrate with a low osmolality (Caloreen) may be of assistance, or it may be enough simply to thicken the mixture with arrowroot or cornflour.

In feeding unconscious patients, Day and Buckell (1971) recommend that when the stomach tube has been passed 30 ml of water should be put down the tube and an hour later the stomach aspirated. If this water has been absorbed another 30 ml is given and the stomach again aspirated after a further hour, 120 ml of 5 per cent glucose solution is then given. After 3 hours the stomach is aspirated to see if this has been absorbed and aspiration is repeated before every subsequent feed. If a feed is not absorbed then the next feed should be weaker. Otherwise the strength of the feeds is gradually increased.

Gastrostomy and Jejunostomy

Although in general a gastrostomy is simpler to make and maintain than a jejunostomy, jejunostomy feeding has some advantages over gastrostomy feeding. Filling the stomach with a feed causes various subjective sensations which are not found with jejunostomy feeding. Moreover, there is much less risk of regurgitation of feeds from a jejunostomy, whereas reflux of gastrostomy feeds is not uncommon and in the unconscious patient is liable to be followed by aspiration into the respiratory passages. In jejunostomy there is more liability for the tube to perforate the wall of the intestine and occasionally it may become kinked and turn back on itself. Gastrostomy tubes are usually of wider bore than jejunostomy tubes and rather less likely to perforate the wall of the stomach but in both cases it is important to see that the tube is made of material which is not 'cured' by the gastrointestinal secretions, as this causes hardening which greatly increases the risk of perforation of the wall of the intestine or stomach.

There is a good deal of prejudice against the use of jejunostomy feeding, and it is too seldom employed. In oesophageal obstruction it avoids the necessity for interference with the obstructing lesion either by dilatation or intubation, and allows of the maintenance of a high intake of protein and calories. It is said to interfere with the free choice of a loop of jejunum for anastomosis to the oesophagus after resection of the obstructed segment. This difficulty can be avoided by making the jejunostomy in a loop lower than usual. Feeding does not have to be interrupted during the immediate postoperative period. In patients with gastric, duodenal, biliary or pancreatic fistulas, in addition to enabling food intake to be continued it has the immense advantage that collected discharges from the fistula can be replaced in the intestine through the jejunostomy and disturbances of body equilibrium are largely avoided.

The jejunum is intolerant of fat, and the fat content of feeds should be kept low. The caloric value of whole milk is too low for adequate nutrition to be maintained on this alone. Since there is no impairment of the digestive capacity of the intestine, there is no reason to use protein hydrolysates in jejunal feeding.

With both gastrostomy and jejunostomy the first feed of 120 ml of 5 per cent glucose solution should be injected as soon as the operation has been completed, and thereafter 2 hourly feeds are given. At first 60 ml of milk mixture, followed by 60 ml of 5 per cent glucose solution or water, are run in from the funnel under gravity. After 12 or 24 hours it is usually possible to increase the quantities to 90 ml and then to 120 ml of milk mixture, followed on each occasion by an equal volume of water or glucose solution. The total water intake amounts to 2800 ml in 24 hours, and when 5 per cent glucose solution is used to wash the tube after a feed an additional 260 calories are provided. Such a large water intake is desirable in all patients whose intake of protein is high, regardless of the manner in which they receive the protein; when the water intake is too low for the complete excretion of the end-products of metabolism there may be a deterioration in the clinical condition of the patient with elevation of the extracellular concentration of urea, sodium and chloride; improvement follows an increased water consumption and the reduction of the protein intake. If jejunal feeding is continued for more than a week, a complete vitamin supplement should be administered, preferably as a compound mixture in syrup, which is diluted with water to avoid jejunal irritation. When there is potassium deficiency, up to 12 g potassium chloride (156 mEq potassium) and 2 to 3 g magnesium chloride or sulphate (33 to 50 mEq) may be added in each 24 hours period to the water used to wash the tube after feeds. The addition of sodium chloride to the feeds usually causes severe diarrhoea. Fluid collected from fistulas or by gastric aspiration can be run into the jejunostomy in the intervals between feeds; when this is done, to reduce the risk of blockage the tube should be washed clean with water before the milk mixture is run in.

Elemental Diets

An elemental diet consists of pure and usually synthetic amino acids with glucose as the main source of calories and a small quantity of essential triglyceride and a complete provision of vitamins, mineral salts and trace metals. The advantage of such a diet is that almost all the constituents are absorbed in the upper small intestine leaving almost no residue. In 1800 ml it is possible to provide 1800 calories including 38 g of protein (8·5 per cent of total calories) 2·6 g of fat and 407 g of carbohydrate (90·2 per cent of total calories); such a solution has a high osmolality and may cause diarrhoea. Although the taste and odour of such preparations have been much improved they are still too nauseating for some patients.

An elemental diet has been shown to support reproduction, growth and lactation in rats (Schultze, 1956) and has been the sole food intake for adult men for 22 weeks (Winitz *et al.*, 1970). The main clinical use of such a diet has been in patients with intestinal fistulas, Crohn's disease (Stephens *et al.*, 1972) ulcerative colitis (Wall and Kirsner, 1971) and before operation on the large bowel. Because so much of the intake is absorbed faeces are small in quantity and infrequently passed. It is unfortunate that too high a content of sodium still makes this kind of preparation unsuitable for use in neonates and infants, although it is satisfactory for older children and adults.

INTRAVENOUS FEEDING

Sir Christopher Wren was probably the first person to suggest in 1657 that animals and man might be kept alive by the intravenous injection of nutrients of various kinds and soon afterwards his friend Dr Robert Boyle injected opium in warmed sack into the veins of a dog (Boyle, 1663). It was more than 200 years, however, before the widespread clinical adoption of the continuous drip intravenous infusion prepared the way for the introduction into clinical practice of the intravenous infusion of protein hydrolysate and fat emulsions. It was not until 1913 that Henriques and Anderson maintained a goat in nitrogen equilibrium by the intravenous infusion of amino acids derived from the enzymic hydrolysis of goat muscle as the sole source of nitrogen.

Intravenous feeding implies the provision of the complete daily requirements of energy, protein components, mineral salts, trace elements, essential lipids and vitamins by intravenous infusion. Clinical practice usually falls short of this objective. Even the provision of energy alone in the form of carbohydrates or fat is subject to great variation and is often far from adequate. It is of most value in the prevention of starvation and the maintainance of an adequate intake of calories and protein components during the prolonged inability to take food by mouth, by tube or by some form of gastrostomy or jejunostomy. Its most common use is in a patient with a fistula of the alimentary tract; with persistent diarrhoea, due to infection with *E. coli* or other organisms or to disaccharide intolerance; in some kinds of peritonitis or in renal failure. It is not usually indicated in patients with head injuries who are suffering from prolonged unconsciousness who can be fed more simply and cheaply by tube. The replacement of losses of gastrointestinal secretions is a separate problem and should always be treated as such.

THE PROVISION OF WATER. The normal minimum daily water requirement of a healthy adult is 1500 ml. When oral intake has been stopped this may be supplied by the intravenous infusion of a 5 per cent solution of glucose, up to 2 litres being administered in each period of 24 hours. Such a solution is usually acid in reaction, but apart from its irritant effect on the vein used, this acidity does not seem to matter. The administration of glucose solution requires careful control: the volume should not exceed the estimated requirements of water for insensible loss by vaporisation and for urine formation; glucose solution is not of any use to replace gastro-intestinal secretions. The value of glucose solution as a replacement for loss of body fluids by sweating is limited by the losses of sodium and chloride in the sweat. The daily administration of 2 litres of glucose solution for several days after major operations does not reduce the eventual loss of weight and body constituents, and does not relieve thirst. Glucose solution should not be administered intravenously to patients with anuria, except when, during the diuretic phase, persistent vomiting prevents the replacement by drinking of water lost in the urine. It is liable to produce water intoxication when there is oliguria after surgical operations or in the presence of severe infection of any kind, especially in elderly patients or when renal function is impaired by chronic renal disease.

THE PROVISION OF CALORIES. In an ideal mixed diet there should be sufficient protein to provide 12·5 per cent of the total calories (70 g in a 2240 calorie intake). It is well established that the full utilisation of dietary protein depends on the simultaneous provision of an adequate supply of non-protein calories, in the absence of which some, or even all, of the protein is used for energy purposes and so is wasted as a source of protein components. This principle applies equally to the use of protein or protein components in intravenous feeding; unless the protein is accompanied by a source of calories it will be deaminated, the nitrogen will be converted to urea and the residues used as a source of calories.

A healthy adult at rest in bed probably requires about 2100 calories per day, but after injury the requirement is higher. In clinical practice the chief limiting factor in the parenteral supply of a complete daily quota of calories is the volume of fluid which can be tolerated when administered by intravenous infusion. In the normal uninjured adult the diuretic response to the infusion of 5 or 6 per cent *glucose* solution is rapid and complete, but after injury the ability to excrete water is limited, and not more than about 2·5 litres of glucose solution per day can be safely administered without some water being retained. When 5 per cent glucose solution is employed, only 125 g of glucose providing 500 calories can be supplied by the infusion of 2·5 litres of solution, but this is sufficient to reduce protein catabolism due to starvation to the minimum.

When strong solutions of glucose are used up 30 per cent or more of the glucose may be lost in the urine. The former practice of administering glucose solutions rapidly for short periods of three or four hours several times a day also leads to sudden rises in blood sugar concentration and glycosuria and the loss or catabolism of part of the administered amino acids. To be most effective intravenous feeding must be maintained steadily throughout 24 hours and the protein components must at all times be adequately covered by non-protein calories.

For solutions of similar strength, glycosuria is less marked when *fructose* is employed (Weinstein and Roe, 1952) because of the more rapid removal of fructose from the blood. Sorbitol and fructose are both metabolised independently of insulin but sorbitol has the additional advantage that it can be autoclaved without being caramelised, is even less irritant to venous endothelium than fructose and can be used in 20 per cent or 30 per cent solutions. The urinary loss of carbohydrate is reduced by a slow rate of infusion, because the blood concentration is lower, but the incidence of thrombophlebitis is increased as the duration of a glucose infusion is prolonged. The slow infusion of concentrated glucose solution (50 per cent) into the great veins offers one means of providing 1500 calories per day in a volume of less than 1 litre, but this method of administration is unsuitable for routine postoperative use and should be reserved for the critical circumstances of the anuric patient.

Heat sterilisation of glucose and fructose lowers the pH to 5·0 or even lower and it should be recognised that nearly all the solutions in use are acid in reaction and undesirably large quantities of sodium bicarbonate would be needed to bring them to neutrality. Metabolic acidosis is not uncommon when fructose is infused and has been attributed to the production of lactic acid from the fructose. It is wise therefore, especially in infants and whenever there is a liability otherwise to metabolic acidosis, regularly to measure the base excess and to use other sugars or fat emulsions if possible.

The intravenous infusion of *ethanol* is another means of providing calories; each gram of ethanol yields 7 calories on oxidation. Ethanol can replace fat and carbohydrate in the diet (Atwater and Benedict, 1902) and its rate of oxidation is increased by 15 to 30 per cent by the consumption of fructose and reduced by the previous consumption of a high fat diet or by starvation; even hard physical exercise has no effect on the rate of oxidation of ethanol consumed by mouth (Pawan, 1972). Although 2 to 10 per cent is eliminated by the lungs and in the urine the remainder is oxidised mainly in the liver at the rate of 50 to 180 mg per kg body weight per hour (Thompson, 1956). Following the oral consumption of ethanol there is a rapid initial rise in blood ethanol concentration, which then slowly declines in a linear fashion (Mellanby, 1919). When ethanol is administered at a steady rate by intravenous infusion, the blood ethanol concentration rises slowly to a degree dependent on the rate of infusion (Eggleton, 1940); provided this rate does not exceed the usual rate of oxidation of 8·0 g (10 ml) per hour there are no adverse effects such as inebriation, excitement or restlessness (Moore and Karp, 1945; Wilkinson, 1955). Up to 192·0 g (240 ml) of ethanol can be safely administered by intravenous infusion in 24 hours, which will provide over 1300 calories, and 3 litres of a solution containing 6 per cent of ethanol (180 ml) have been repeatedly administered over 24 hour periods to severely ill and wasted patients without adverse effects (Table XXIII).

TABLE XXIII

Quantities of fat, carbohydrate and ethanol necessary to supply 2000 calories per 24 hours

	Calories/g	*Solution %*	*Litres per 24 hours*
250 g fat	8·0	20	1·25
		5	10·0
500 g glucose or	4·0	10	5·0
fructose		50	1·0
285 g ethanol (356 ml)	7·0	6	4·75

A fat emulsion is a compact source of calories for intravenous administration, can be used repeatedly and does not cause thrombophlebitis as do strong sugar solutions. Fat emulsions do not exert any osmotic effect and so can be employed at high concentrations without withdrawing water from the tissues as strong glucose solutions do. The commercial fat emulsions now available are mostly made from soybean oil and there is abundant evidence of their safety (Schuberth, 1964). These emulsions contain 10 or 20 per cent fat and varying concentrations of glucose, sorbitol or glycerol to maintain tonicity, and some kind of phosphatide as an emulsifier. The fat disappears more rapidly when the metabolic rate is high, for example in thyrotoxicosis, and more slowly in patients with impaired renal function. Upjohn *et al.* (1957) found that when a fat emulsion was added to an otherwise adequate intake of calories there was an increase in nitrogen retention. The optimum intake for the post-operative patient of 0·2 g nitrogen and 35 or more calories per kg body weight per day (Abbott *et al.*, 1957) would require the administration of 500 ml of 20 per cent fat emulsion and 1·75 litres of 5 per cent amino acids with fructose and ethanol. There seems to be no reason to depart from the well-established nutritional tradition that the protein content of a diet should not account for more than 12·5 per cent of the total caloric intake even when the materials are to be injected into a vein rather than consumed as food. In malnourished patients the degree of the nitrogen retention seems to depend on the basal protein intake and the degree of nutritional depletion. Stare and his colleagues (Van Itallie *et al.*, 1952) kept a severely injured man alive for 67 days by infusions of fat emulsion, glucose and protein hydrolysates. Abbott *et al.* (1957) gave fat emulsions combined with amino acids, glucose and ethanol to well-nourished patients who had been submitted to partial gastrectomy, and were able in this way to abolish starvation during the first postoperative week.

The same care to avoid bacterial contamination is needed with fat emulsion as with amino acid solution or blood. The fat emulsion should never be mixed with other solutions before administration. Separate infusion sets can be connected by a Y junction so that the emulsion and the amino acid and carbohydrate mixture enter the vein together.

Pyrexia is the most frequent complication, the temperature beginning to rise during or just after the fat infusion, reaching a peak within an hour or two and returning to normal within 8 hours. Sometimes the rise in temperature is accompanied by headache or nausea and more rarely vomiting, loss of appetite or even diarrhoea. These reactions usually subside rapidly when the infusion of fat is stopped; after a short interval there is seldom any objection to restarting the infusion at a rather slower rate. Pain in the back and urticaria are very rare, but anaemia is common when repeated daily infusions are given. Although a mild degree of liver damage is not a contraindication to the use of fat emulsion, during prolonged treatment liver function should be regularly tested, and when impairment is progressive the administration of fat should be reduced or stopped. To be certain that injected fat is being satisfactorily cleared from the blood stream a specimen of citrated blood should be centrifuged at 1500 rev/min for 10 minutes and the plasma examined for opalescence. Usually the fat is completely cleared in 12 hours after the administration of 2 to 3 g fat per kg body weight. If the plasma is not clear the infusion should be delayed. Heparin (0·5 IU) will accelerate the clearance of fat from the plasma (Borresen *et al.*, 1970) but does not necessarily have any further effect on its metabolism.

Reactions and side effects are much less common with modern fat emulsions, especially those made from soybean oil, than with the earlier preparations. In the past repeated infusions for several weeks caused anorexia, loss of weight, vomiting, bleeding into the alimentary tract, the skin and subcutaneous tissue, impaired liver function, thrombocytopenia and prolonged coagulation and prothrombin times. The fat particles in some fat emulsions are taken up by the reticulo-endothelial system which is partially blocked and the formation of antibodies is thereby impaired. Fat emulsions, unlike strong solutions of glucose and other carbohydrates, do not have any osmolar effects. The rate at which a soybean oil emulsion is removed from the blood stream depends on the dose, the rate of infusion and the nutritional state of the patient. It is higher in the starving subject and after injury (Hallberg 1965). Up to 2 g fat per kg body weight has been given without severe reaction for long periods. In general fat emulsions should provide about 40 per cent of the total calorie intake.

THE PROVISION OF PROTEIN. Whole protein other than plasma must be hydrolysed to amino acids and small peptides before it can be administered by intravenous infusion. Protein hydrolysates for this purpose may be prepared by the acid or enzymatic hydrolysis of milk or meat protein, care being taken to ensure that any deficiencies of 'essential' amino acids in the resulting mixture are made up by the addition of supplements. Solutions of synthetic L-amino acids in theoretically desirable and nutritionally adequate proportions and concentrations are now available and some also contain vitamins and various mineral salts.

The daily requirements of proteins have been reviewed by Munro (1972), who concluded that a minimum intake of 0·6 g per kg body weight was necessary to cover all the needs and losses in an average adult and to achieve nitrogen equilibrium. When taken orally proteins of different amino acid composition are probably used with similar efficiency and this suggests that there is a need for amino nitrogen rather than 'essential' amino acids, for which the maintenence requirements are relatively small in adults. In infants growing optimally on milk protein, however, the requirements are 2·4 g per kg per 24 hours during the first month and 1·5 g per kg during the fourth to sixth months of life (Fomon and May, 1958), and for older children are lower and nearer to those of adults. In adults eight amino acids, leucine, isoleucine, lysine, methionine, phenylalanine, threonine, tryptophan and valine, are 'essential'; but infants also require histidine, as well as all the other eight in quantities which will support optimal growth. In normal adult subjects the basal daily requirement per 1·73 m^2 body surface is of the order of 10 g nitrogen and 1600 calories; average basal figures for clinical use are 70 to 80 g protein (11·2 to 12·8 g nitrogen) and 1800 to 1900 calories.

Provided it has been stored at room temperature for 6 months the administration of human *plasma* no longer carries the risk of causing infective hepatitis (Allen, 1955). There is therefore less objection to using human plasma as a source of protein in malnourished patients. Stemmer *et al.* (1955) have shown that when injected intravenously plasma protein is as adequate for maintaining the growth of puppies as the consumption of an equal quantity of horse meat. In their experiments, as in human nutrition, the most important limiting factor seems to have been the quantity of plasma which it was reasonable to inject each day in addition to a parenteral source of adequate non-protein calories. They also confirmed the earlier observation of Allen *et al.* (1948) that anaemia appears within a week of beginning the daily infusions of plasma, which may have to be interrupted while packed cells are transfused to correct the anaemia. It cannot be too strongly emphasised, however, that the intravenous use of human plasma as a source of protein is completely unjustified, and almost certainly valueless, unless at the same time an adequate quantity of non-protein calories is also injected or consumed; for the typical 70 kg adult male an adequate quantity is at least 1800 calories per day or 75 calories per hour. Moreover, 'the futility of attempting to transfuse enough serum to replace deficits of disease impresses all who try it, the only practical way to meet the demands of the body for protein is in the diet' (Weech 1938).

Some of the solutions which may be used for parenteral feeding are shown in Table XXIV. In solution A 3·3 per cent amino acids combined with 5 per cent glucose provide 332 calories per litre, of which 42 per cent come from protein, and 53 mEq of sodium and 43 mEq of chloride but only 0·15 mEq of potassium. When 3·3 per cent amino acids are combined with 2·5 per cent ethanol and 15 per cent fructose (B) the total calories rise to 907 per litre and the percentage derived from protein falls to 15 per cent. Amino acids are also available in 10 per cent solution but wastage in the urine may reduce the potential advantage of using such a concentrated solution. With 10 per cent amino acids it is essential that an adequate intake of non-protein calories is provided at the same time and this usually means that a fat emulsion must be used. The combination of a solution such as B with a 10 per cent fat emulsion (D) will provide 1700 calories of which only 8 per cent come from the amino acids and the volume of water injected is only 1700 ml out of the 2 litres of solution infused, which contains 53 mEq of sodium and 43 mEq of chloride but only 0·15 mEq of potassium.

Although the sodium content of commercially available solutions of amino acids is probably suitable for adults it is usually far too high for prolonged use with safety in neonates. The quantity of potassium in such solutions is usually too small in proportion to nitrogen and some do not contain any magnesium. It is hard to imagine how the amino acids can be converted to protein tissue in the absence of enough potassium, and it is known that the cellular content of potassium depends on the presence and availability of sufficient magnesium. The normal relation in muscle of 1 g of nitrogen to 2·5 to 3·5 mEq of potassium and 5·75 mEq of potassium to 1·0 mEq of magnesium implies that in a litre of a solution containing 7 per cent amino acids there should be 70 g amino acids, equivalent to 11·2 g of nitrogen, with 28 to 39 mEq potassium and 4·8 to 6·7 mEq magnesium.

TABLE XXIV

Solutions used for intravenous feeding

		g per litre	*Calories per litre*	*% total calories*	*Water ml per litre total volume*
A	5% glucose	50	200	60	950
	3·3% amino acids	33	132	40	—
			—		
			332		
B	3·3% amino acids	33	132	14·5	850
	2·5% ethanol	25	175	19·3	—
	15% fructose	150	600	66·1	—
			—		
			907		
C	10% amino acids	100	400	—	950
D	10% fat emulsion	100	800	—	850
E	20% fat emulsion	200	1600	—	700

In adults a litre of amino acid, fructose, ethanol should be administered over a period of at least 5 or 6 hours and the same rate (60 drops per minute) should be employed for fat emulsion. Thrombophlebitis can be largely avoided if the vein used for the infusion is changed every day. It is safer to use superficial veins in the limbs rather than to give prolonged infusions into the vena cava.

We do not understand how anabolism occurs in one tissue or organ while catabolism strips the protein from the skeletal muscles, nor the factors which will determine the use made of amino acids and other protein moieties infused into the patient's vein. The parenteral administration of adequate quantities of glucose or fructose combined with fat will prevent that part of the destruction of endogenous protein which is due to starvation (Abbott and Albertsen, 1963). In general the discomforts, limitations of freedom of movement and risks of thrombophlebitis and infection associated with parenteral feeding are not justified except in the few circumstances in which the patient is unable to digest food for more than a week. In other situations, and especially during uneventful recovery from even major abdominal operations, emphasis on the return to the consumption of a good mixed diet as soon as possible is much more important to the patient's well-being and survival.

THE REPLACEMENT AND MAINTENANCE OF ELECTROLYTE CONTENT

Before the administration of solutions of electrolytes (Table XXV) is begun, an attempt should be made to estimate the total loss of cations and water and the type of accompanying anion disturbance, as well as the probable normal and abnormal daily requirements of the individual patient.

Sodium

ISOTONIC (0·9 PER CENT) SALINE contains 153 mEq per litre each of sodium and of chloride and is therefore not strictly isotonic with the concentrations of sodium (about 140 mEq per litre) or chloride (about 103 mEq per litre) in extracellular fluid. This solution, however, is nearly isotonic with the total cation and anion of extracellular fluid (about 155 mEq per litre). When isotonic (0·9 per cent) saline is used to replace a loss of extracellular fluid, its most important effect is to increase the quantity of sodium and water; although it provides an excess of chloride, this is usually compensated by an increased renal excretion of chloride. Isotonic saline is used for the replacement of acute losses of extracellular fluid by vomiting or by diarrhoea. The administered fluid is rapidly distributed throughout the extracellular fluid. Thus although some increase in plasma volume accompanies the rapid infusion of saline, this increment is short-lived, since about three-quarters of the administered saline is eventually distributed in the interstitial fluid

TABLE XXV

Composition of solutions used for electrolyte replacement

	Constituents	*g/100 ml*	*Concentration of components (mEq/litre)*				
			Na	K	Cl	HCO_3	Lactate
Extracellular fluid			140	5·0	103	25	—
Isotonic (0·9 per cent) saline	NaCl	0·9	153	—	153	—	—
Hypotonic (0·45 per cent) saline	NaCl	0·45	76·5	—	76·5	—	—
1/5 normal (0·18 per cent) saline	NaCl	0·18	30·6	—	30·6	—	—
Hypertonic (5·85 per cent) saline	NaCl	5·85	1000	—	1000	—	—
Sodium lactate (1/6 M)	Na lactate	1·86	167	—	—	—	167
Saline lactate (Hartmann or Darrow)	NaCl	0·6	102	—	102	—	—
	Na lactate	0·62	56	—	—	—	56
			158	—	102	—	56
Ringer lactate	NaCl	0·6	102	—	102	—	—
	Na lactate	0·31	28	—	—	—	28
	KCl	0·03	—	4	4	—	—
	$CaCl_2$	0·02	—	—	4	—	—
			130	4	110	—	28
Darrow's solution (K lactate)	NaCl	0·4	68	—	68	—	—
	Na lactate	0·62	56	—	—	—	56
	KCl	0·27	—	36	36	—	—
			124	36	104	—	56
Balanced electrolyte (Fox)	NaCl	0·5269	90	—	90	—	—
	KCl	0·037	—	5	5	—	—
	$MgCl_2$	0·014	—	—	6	—	—
	Na acetate	0·2229	27	—	—	27	—
	Na gluconate	0·502	23	—	—	23	—
			140	5	101	50	—

and only one-quarter in the intravascular fraction of the extracellular fluid.

GLUCOSE SALINE. The combination of 5 per cent glucose and 0·9 per cent sodium chloride as glucose saline results in a hypertonic solution, since both constituents are present in an isotonic concentration.

HYPOTONIC SALINE. Solutions of sodium chloride weaker than 0·9 per cent may be used when the need for water exceeds that of sodium and it is desired to prescribe only one solution for use throughout the 24 hours. This method has the advantage of steady administration of a particular mixture and avoids the sudden loading of the body with a large quantity of sodium chloride during a brief period followed by a long infusion of glucose solution. So-called 'half normal saline' (0·45 per cent) is prepared by mixing equal volumes of 0·9 per cent saline and 5 per cent glucose solution. 'Fifth normal saline' containing 0·18 per cent sodium chloride is widely used in continuous infusions in paediatric practice. In effect, the same end is achieved by those who employ for routine post-operative infusions in adults the daily ration of 2 litres of 5 per cent glucose solution and 500 ml of 0·9 per cent saline.

HYPERTONIC SALINE. This is of value in water intoxication, or when an excessive volume of water has been administered to a patient with sodium depletion. A 5·85 per cent solution has the advantage that, being a molar solution containing a gram molecular weight of sodium chloride (58·5 g per litre, 994·5 mEq), each millilitre of solution contains almost one milliequivalent of sodium and of chloride and the regulation of the dosage is therefore much easier. It is injected slowly under close supervision, since the too rapid intravenous injection of hypertonic saline causes cardiac arrest.

SODIUM LACTATE. A solution of sodium lactate is used to provide sodium with a disposable anion either when sodium deficiency predominates, or by the addition of sodium lactate to another solution to increase the content of sodium in the resulting mixture. This provision of an excess of sodium, free of anion, is possible because the lactate is metabolised in the liver. Sodium lactate solution alone has a limited field of use to reduce the severity of the hyperpnoea in severe acidosis, for example in severe and advanced infection, but great care must be exercised in its administration. An 'isotonic' solution (one-sixth molar or 1·86 per cent) contains 167 mEq of sodium and lactate per litre.

SODIUM BICARBONATE. As an alternative to sodium lactate a 4·2 per cent solution of sodium bicarbonate may be used. This solution contains 0·5 mEq of bicarbonate per ml.

Potassium

Potassium chloride is used in the treatment of potassium deficiency, due either to vomiting, when it is associated with alkalosis, or to loss of intestinal secretions, when there is usually an accompanying acidosis. An isotonic solution of potassium chloride contains 1·11 per cent potassium chloride (149 mEq potassium per litre), and this is too great a concentration of potassium for safe use. By mixing equal parts of such an isotonic solution of potassium chloride with 5 per cent glucose solution a safe concentration of potassium (74 mEq potassium per litre or 0·55 per cent potassium chloride) is achieved. Alternatively, 20 ml of a 10 per cent solution of potassium chloride are added to 500 ml of a 5 per cent solution of glucose to make a solution of 0·4 per cent potassium chloride (54 mEq potassium per litre). Solutions of potassium chloride are commercially available which contain 10 or 20 mEq potassium, as potassium chloride, in 10 ml of solution. In acute potassium deficiency 2 g of potassium chloride (27 mEq potassium) may be administered by intravenous infusion during a period of 4 hours.

Magnesium

Magnesium chloride or sulphate is usually used for replacement of magnesium and can be added to solutions used for intravenous infusion or may be given by deep intramuscular injection. These salts should be made up in sterile solutions in ampoules which contain 1mEq of magnesium per ml. The usual dose is 0·5 mEq per kg body weight per 24 hours.

Mixed Electrolyte Solutions

The solutions which have been described so far replace only water, one cation and one anion. By combining several salts in appropriate concentrations in a single solution it is possible to replace more accurately the complicated losses of electrolytes which are commonly incurred in clinical practice. A good example of such a combination is the solution introduced by Darrow (1946), the beneficial effects of which in infantile gastroenteritis are described on p. 58.

SALINE LACTATE (Hartmann's solution). In this solution the

excessive quantity of chloride in proportion to sodium in isotonic (0·9 per cent.) saline is reduced by the addition of sodium lactate. It contains in one litre 6·0 g of sodium chloride and 50 ml of molar sodium lactate solution (158 mEq sodium, 102 mEq chloride and 56 mEq lactate per litre). The same solution can be prepared by adding one volume of one-sixth molar sodium lactate solution to 2 volumes of 0·9 per cent saline (Darrow *et al.*, 1949).

RINGER LACTATE. This solution contains potassium chloride and calcium chloride in addition to the sodium chloride and sodium lactate in Hartmann's solution, and is intended for use in patients with acidosis and potassium deficiency. It contains too little potassium and rather more sodium than are desirable for the treatment of potassium deficiency.

DARROW'S SOLUTION (K LACTATE). This solution was originally introduced for the treatment of the losses of gastrointestinal secretions in infantile diarrhoea. When administered by intravenous infusion to babies, Govan and Darrow (1946) recommended that the solution should be diluted with 5 or 10 per cent glucose solution, but in adults this is not necessary. It contains 4·0 g sodium chloride, 2·7 g potassium chloride and 50 ml molar sodium lactate per litre (124 mEq sodium, 36 mEq potassium, 104 mEq chloride and 56 mEq lactate per litre). This solution can be used in the treatment of potassium deficiency provided there is an adequate output of urine. It was designed to correct extracellular fluid depletion (by the administration of water, sodium and chloride) as well as potassium deficiency-and acidosis (by the administration of lactate). The potassium content of Darrow's solution is relatively low and its use is correspondingly safe, but the rate of administration should not exceed 1 litre in 4 or 5 hours. As soon as possible the oral administration of potassium salts should be started.

Solutions containing magnesium and phosphate in addition to sodium and potassium chloride have been devised (Butler *et al.*, 1946; Butler, 1950; Fox *et al.*, 1952), and represent a further advance in the replacement of lost constituents of intracellular fluid.

The balanced electrolyte solution recommended by Fox *et al.* (1952) contains sodium, potassium and chloride and bicarbonate in concentrations similar to those found in normal extracellular fluid. Bicarbonate is present at twice the normal extracellular concentration. Both calcium and magnesium are included to maintain their extracellular concentrations when extracellular volume is being increased and the calcium removes some of the risk associated with the high potassium concentration. Acetate is used in preference to lactate because it is more rapidly converted to bicarbonate, and unlike bicarbonate is easily sterilised by boiling or in the autoclave and yields a neutral pH after administration. The use of citrate in the original prescription to reduce clotting in slow infusions was perhaps the least valuable feature of the mixture. This solution does not result in the elevation of chloride and depression of bicarbonate concentrations in the plasma which follow large infusions of 0·9 per cent saline. In spite of its potassium content this solution has been used safely in patients with impaired renal function. It is probably safer as a replacement solution than Darrow's solution in children and extra supplements of magnesium and potassium salts can be added when deficiencies of these ions exist. This solution is not a substitute for bicarbonate or lactate in the treatment of metabolic acidosis.

There are several similar solutions which contain mixtures of salts suitable for specific types of deficiency. Rather than relying on such preparations some clinicians prefer to try to make up solutions which will replace the measured losses of an individual patient, by adding to a basic solution such as 0·9 per cent saline or 6 per cent glucose solution small quantities of concentrated solutions of sodium bicarbonate or potassium or magnesium chloride.

COCONUT WATER. Coconut water is a sterile pyrogen-free fluid which contains 2·5 to 5·9 g of carbohydrate per 100 ml of fluid mainly as glucose and fructose. The carbohydrate content diminishes as the nuts mature (Eiseman, 1954). It contains also potassium, magnesium, calcium, chloride and phosphate, but little protein.

Rajasuriya and Hamza (1954) have described the use in Ceylon of coconut water derived from the king coconut and the green coconut. After sterilising the exterior of the nut by washing with soap and water the two ends of the nut are cut off and the cut surfaces are washed with Cetavlon and surgical spirit. The nut is then punctured at each end with a sterile trocar and cannula and fluid is withdrawn into a transfusion bottle. The young king coconut holds between 480 and 850 ml of fluid which is opalescent. The young green coconut holds about 600 to 900 ml of fluid. The fluid from both nuts is a good medium for bacterial growth and should be used as soon as possible after extraction. The fluid contains about 12 mEq of calcium per litre,

17 mEq of magnesium, 49 mEq of potassium, 5 mEq of sodium, 66 mEq of chloride, 8 mEq of phosphate and about 1 per cent of protein. Rajasuriya and Hamza administered this fluid by intravenous infusion into 26 patients who were suffering from dehydration due to severe diarrhoea. No ill effects were observed after the infusions apart from a rise in temperature in the first patient treated, possibly because of the poor aseptic precautions observed in the extraction of the fluid from the nut. In spite of repeated infusions there was no evidence of sensitisation and the age of the patients varied from 7 days upwards. The rate of infusion was about 1 pint every 2 or 3 hours in an adult and half this rate in children. The cost of the fluid is much less than that of any sterile commercially prepared intravenous solution but there has not been any subsequent report of the use of this fluid in patients in Ceylon or elsewhere. It is of considerable advantage in the treatment of extracellular fluid depletion due to diarrhoea in the Tropics because of its high potassium content but the low sodium content is a serious disadvantage. It has also been administered by subcutaneous infusion but this causes some local reaction (Pradera, Fernandez and Calderin, 1942).

INTRAVENOUS INFUSIONS

To the patient an intravenous infusion is always a disturbing and often an alarming complication of his primary disease. Before an infusion is started, some explanation of the need and nature of the procedure should be given, and when complications arise, such as leakage or thrombophlebitis, these also should be openly recognised, fully explained and promptly treated. An intravenous infusion should be continued for as short a period as possible. Immobilisation of the patient by the apparatus should be reduced to a minimum, and in this comfort and efficiency are closely linked.

Whenever possible the infusion should be administered through a needle inserted into an accessible superficial vein. Cannulation should rarely be necessary except in severely shocked patients. For the slow infusion of thin fluids, such as electrolyte or glucose solutions, fine needles are adequate, but when there is a possibility that more viscous fluids such as blood or dextran are to be employed, the widest-bore needle or polyethylene tubing that can be inserted into the vein should be used. Doubling the diameter of the needle increases the rate of flow 16 times, whereas quadrupling the head of pressure on the fluid only doubles the rate of flow (Melrose and Shackman 1951). It is also important to reduce the resistance to flow by ensuring that the narrow segments of the delivery set are as few and as short as possible. When polyethylene tubing is used instead of a metal needle, the length of the tubing should not exceed 6 inches unless concentrated solutions are to be injected into the great veins near the heart.

There are several types of combinations of needle and polyethylene tubing by which the polyethylene tubing can be inserted into a peripheral vein and advanced for a suitable distance. At times when a sufficiently large peripheral vein cannot be found or entered it is necessary to cannulate a vein after surgical exposure. The skin over the vein and the fatty tissue round the vein should be infiltrated with local anaesthetic. Through a transverse incision $\frac{3}{4}$ inch in length the vein is then exposed and cleared for half-an-inch and two short lengths of 00 catgut are passed behind the vein, the distal ligature is tied, and one throw of a reef knot is loosely put on the proximal ligature. The vein is then opened between the ligatures by a transverse cut with small straight scissors which must be capable of cutting cleanly at the very tip of the blades. The cannula is then inserted into the vein and fixed by drawing the proximal ligature tight and completing the knot. The catgut ligatures are cut short and the skin incision is closed with fine silk sutures. The use of catgut for tying the vein is more expensive than linen or silk, but allows the vein to reopen after absorption of the catgut. Alternatively the polythene tubing can be pushed through a wide-bore needle which is inserted into the exposed vein and ligatures are not used at all thus reducing the risk of thrombophlebitis since blood continues to flow past the tubing from the periphery.

Because of the persistent disability which may follow superficial thrombophlebitis of the internal saphenous vein, the forearm veins should be used; leg veins should not be used in patients who have abdominal or lower limb injuries, intestinal obstruction, peritonitis or ileus. The most useful vein of all is that which runs obliquely across the forearm from the lower end of the radius towards the middle of the cubital fossa, and it is as constant in position as the internal saphenous vein. When blood volume is low, this vein is not always easy to enter with a needle; it is then better to insert a cannula; this is also the wisest course to adopt in obese patients. The large veins in the cubital fossa can nearly always be entered even with a large needle, but should be used only in emergency and for infusions of short duration; the risk of damage to these veins and of displacement of the needle by movement of the arm is not entirely avoided even by firm splinting, which is uncomfortable. When the cephalic vein in the middle of the forearm is used, the forearm lies comfortably in pronation on the bed on a pillow and little fixation is necessary. The veins on the back of the hand are not suitable for prolonged infusions, and leakage in this situation is particularly uncomfortable, and the bruising which follows leakage of blood after withdrawal of the needle is often very distressing to the patient and the relations.

In severely shocked patients, vasoconstriction markedly slows the rate of flow of fluid in the peripheral veins, and it is often an advantage to insert the needle for transfusion near the trunk. In general, the median cubital vein is the best for this purpose, but the internal saphenous vein at the mid-thigh level may be an even better site. Although it lies largely beneath the deep fascia, its constant position makes the cephalic vein of value when the more commonly used veins have been thrombosed by infusions; the external jugular vein also may be used when others are thrombosed.

For prolonged intravenous feeding, especially with hypertonic solutions of glucose, the superior vena cava has often been recommended. To insert a cannula into the superior vena cava through the subclavian vein the patient should be lying supine, slightly head down with a small sandbag under the upper thoracic spine. The skin over the upper chest, neck and shoulder should be prepared as for an ordinary surgical operation but in addition the fat should be removed from the skin with ether and the skin then painted with a suitable antiseptic such as 0·5 per cent hibitane in spirit, or an iodine solution. After infiltration of the point of skin puncture and the track of the needle with a suitable local analgesic a 14 gauge needle is pushed through the skin at the lower border of the midpoint of the clavicle and advanced towards the back of the suprasternal notch in a horizontal plane. When the subclavian vein is punctured blood flows freely into the attached syringe while the patient holds his breath. The syringe is removed and a 16 gauge radio-opaque catheter, 20 cm in length, is inserted to the full length of the needle. When it enters the vein, blood should flow freely from the cannula, the needle can be withdrawn so that 1 cm of cannula is exposed between the skin and the end of the needle. The intravenous infusion set is attached to the cannula butt and flow is started, the catheter should be fixed to the skin near the puncture with a silk stitch, antibiotic ointment should be applied to the puncture which is then covered with a sterile dressing. The end of the intravenous infusion set should be fixed to the chest. The insertion of the needle and cannula should be carried out in an operating theatre with full aseptic precautions. The region round the puncture and the point of entry of the cannula should be redressed two or three times a week, the area again being cleaned with ether and hibitane and then antibiotic ointment is reapplied and covered with a dressing. Although with these precautions it is possible to use one cannula for 30 days, sometimes much longer peroids can be achieved but the chance of infection increases considerably after the site has been used for 30 days and it is probably better to change to the opposite side once a month. In small babies the catheter should be passed through the internal jugular vein exposed through the middle third of the sternomastoid muscle, the cannula is then led up under the skin of the neck to come out on the scalp, well above the ear and the exit wound should be treated in exactly the same way as for the subclavian cannulation.

The intravenous administration of concentrated (40 or 50 per cent) solutions of glucose into the inferior or superior vena cava is not as free from the risk of infection and thrombophlebitis as some have suggested but does allow of the administration of large quantities of glucose in small volumes of solution. The relative advantage of this has been much reduced by the use of combinations of the safe new fat emulsions with alcohol and fructose. A soft polyethylene tube of suitable length may be inserted under local analgesia through an incision in the median cubital or internal saphenous vein and pushed in until the end of the tube has been advanced far enough into the chosen great vein. The tubing is then tied into the vein with a catgut ligature and should also be firmly fixed to the skin close to the incision, preferably by a silk stitch.

There are three main causes of stoppage of an intravenous infusion:

1. Damage to the vein wall by the sharp end of the needle. This is due to movement of the needle, usually because the needle has been inserted too near to a flexure or has not been properly fixed.

2. Displacement of the needle out of the vein—due to inadequate fixation.

3. Chemical thrombophlebitis—due to the irritation of the superficial veins by the infusion into them of solutions of glucose or fructose. The irritation is due to the low pH of the solution, which is

reduced from about 6·5 to about 5·0 or even less during sterilisation by heat. The incidence of thrombophlebitis is closely related to the duration of the infusion and can be almost completely prevented by stopping the infusion of glucose after 8 hours. The skin overlying an affected vein becomes reddened and the wall of the vein becomes thickened and tender. When the veins of the leg are involved, a good deal of prolonged disability may result. It has been claimed without good evidence that the addition of a small quantity of heparin to the glucose solution prevents thrombosis.

The risk of infection of the wound in a cut-down infusion or even of the puncture when a needle is used is often too lightly accepted. The prevalence of virulent organisms which are resistant to most if not all antibiotics makes the strict observance of meticulous aseptic techniques more necessary than ever before by all who institute intravenous infusions. There is also a lack of care about the way in which other substances are added to commercial preparations for intravenous use. Some antibacterial drugs such as the semisynthetic penicillins are unstable at the pH of 5 per cent dextrose, and so is heparin which also is incompatible with hydrocortisone. There is considerable risk of inaccurate dosage unless great care is exercised in the prescription as well as the administration of drugs by intravenous infusion. Modern disposable intravenous infusion apparatus is expensive but there should be no hesitation about reducing the risks of infection by changing the set sufficiently often, for example after using blood and at least every 24 hours when giving mixtures of amino acids, dextrose and fat emulsion. When superficial veins are used the site of the infusion should be changed before phlebitis occurs, and infusions into the great veins should be avoided as far as possible.

CHAPTER THIRTEEN

Disturbances During Infancy and Childhood

During childhood and especially infancy, disturbances of fluid and electrolyte balance are less common, but usually more critical, than in adult surgical patients. In the newborn period while the causes and the effects of such disturbances resemble those in older children and adults, the structural and functional peculiarities, especially of the premature baby, are so considerable that diagnosis, assessment and treatment must be based on different standards to those used after the first few months of life. The newborn of all species have their own biological limitations and peculiarities and it is not enough simply to regard the newborn baby as 'just a little adult', and to scale down adult treatment quantitatively on a weight basis, without allowing any qualitative differences.

Disturbances of fluid equilibrium are relatively easier to produce in infants and may cause severe functional disturbances. The requirements for growth, a high metabolic rate and interference with the intake of food, combined with differences in the internal environment and in the functions of the kidneys, make the physiological background to losses by vomiting and diarrhoea different to that found in adults and older children. It is unfortunate that some paediatricians still base their recommendations for the treatment of surgical patients on the same principles which they use for the treatment of the effects of diarrhoea and vomiting in gastroenteritis, and ignore the differences in the underlying disturbances in babies after major surgical operations.

BODY COMPOSITION

The successful surgical treatment of premature babies weighing as little as 1·5 kg (3·3 lb) has shown that such infants can adjust successfully to an independent extrauterine existence more than two months before the normal time in spite of the great differences in composition and functional development of their bodies compared with those of full term babies.

Fat Content

By the analysis of whole bodies Widdowson and Spray (1951) showed that the water content of the fat-free tissue of the foetus fell from over 90 per cent at a weight of 200 g to 81 to 84 per cent at more than 3 kg. The fat content at birth weights of more than 3 kg was from 12 to 16 per cent of body weight, about the same as that of protein. It is remarkable that the human infant contains so much fat at birth since most newborn mammals contain only 1 to 2 per cent; the high content in the human baby enables it to maintain a more stable body temperature and to have greater individual independence, both of advantage in single births. The premature baby weighing only 1·5 kg (3·3 lb) contains only one-eighth the quantity of fat it would have at full term, and being less well insulated is more vulnerable to cold.

Hatai (1902) first drew attention to the similarity between the interscapular gland of hibernating animals and the brown fat of the cervical and dorsal fat masses of the human foetus. It has now been shown that these masses are the site of heat production when newly born mammals are exposed to cold (Dawkins and Hull, 1963; Smalley and Dryer, 1963). This response enables the animal or the human neonate to maintain body temperature without shivering.

Water Content

The increasing fat content during the last half or third of pregnancy is related to the reduction in water content from 82·5 per cent of body weight at 1·5 kg, to 77 per cent at 2·5 kg, and 68·8 per cent at 3·5 kg (7 lb). The most accurate method of measuring the water content of babies is by the dilution method using heavy water and the infrared absorptiometer. Tsingoglou *et al.* (1972) used this method in 55 neonates who had been admitted for the treatment of various congenital anomalies. The mean weight of the group was 2·588 kg (range 1·160 to 3.851 kg) and the mean total water content was 77·03 per cent of body weight (range 67·4 to 88·6). Total body water expressed as a percentage of weight decreased by 5·2 per cent per kg over the range of 1·160 to 3·851 kg. Edelmann *et al.* (1952) also found similar high values in the first month of life, ranging from 71·6 to 83 per cent (mean 76·7 per cent). During the first six months after birth the body water content falls to about 60 per cent of body weight, at which it remains regardless of sex until puberty.

It must be recognised that there are wide variations in body composition between individual newborn infants, due for example to differences in the size of the skeleton and thus in the proportions of bone and soft tissue as well as in fat content, and that infants with the same body weight do not have identical daily requirements for calories, water or minerals, or present exactly the same therapeutic problems. The use of so-called standard values for the calculation of the total body contents of sodium, potassium or water from the weight is also liable to be misleading, although it is the only way in which most clinicians can obtain any idea of the normal range of composition of their patients. The good correlation between total body water and body weight suggests that there is not much disturbance in total water content in neonates with anomalies of the alimentary tract. Widdowson (1960) calculated that the starving neonate loses water and solids in about the same proportions as those in which they are present at birth in both premature and term babies.

Distribution of Water

The distribution as well as the total quantity of water in the body undergoes a series of changes with increasing age. Maclaurin (1966) observed an increase in the extracellular fluid volume during the first three days after birth, largely due to the transfer of water from the cells. Fellers *et al.* (1949) found that the extracellular fluid volume decreased rapidly during the first weeks of life and again at adolescence. At birth weights of 2 to 5 kg the extracellular fluid was equal to just over 40 per cent of the body weight and fell to 32 to 35 per cent at body weights from 5 to 20 kg and to 23 to 27 per cent in adults. Thus in the newborn the extracellular fluid volume is in proportion nearly 80 per cent larger than in an adult, and this is of course associated with a smaller proportion of cellular material in the infant than in the older child or adult. The intracellular fluid amounts to only about 30 per cent of body weight in the newborn, compared with over 40 per cent in adults, and the total solids of the newborn equal about 20 per cent of body weight instead of 30 per cent in the adult. These variations are associated with differences in sodium and potassium content; at birth per kilogram body weight the sodium content of the body is 50 per cent higher and the potassium content is 20 per cent lower than in adults (Table XXVI).

TABLE XXVI

	3·5 *kg Neonate*				70 *kg Adult*			
	Total	*ECF*	*ICF*	*Bone*	*Total*	*ECF*	*ICF*	*Bone*
Sodium (mEq)	240	215	17·4	7·6	3900	1720	340	1840
Potassium (mEq)	156	7·0	128	21	3400	60	3340	—
Magnesium (mEq)	63	2·6	27·6	33	2000	20	1980	1000
Water (% body wt)	77	43·9	33·1	—	60	17	43	—
litres	2·7	1·54	1·16	—	42	12	30	—

Table to show the distribution of sodium, potassium, magnesium and water in a 3·5 kg neonate and a 70 kg adult based on calculation from standard values, assumed or measured, for total body water, sodium, potassium and magnesium contents. Non-exchangeable sodium has been assumed to be 25 per cent of total sodium and 55 per cent of bone sodium.

WATER BALANCE

A large loss of weight, amounting to 10 per cent or more of birth weight, is a constant feature of the first few days of life. In full-term infants this loss of weight is related to the duration of the restriction of water intake and can be reduced by starting the water intake soon after birth. Premature infants may lose 20 per cent or more of their birth weight without apparent harm and lose more water, sodium and potassium in larger daily volumes of urine for longer than do full-term babies.

Insensible Water Loss

When a 3·5 kg (7 lb) baby loses 10 per cent (350 g) of its birth weight in 3 or 4 days, only 20 to 30 per cent (70 to 105 ml) of this loss can usually be accounted for by the quantity of urine which is passed during this time. Some of the remainder is due to the consumption of tissue to provide for the continuing energy requirements of the body, but the bulk of the lost weight is caused by the insensible loss of water in the expired air and through the skin. While the rate of insensible water loss may be influenced by the temperature and humidity of the environment, there is reason to believe that, as in adults, the insensible water loss (p. 18) is responsible for the dissipation of about 25 per cent of the total heat production of the body (Levine and Marples, 1930). At an *energy consumption* of 60 calories per kilogram per 24 hours (Butler and Talbot, 1944) an infant weighing 3·5 kg would metabolise 210 calories per 24 hours and this would impose on it an insensible water loss of 90 g per 24 hours, a figure which conforms well with the results of clinical observations. McCance *et al.* (1954) found that the average extra-renal water loss of 10 babies was 1·15 g per kg per hour, or about 96 g per 24 hours, but Benedict and Root (1926) estimated the hourly loss might be as high as 1·3 g per kg, or 109 g per 24 hours for a 3·5 kg child.

Zweymüller (1970) found that the insensible water loss of the newborn baby under basal conditions was 390 to 460 mg per kg per hour, or 32·6 to 38·6 g per 24 hours for a 3·5 kg baby, was increased by crying and other activity and was less in those who slept much of the time than in those who were more awake. Such a low rate of loss of water during the first 24 hours of life is related to the low oxygen consumption at that time and to the basal conditions under which the measurements were made. Hill (1965) showed that in a neutral thermal environment oxygen consumption rose gradually from just under 7 ml per minute per kg body weight 30 hours after birth to just over 7 ml at the age of 7 to 10 days. In a 3·5 kg baby this is equivalent to an oxygen consumption of about 35 litres per 24 hours, or an energy expenditure of 170 calories per 24 hours. This is less than 75 per cent of the estimate of 210 calories of Benedict and Talbot (1915) and is perhaps another illustration of the way in which a neutral thermal environment reduces energy expenditure and oxygen requirements.

The direct measurement of oxygen consumption is difficult; it is much easier to collect the whole output of urine, faeces and any other losses from the body and to weigh the child accurately, and thus to arrive at a reasonable estimate of insensible water loss plus the weight of tissue consumed for the provision of energy.

TEMPERATURE REGULATION

To a varying extent the newborn baby is at the mercy of its environment and cannot complain as older children and adults do when conditions are unfavourable. Those skilled in the care of babies know the signs of restlessness and undue activity which indicate that the baby is being subjected to an uncomfortable environment, and it needs little skill or experience to recognise the sublime peace and obvious well being of the baby who is in the ideal and favourable environment.

The young of some species, such as mice and rats, are poikilothermic and as they cool their oxygen consumption and heat production fall. They have no inherent capacity to maintain body temperature and must huddle together or against the body of their mother if they are not to lose heat so rapidly that they will cool too much and die. Puppies and kittens also have little control over their body temperature at birth, but newborn pigs are homeothermic in the sense that cooling stimulates their metabolism so long as they are fed. The newborn baby is also homeothermic to a limited degree but the capacity to respond to cooling is limited; its greater size also gives it an advantage over many small mammals, since the surface area of bodies of similar shape varies inversely with their size. Only about 25 per cent of the total loss of heat from the surface of the human body is due to the insensible loss of water, the remainder being by conduction, convection and radiation, but the surface loss of both water and heat depends to a large degree on the environmental conditions and clothing. Day (1943) showed that in the premature infant heat production increased when the environmental temperature fell but that heat loss was mainly due to radiation. It has been suggested that premature infants cool more quickly than full-term babies because they have a smaller fat content and therefore are less well insulated from their environment. It seems likely that because of their smaller lean tissue mass and larger extracellular fluid volume they are incapable of maintaining as high an energy output per kg body weight as full-term babies.

The high specific heat and poor thermal conductivity of water confer remarkable physical advantages on the multicellular organism, more than 60 per cent of which is composed of water. But these advantages are not quite enough to insulate the warm-blooded organism from its more variable environment. In addition to a layer of fat of which the thickness depends on many factors and the heat-insulating capacity has been widely accepted, the skin forms the ultimate boundary layer and physical defence. Heat loss through the skin can be increased or reduced by changes in the quantity of blood circulating in the potentially vast cutaneous capillary network.

The skin of the newborn is capable of great change in colour and temperature, but control of the calibre of the capillaries and of the rate and total volume of blood flow appears to be poor.

These are not the only factors concerned. The *surface area* of the newborn infant is 15 per cent of that of an average adult (70 kg), but its weight is only 5 per cent of the adult's, so that the infant has three times as much surface area per kilogram as an adult. Benedict and Talbot (1915) found an average heat production of 1·75 calories per kg per hour during the first day of life, which is nearly 60 per cent more than the adult rate of 1 calorie per kg per hour but only 85 per cent of the rate of 2 calories per kilogram per hour between the ages of one and three years. The period of greatest metabolic activity is from six months to two years at body weights of about 11 to 33 lb (5 to 15 kg) (Holliday and Segar, 1957). When heat production is expressed against surface area, the larger surfaces of smaller bodies change the picture. Benedict and Talbot (1915) showed that in the first week of life heat production was 25·5 calories per square metre of body surface per hour, at two years of age Levine and Marples (1930) found it was 50 calories per square metre per hour compared with the adult rate of 35 to 40 calories per square metre per hour (Dubois, 1936). That is to say the infant's heat production per unit area is half that of a two-year-old child and 60 per cent that of an adult.

It is usually assumed that there is a close relationship between surface area, metabolic rate and basal daily water requirements. As Oliver *et al.* (1958) pointed out, the 37 formulas for the calculation of surface area are based on only a few direct measurements of surface area in children. It is just in those children for whose management the information is most important that the errors are largest and direct evidence most lacking. When Boyd (1935) plotted all the recorded measurements of surface area against the surface area of the same subjects calculated from the equations of DuBois and DuBois (1916), she found a standard deviation of 7·5 per cent at weights above 3 kg, 10 per cent when infants of less than 3 kg, were included and 18·6 per cent for infants weighing less than 3 kg. Benedict and Talbot (1921) showed that when the heat production of children is referred to surface area there is a progressive increase in heat production up to about 1150 calories per square metre for bodies with a surface area of 0·5 to 0·6 square metres, a gradual decrease to about 1000 calories per square metre in those with surface areas of 1 square metre, and a further reduction in larger bodies towards the revised estimate of Rubner (1931) of about 615 calories per square metre.

Costeff (1966) has derived a formula for the calculation of surface area from weight

$$\text{surface area} = \left(\frac{4W+7}{W+90}\right)$$

which is as accurate as the DuBois formula but less so than that of Boyd (1935). It is good enough for those who wish to use surface area for the calculation of dosage of drugs and fluids.

There is a need, however, for much more information about the behaviour of the neonate, and especially of the premature child. Ylppo (1919) showed that the survival rate of premature babies could be increased by reducing their heat loss during the first five days of life. It is interesting that when Silverman and Blanc (1957) increased the relative humidity of the environment from 30 to 60 per cent to 80 to 90 per cent at a temperature of 84° F (28·9° C) more of their premature neonates, whose body temperature was higher at the higher humidity, survived.

The main effect of a high environmental humidity is presumably to reduce the heat loss from the body by diminishing the gradient for insensible water loss, although it has been speculated that respiration also is made easier. There is a theoretical limit to the degree to which environmental humidity can be raised without causing hyperpyrexia, and it may be fortunate that it is seldom possible to achieve 100 per cent relative humidity in incubators in clinical use. An atmosphere of low relative humidity is most commonly encountered during winter in continental countries with extreme ranges of temperature, but in a temperate island climate such as that of Great Britain it is rather uncommon.

Even in conditions which are comfortable for the adult, the neonate, because of small size and poor heat insulation, is at a considerable disadvantage. When attempts are made to maintain a neutral thermal environment in an incubator it is essential to watch the deep body temperature of the baby very closely, especially for very small babies, since overheating may be as harmful as cooling them.

A newborn baby can maintain its body temperature when the difference between rectal and environmental temperatures does not exceed 2 to 3° C. When the difference is greater extra heat must be generated and this is associated with a rise in oxygen consumption. Hill and Rahimtulla (1965) and Scopes (1966) have shown that when the environmental temperature of a naked premature infant falls 2°C an increase of 25 per cent in heat production and oxygen consumption may be necessary to prevent a fall in body temperature. The rate of radiant heat loss can be reduced by clothing the infant, but this prevents close observation of the whole baby which is necessary in many ill neonates, or by having a double-walled hood on the incubator; the latter is most easily achieved by inserting a thin perspex baffle inside the perspex hood. In a neutral thermal environment air flow, relative humidity and the temperature of the air and the skin of the baby are so combined that the core temperature is within the range of 36·5° to 37·5° C yet the heat production indicated by oxygen consumption is minimal. The range of neutral temperature is higher in infants (32° to 34° C at 50 per cent humidity: Bruck, 1961; Oliver and Karlberg, 1963) than in adults (26° to 31° C).

When treating neonates it is very important to ensure that the air temperature inside the incubator is within the neutral range in which heat loss is at a minimum, and therefore there is no need to increase heat production above the basal level in order to maintain a deep body temperature of 37° C. The lower margin of the neutral thermal zone is called the critical temperature and below this heat production of the baby must be increased to maintain body temperature. When the air temperature in the incubator approaches or is above 37° C heat loss must be raised by increased evaporation of water through the expired air and by sweating, and the neonate has a limited capacity to do either. The neutral range of temperature varies with the size of the baby. If the thermometer is mounted too close to the wall of the incubator canopy the temperature it records may not accurately indicate the average temperature inside the incubator.

Extensive heat loss by unnecessary exposure of the baby to cold air must be avoided, especially when the baby is small. This is most likely to occur when the lid or ports of the incubator are opened for something to be done to the baby, during transfer of the baby from the incubator to the operating table if the baby is not first wrapped in a warm towel or cotton-wool, and during thoracotomy or laparotomy, especially when the intestines are exposed to the air. During operation the baby should also lie on an electrically heated mattress and the limbs should be wrapped in cotton wool or aluminium cooking foil; this avoids the need to heat the theatre air to 85° F (29·4° C) which is uncomfortable for those working in it. The core temperature of the baby should be measured during operation with a thermal electrode placed either in the rectum or the oesophagus, or more conveniently and safely with one placed in the axilla with the arm strapped to the trunk. The temperature in the axilla measured in this way is only 0·2° C lower than that in the rectum or the oesophagus (Tsingoglu and Wilkinson, 1971).

Hey and Mount (1967) have recommended that babies should be covered even when nursed in an incubator and believe that by doing this oxygen consumption and energy requirements can be reduced by 25 per cent. Hey and O'Connell (1970) found that the critical temperature is lower for clothed than for naked babies and that in the first month of life a draught-free temperature of 24° C (75° F) will provide a neutral thermal environment for a clothed baby in a cot. It is obvious that a clothed baby in a cot is much safer than a naked baby in an incubator for which the standard of supervision must be much closer and more accurate.

WATER REQUIREMENTS

The recommended theoretical water requirements for infants vary even more widely than do those for adults and it is particularly unfortunate that so little attention or recognition has so far been given to the effects of climate on the real daily requirements for water. These arbitrary estimates of water requirements have usually been based on calculated surface area or on body weight. The possible error in calculating surface area has already been mentioned (p. 270) and compares very unfavourably with the error in weighing a baby, provided a few elementary precautions are observed. Each time the child should be weighed in the same type of clothing or covering before being fed. An error of one ounce in 10 lb amounts to only 0·6 per cent. The range of recommended daily intake is commonly too wide. Oliver *et al.* (1958) suggested an allowance of 60$\pm$ 15 ml per lb body weight per day; for a 10 lb (4·54 kg) baby this amounts to a variation of 300 ml over a range of 450 to 750 ml. They suggested that this allowance be applied to babies weighing from 5 to 22 lb (2 to 10 kg), but a variation of 150 ml over the range of 225 to 375 ml at a weight of 5 lb (2 kg) seems too large.

RENAL FUNCTION

In spite of much individual variation during the first week after birth the volume and osmolality of the urine follow a fairly consistent pattern. Urine present in the bladder at the time of birth which has been produced before birth is invariably dilute; the urine passed during the first day of life usually includes a large proportion of this antenatal urine, and is usually of larger volume and more dilute than urine produced during the next two days. The volume of urine is only about 20 to 30 ml per day on the second and third days of life, but then as the consumption of milk and water rises so does the urine volume which may reach 120 to 150 ml by the seventh day. Even when breast milk is fed from the first day, Thompson (1944) found that only small quantities of urine were passed on the second and third days. Before birth urine osmolality is about 50 mosmol per litre and rises to 400 to 500 mosmol per litre during the first three days after birth and falls again to about 100 mosmol as the water intake rises at the end of the first week (McCance, 1950). Human breast milk imposes a much smaller osmotic load (about 12 mosmol per 100 calories) on the kidneys than does cow's milk (about 30 mosmol per 100 calories).

Hansen and Smith (1952, 1953) compared the effects of giving and withholding water during the first three days after birth. They found that when water was withheld the weight loss was greater and urinary volume was smaller; the total losses of sodium and chloride in the urine did not vary although those of potassium and nitrogen did, and the serum concentrations of sodium and chloride and the haematocrit rose. They compared these changes with those in adults treated in a similar way, and showed that the losses of weight were similar whether water was given or withheld. With an ample water supply, the losses of sodium, potassium and other ions were less in full-term or slightly premature infants than in adults; the newborn infants losing only a quarter as much sodium and potassium expressed per litre of body water as an adult or a baby more than a month old. One of the most remarkable features of renal function during the first week of life is the remarkable capacity of the kidneys of the newborn to restrict the excretion of sodium and potassium in the urine to concentrations of less than 20 mEq per litre of urine within 48 to 72 hours of birth.

Although the kidneys in the newborn cannot concentrate urine to the degree which is achieved later in life, and this seems to impose a larger loss of water in the urine than is necessary in older subjects, renal conservation of sodium and potassium is usually very efficient even during the first week after birth. This adds to the interest and significance of the effects observed when the newborn premature or full-term infant is loaded with water or saline. Lasch (1923) showed that during the first month of life infants could excrete only 55 per cent of a water load; the remainder was only partly accounted for by extrarenal losses and in spite of the retention of water the rate of urine formation fell. McCance *et al.* (1954) gave infants 6 to 18 days old a dose of water equal to 6 per cent of their body weight and found that at first urinary volume rapidly increased to a degree comparable to that in adults, provided the volumes were compared on the basis of 42 litres of body water. At the peak of the diuresis glomerular filtration rate and tubular reabsorption were very similar per unit of body water and the urine was as dilute in infants as in adults loaded to a comparable degree. The infants, however, could not excrete within four hours as the adults did, a volume of urine equal to the dose of water.

The capacity to produce a diuresis increases with age. Ames (1953) found that regardless of whether the water was given orally or by intravenous infusion in the first three days of life there was no diuresis. From 2 weeks in some and 4 weeks in all babies the equivalent of the whole of a water load of 3 to 5 per cent of body weight was excreted within 3 hours in both premature and term infants.

The urine of infants is hypotonic compared with that of older children and their renal clearances of urea, sodium, potassium and chloride are always low even when plasma concentrations are raised. Glomerular filtration rate and renal clearances rise during the first year to reach adult levels after 12 to 18 months, but vary widely between individuals and with hydration (McCance and Young, 1941). In spite of such obvious limitations during experiments under abnormal conditions, the range of function of the infantile kidneys is undoubtedly adequate for the peculiar circumstances of normal neonatal life. When, however, large quantities of glucose solution or saline are administered, especially by intravenous infusion, the limited capacity to excrete a water load and the low renal clearances of sodium and chloride may lead to the retention of undersirably large quantities of such fluids (Fig. 12). It is always difficult to decide exactly how much water, minerals and calories should be given to each child, especially during the neonatal period when the margin between enough and too much is so small.

THE METABOLIC EFFECTS OF INJURY

After the first year of life the metabolic disturbance which

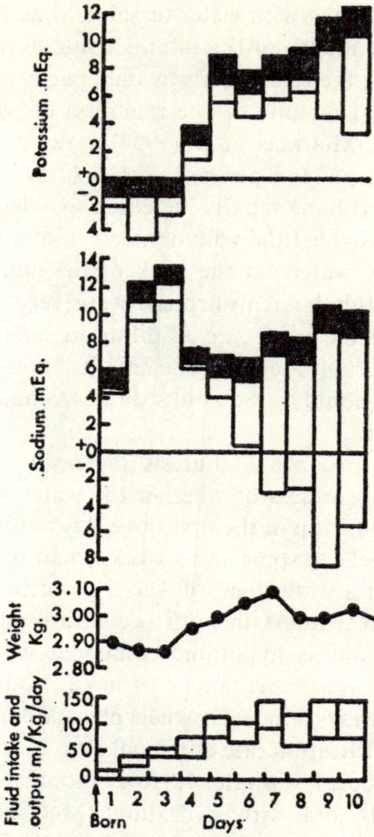

FIGURE 12. Sodium and potassium balances in newly born baby who weighed 2·9 kg and was admitted because of bilateral complete cleft palate and lip with small lower jaw and was given dilute glucose saline for 4 days and milk from the fourth day. The large positive balance of sodium which accumulated during the first 4 days was excreted from the sixth day onwards and this led to a negative sodium balance and loss of weight. This is an example of the slow excretion of sodium by the neonate even when the sodium is administered by mouth (Wilkinson, 1966).

(Reproduced by kind permission of the Editor of the *Annals of the Royal College of Surgeons of England.*)

characteristically follows injury resembles exactly that invariably exhibited by well-nourished adults. The capacity to produce this adult pattern of response is acquired early during the first year of life, and often within two or three months of birth, although what is regarded as full maturity of renal function, the attainment of the adult range of clearance and concentrating capacity, is not reached until the age of a year or eighteen months. During the birth of a baby a varying amount of injury is inflicted, and this probably has some effect on renal function. It is still difficult to describe in detail a normal range of urinary composition for the newborn child with the modifications imposed by different degrees of prematurity or postmaturity, and when the exact length of gestation is often in doubt. Until a reliable means of dating every pregnancy is obtained, some doubt about the exact age of the child at birth must remain and it will be necessary to allow for a wider range of normal than is really desirable.

Even normal babies may starve for up to four days after birth and it used to be thought that this was due to a delay in the establishment of lactation. It has been shown, however, that even when a liberal supply of expressed human milk is provided for newly born babies they do not all start to feed at the same time, and that this variable delay is due to some factor in the baby which determines whether the baby takes milk or not (Wilkinson *et al.*, 1962). When allowance is made for this delay in starting to feed there is a remarkable resemblance in metabolic behaviour between individual babies. A week after birth a normal neonate may be taking as expressed breast milk about 7 g of protein (1100 mg nitrogen), 5 to 6 mEq sodium and 7 to 8 mEq potassium, and will absorb from the

TABLE XXVII

Comparison of the intakes (total and per kg body weight), urinary output and daily balance in an adult weighing 70 kg and a baby weighing 3·5 kg

	70 kg Adult			*3·5 kg Baby*			
	Intake		*Output*	*Intake*		*Output*	*Balance*
	Total	*Per kg*		*Total*	*Per kg*		
Protein (g)	70	1	—	7	2	—	—
Nitrogen (g)	11	0·157	11	1·1	0·31	0·4	+0·7
Potassium (mEq)	80	1·14	80	8	2·28	2·8	+5·2
Sodium (mEq)	120	1·7	120	5	1·43	1·75	+3·25
	Equilibrium			Growth			

bowel 85 per cent of this intake and retain 65 per cent of it in the body, where it will be incorporated in new tissue. Thus a week after birth the normal neonate consumes per kg body weight twice as much protein and potassium and three-quarters as much sodium a the adult, and retains 60 per cent of these intakes, equivalent on a weight basis to the whole adult intake of potassium and nitrogen (Table XXVII). Of this large intake only about 20 per cent has to be excreted in the urine, just over 1 mEq potassium, less than 1 mEq of sodium and about half a gram of nitrogen per day, and so the neonate needs only 10 per cent of the adult renal capacity. In normal circumstances in the early weeks after birth, on a diet of breast milk, the renal functional capacity of the human child is amply fitted for the normal functions it has to perform. When these very small normal excretory requirements are remembered it is hardly surprising that the capacity to excrete large loads of water and mineral salts is limited, and that great care should be taken to ensure that when fluid is administered to a neonate it should resemble as closely as possible, both qualitatively and quantitatively, the losses which have been sustained.

In the past the comparatively poor concentrating capacity of the neonate's kidneys has been misinterpreted. It has been suggested that since to excrete a given solute load the infant needs more water than an older child or adult, the neonate will be dehydrated more quickly by excreting a solute load if enough water is not also provided (Calcagno *et al.*, 1955; Colle and Paulsen, 1959). In fact, the naturally poor concentrating capacity is related to the small osmotic excretory requirements on a diet of human milk, and inadequate excretory capacity arises mainly when the body is unwisely loaded with mineral salts, in attempted replacement of real or imaginary losses of body constituents. Retention of materials may also result from water lack when renal function is normal, and is not simply due to the functional limitations of the neonatal kidneys.

The normal neonatal metabolic pattern as shown by dietary intake and faecal and urinary losses is shown in Figure 13 (*a*). There are very small urinary losses of sodium, potassium and nitrogen during the first week. As soon as the intake of milk is sufficiently high, positive balance is achieved.

Some of the typical features of urinary composition and renal function are shown in Figure 13 (*b*). There is a characteristic sharp reduction in the concentrations of sodium and potassium as soon as the milk intake rises enough. As in adults this conservation of sodium is partly dependent on the provision of sufficient calories in the form of carbohydrate. The urinary concentrations of sodium and potassium subsequently remain low for more than a week and then gradually rise as the milk intake rises. The urinary nitrogen concentration falls more slowly than that of either potassium or sodium. The osmolality of the neonate's urine is low by adult standards, even on the first day, but thereafter falls progressively, usually to less than 100 mosmol per litre. Although the fractions of the total osmolar activity in the urine which are accounted for by the nitrogen, sodium and potassium resemble those found in an adult (Fig. 6) the total osmolality is many times higher in adult urine, both in starvation and after injury, and rises rather than falls during the first week.

When four groups, each of five neonates, were studied by metabolic balance the only statistically significant difference between those who were normal and those who suffered from foetal distress or duodenal or oesophageal atresia was that there was a high retention of sodium by babies with foetal distress. Foetal distress seems to be a more severe and more lasting disturbance to the neonate than a laparotomy or a thoracotomy (Wilkinson, 1966). Between the groups there was a closer resemblance of the retentions of nitrogen and potassium than of sodium. It must be remembered that in the neonate milk feeds are usually started 24 hours after operation and metabolic balances rapidly become positive, perhaps to such a marked degree that the catabolic aspect of metabolism is obscured.

When the effects of an operative injury are added within two or three days of birth, the decline in urinary sodium and potassium concentrations may be delayed for a day or two but very low concentrations may persist for several days longer than in the normal; the urine volume also may be low for more than the usual three or four days. The kidneys of a newborn child can reduce the concentration of sodium from around 140 mEq per litre in glomerular filtrate to less than 10 mEq per litre in the urine as passed from the fourth to the seventh to tenth days after birth. These kidneys excrete little potassium until some time after the intake of milk is started, but whenever an excessive potassium load is added to the body, are capable of responding by excreting potassium at a concentration of up to 50 to 60 mEq per litre.

When quantities of sodium chloride are administered by continuous intravenous infusion, in large excess of the requirements of the body, the outputs of water and sodium in the urine increase in spite of the retention of some of the administered sodium in the body (Colle and Paulsen, 1959). In the artificial circumstances

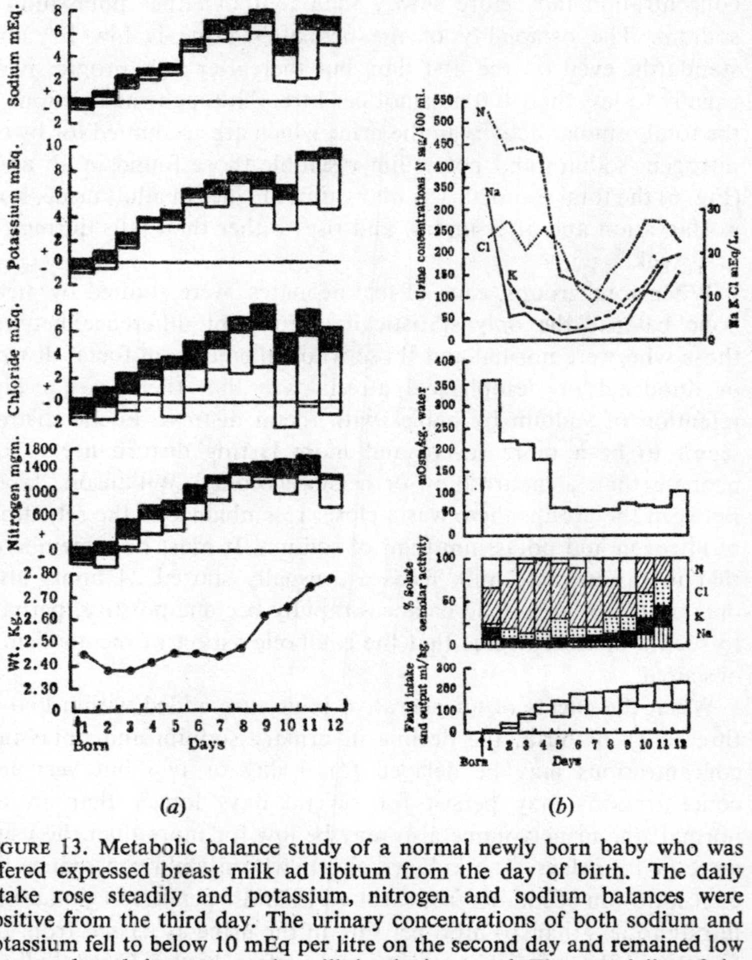

(a) (b)

FIGURE 13. Metabolic balance study of a normal newly born baby who was offered expressed breast milk ad libitum from the day of birth. The daily intake rose steadily and potassium, nitrogen and sodium balances were positive from the third day. The urinary concentrations of both sodium and potassium fell to below 10 mEq per litre on the second day and remained low for a week and then rose as the milk intake increased. The osmolality of the urine which was mainly due to urea fell from 350 mosmol per litre to less than 100 mosmol on the fifth day when there was a large increase in urine volume (Wilkinson, 1966).

(Reproduced by kind permission of the Editor of the *Annals of the Royal College of Surgeons of England.*)

of water and sodium loading by the intravenous infusion of saline, the infant kidneys lack some of the specific capacities of older kidneys. Soon after birth the baby is incapable of responding to a sudden water load by a rapid and complete diuresis and when loading is continued for several days by intravenous infusion, sodium conservation may be impaired by the continued passsge of larger volumes of urine than would be the case if only sufficient glucose solution to satisfy the theoretical insensible water loss and urinary output of the baby were infused. The newborn tolerates well the restriction of water intake, and excretes very little sodium or potassium for some days after the first day of independent life. The object of postoperative treatment should be to establish oral feeding as soon as possible and to avoid the use of intravenous infusions. Nevertheless, when acute losses of water and sodium occur, the surgeon should be ready to employ the rapid infusion of an adequate volume of 0·9 per cent saline or some other more suitable fluid without hesitation. Some babies who have not been fed are unable to clear infused glucose from the blood stream at a normal rate (Elphick and Wilkinson, 1965). The prolonged intravenous administration of glucose to such babies would cause severe hyperglycaemia.

There is little place for the slow continuous intravenous infusion of hypotonic saline and glucose solution which is too often used simply because of a desire to maintain a needle in a vein and some kind of fluid intake. Those who have the care of neonates should be capable of inserting a needle or a cannula into a peripheral vein whenever this is needed and should not have to inflict the risk of a continuous infusion on their patients.

An infant weighing 3·5 kg (7 lb) with an insensible water loss of 90 ml and a urinary output between 30 and 100 ml per 24 hours is losing 120 to 190 ml water per day. The common belief that babies need 2½ oz water per lb body weight per day (165 ml per kg) does not apply to the newborn; on this scale the 3·5 kg infant would receive 500 ml per day. Gross (1953) wisely recommended that the total intake of fluid in a premature baby should not exceed 30 ml per lb per day (66 ml per kg). If this fluid is to be injected subcutaneously or intravenously it should be given in two or three parts at intervals of 12 or 8 hours.

The use of 5 per cent glucose solution and of a mixture of 4·3 per cent glucose and 0·18 per cent sodium chloride has been commended because the glucose provides calories; 200 ml of 5 per cent glucose solution will provide only 10 g of glucose (40 calories), which cannot do more than take the edge off the effects of starvation, spare a little protein and help to make the oxidation of fat more complete. The newborn baby weighing 3·5 kg (7 lb) contains about 128 mEq of potassium in its 1·15 litres of intracellular fluid and about 190 mEq of sodium in 1·4 litres of extracellular fluid. There are 153 mEq each of sodium and chloride in one litre of isotonic (0·9 per cent) saline and 31 mEq of each in a litre of 0·18 per cent ('one-fifth normal') saline. Although it may seem that a solution containing only 0·18 per cent sodium chloride confers an admirable degree of safety when used for infants, the dangers in administering the accompanying large volume of water have already been emphasised. Even in 200 ml of 0·18 per cent saline there are 6 mEq of sodium which is far more than the starving neonate will lose in the urine in a day. The differences in volume, concentration and detailed composition between the fluid lost from the body and hypotonic saline, which the adult may tolerate without much harm during arbitrary therapeutic replacement according to formulas, are too often more than the infant can survive.

It has been shown (Hughes *et al.*, 1964; Wilkinson, 1966) that when sodium chloride solution is administered even by mouth in excess of the real needs of the body it will ultimately be excreted (Fig. 12). Although the administration of large volumes of saline may greatly improve the clinical appearance of the baby by improving the consistence of the skin and subcutaneous tissues and by filling up the hollow sockets of the eyes it may not have any effect on the output of urine.

EFFECTS OF LOSS OF BODY FLUIDS

In children as in adults loss of gastrointestinal secretions is the commonest and most important cause of disturbance of body fluid equilibrium. During infancy accidental injury is a rare cause, and gastroenteritis is only rarely a complication of surgical treatment. The loss may be due to vomiting of gastric secretions in pyloric stenosis, of mixed gastric and intestinal secretions in intestinal obstruction due to atresia or stenosis of the intestine or to volvulus or incarceration of the small intestine in a hernia, or as a result of the accumulation of intestinal secretions in the dilated bowel above an intestinal atresia or in ileus due to peritonitis or operation. The most important components of the lost fluid are sodium and water. The concentration of sodium in the vomited or aspirated fluid varies from 100 to 140 mEq per litre, depending on the amount of water which has been drunk and the origin of the secretions. The fluid thus resembles extracellular fluid in its sodium content, and if sufficient is lost the volume of extracellular fluid, and therefore also of the plasma, falls enough to cause an evident acute circulatory disturbance. Because the normal intake of water and milk and other foodstuffs also is hindered, the patient cannot replace the substances lost by vomiting. In the newborn child starvation is usually tolerated well for up to a week provided blood volume is maintained, if necessary by transfusion during or after operation, and sufficient water and sodium are supplied by infusion to prevent any severe reduction of extracellular fluid volume. When interference with the normal intake of food persists for more than a week it is necessary to provide calories as fat and carbohydrate and some form of protein, either as a hydrolysate or a solution of synthetic amino acids, as well as sufficient water, sodium and potassium salts and vitamins.

Clinical Features

As in adults an accurate history is of primary importance and particular attention should be paid to details of the type and quantity of fluid which has been lost, as well as to the other features of the illness. At first the child frets and is wakeful, thirsty and has a dry tongue and red lips, but the eyes and fontanelle are not sunken and skin turgor is not much altered. As the loss of fluid continues, the child becomes obviously ill, pale, restless and anxious, the eyes and fontanelle are sunken, the lips are pale and may be bluish and the hands and feet are cold and blue although the rectal temperature may be raised. Blood pressure is usually maintained until a late stage even when the pulse rate is raised, but this circulatory compensation may be disturbed by sudden changes in position and unskilful handling of the baby. When water depletion predominates, thirst is intense, the lips and tongue are cracked and dry and only a small amount of urine is produced.

Until a baby is dead there is always hope, and even when the child is mute, ashen grey with dull eyes deeply sunken in their sockets, and pulseless with cold, greyish blue hands and feet, a determined attempt should immediately be made at resuscitation; the astonishing response such an apparently moribund infant will make to the rapid intravenous administration of a suitable fluid is too often not appreciated or given an opportunity.

It is no easier to measure changes in cellular composition or in extracellular fluid volume in ill babies than it is in adults, and chemical analysis of the blood provides information only of the concentrations of the constituents. In babies it is necessary to use micro or ultra-micro methods of analysis, especially for repeated determinations, since the amount of blood which can be withdrawn is limited by the size of the child. In an adult with a blood volume of 5 litres up to 20 ml of blood may be withdrawn for chemical analysis, but this is equivalent to only 1 to 2 ml in a neonate weighing 3·5 kg (7 lb) with a blood volume of 90 to 120 ml per kg. An isolated estimation of any one constituent is not usually of much help because of the wide normal range in infancy. The blood urea concentration in particular may be misleading in babies in whom it is normally high compared with the adult range; because of the low urea clearance rate in infancy high protein feeding, an inadequate water intake or a small reduction in renal functions may each cause an elevation. In infants the plasma sodium concentration is usually within the normal adult range, but potassium is often considerably elevated and concentrations which in adults are believed to be incompatible with life are not uncommonly encountered in infants without apparent ill effects; Smith (1951) has stated that the normal range for infants is up to 9·8 mEq per litre.

Infants tend to become acidotic very readily, with a high serum chloride and low bicarbonate and, as McCance (1950) has pointed out, this can be made worse by feeding fortified milk. The low rate of phosphate excretion by infants may reduce their ability to excrete organic acid in the urine, and this may account for their greater tendency to become acidotic. The infant may not be able to cope with ingested ammonium chloride as well as an adult, and this is an additional contraindication, if any were needed, to its use in pyloric stenosis with alkalosis. The plasma protein concentration and the haematocrit are both high during the first three or four days of life, and during this period a subnormal haemoglobin concentration is therefore an indication of a more severe degree of anaemia than usual. Repeated estimations of the same constituents will sometimes provide worthwhile information of the rate and direction of a change in the composition of extracellular fluid, or perhaps an indication why current treatment is ineffective or is causing deterioration, but far more often the results of serum analysis are of less value in guiding and controlling treatment than close clinical observation.

The complete collection of urine is difficult at any age but experienced nursing staff usually can make good estimates of changes in urinary output from the wetness and colour of the napkins. There are several types of bag, such as that used for collecting discharge from an ileostomy, which can be attached over the penis or vulva for the collection of urine. These have the disadvantage that the area of skin is covered by adhesive is liable to become irritated. However, an ileostomy bag is the best way of all in girls and is the best method for single specimens in boys. A catheter should be passed into the ileostomy bag and sealed in place: urine should be withdrawn from the bag through this catheter whenever it is passed.

Ideally, when a baby is losing gastrointestinal secretions all the lost fluid as well as the urine should be collected, measured and analysed before a decision is made about the nature and quantity of fluid to be administered. Change in weight is more easily measured in small babies than at any other time of life and may give the best indication of the real size of the fluid losses which have been sustained. If changes in weight are to be properly interpreted it is necessary to think carefully about what factors are concerned in the particular set of circumstances. Interpretation is much more accurate when the volumes of the urine and other fluid loss have been measured, and changes in weight always include insensible water loss. When a fluid loss is continuing, the amount and direction of change in weight are very useful indications of the quantitative adequacy of fluid replacement, but when the weight of an infant does not change for several days the normal small daily increase in weight by growth should not be forgotten. It is also very important to remember that, in acute intestinal obstruction and in some forms of chronic intestinal distension, fluid which is within the lumen of the intestine will be included in the body weight, although because of changes in the intestinal wall it is functionally lost to the body.

Causes of Disturbance in Infancy and Childhood

Only those causes which are peculiar to or have particular effects in children will be considered in this section.

Oesophageal Atresia

The consumption of fluid is prevented by the atresia, but when the diagnosis is made early and the obstruction is relieved by operation, the normal period of starvation after birth is increased by only a day or two until the administration of milk is begun either through a fine Portex tube passed across the anastomosis into the stomach or by gastrostomy. We have normally waited for 24 hours after operation before starting to feed the baby by either sort of tube. Then after injecting 5 or 10 ml of 5 per cent glucose solution, hourly feeds of 7·5 to 10 ml undiluted breast or cow's milk are started and increased gradually during the next three or four days. As the volume of each feed rises the frequency of feeding can be reduced. Oral feeding is begun after about seven days and when well established the tube is withdrawn. As in other neonatal emergencies, an intravenous infusion should always be started just before operation, but the rate of infusion should be limited to that necessary to maintain the infusion during operation to allow the injection of anaesthetic agents and in case blood transfusion is needed. Blood loss at operation should be measured by weighing the swabs used and should be replaced promptly if it is large enough, The amount of blood loss which can be tolerated varies according to the weight of the child; in a 3·5 kg neonate it is not usually necessary to replace a loss of less than 10 ml. The intravenous infusion need not be continued after operation because feeding can be started after 24 hours by the transanastomotic tube or by gastrostomy (Fig. 14).

Acute Intestinal Obstruction

There are divergent views about how the child, and especially the neonate, with intestinal obstruction should be treated. Some believe that before operative relief of the obstruction is undertaken the fluid which has been lost by vomiting and into the obstructed bowel should be replaced by intravenous infusion, and that if necessary operation should be delayed for 12 or 24 hours to allow this to be done. In neonates the loss of fluid is estimated from the change in weight since birth and allowance is made for insensible loss and urine. Such estimates are arbitrary and the daily requirements for sodium and water for example may be based on the normal intake in milk feeds and greatly exceed the actual losses from the body. Although the fluid in distended and obstructed loops of intestine is still in some sort of equilibrium with the rest of the extracellular fluid, there is no way of judging the total volume of this fluid until it is removed from the bowel. Replacement of this fluid involves delay in relief of the intestinal obstruction. If the fluid lost by vomiting and constipation into the bowel above the obstruction has resulted in reduction of the blood volume sufficient blood or dextran should be given to restore blood volume to normal before the operation to relieve the obstruction is begun. There is not much evidence to show that the replacement of lost fluid by the infusion of solutions of electrolytes greatly reduces mortality or morbidity and much of the fluid administered in this way is likely to find its way into the

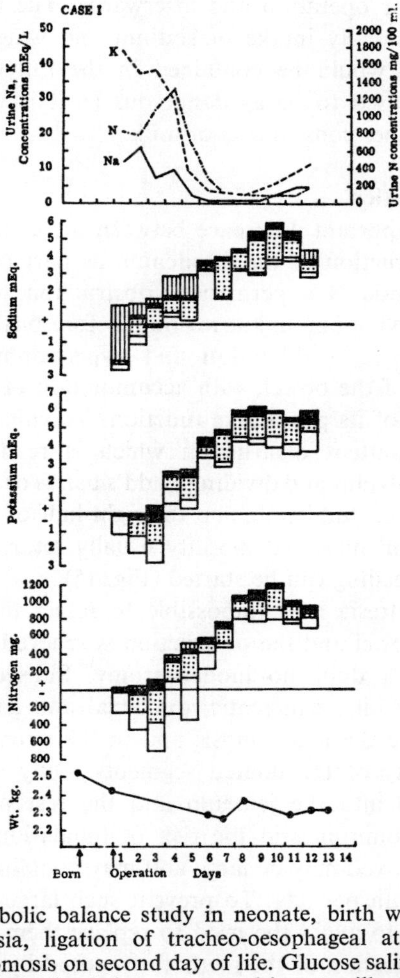

FIGURE 14. Metabolic balance study in neonate, birth weight 2·55 kg with oesophageal atresia, ligation of tracheo-oesophageal atresia and primary end-to-end anastomosis on second day of life. Glucose saline injected through transanastomotic tube for 3 days; expressed breast milk started on 2nd post-operative day. Positive sodium and potassium balances from fourth post-operative day. Large output of nitrogen for 5 days and then positive balance achieved. High urinary potassium concentration for 4 days; very dilute urine from 6th day (Hughes *et al.*, 1965).

(Reproduced by kind permission of the Editor of the *British Journal of Surgery*.)

peritoneal cavity and the lumen of the obstructed bowel and will be sucked out during the operation. Nothing should delay the operation except the restoration of the circulating blood volume. Much less fluid is now administered than was formerly the case, both in preparation for operation and afterwards. The former practice of maintaining a daily intake of sodium and water equal to the quantities which would be contained in the full daily intake of milk is now realised to be as dangerous as it is unsound in the absence of the other constituents of milk.

Duodenal Obstruction

There is an important difference between the effects of duodenal atresia and obstruction of the duodenum as part of a volvulus of the midgut. Atresia is a permanent obstruction which has been present for a varying but unknown time before birth, and as in all other atresias there is dilatation and hypertrophy of the blind obstructed part of the bowel, with accumulation of secretions in it and disturbance of its propulsive function. Volvulus of the midgut causes an intermittent obstruction which is readily relieved by untwisting the volvulus and dividing Ladd's bands or other adhesions in the region of the duodenum and the right half of the colon; after such an operation intestinal motility usually returns to normal in 24 hours when feeding can be started (Fig. 15).

In duodenal atresia it is impossible to resect the dilated blind portion of the bowel and the obstruction is relieved by a duodeno-jejunostomy or a duodeno-duodenostomy. Subsequently for up to 10 to 14 days bile, pancreatic, duodenal and gastric secretions accumulate above the anastomosis and in the stomach because of disturbed motility of the dilated segments. Only a part of these secretions passes into the jejunum and the rest must be sucked off to prevent vomiting and the risk of inhalation. The volumes of fluid thus removed may be large and may contain up to 15 mEq. or more of sodium per day. To prevent such large losses of water and sodium and to avoid the need to replace them by intravenous infusion a modification of the method proposed by Ehrenpreis and Sandblom (1949) may be used. At operation a fine soft Portex tube (No. 6) is passed across the anastomosis into the distal loop of the duodeno-jejunostomy for a distance about 15 cm, the proximal end is passed up the duodenum through the pylorus and out of the anterior wall of the stomach and through the abdominal wall. Beside this tube another of larger size (Malecot 16 Ch.) is passed into the stomach as a gastrostomy and through this tube the gastric contents are sucked off. After operation all the fluid which is sucked from the stomach is preserved. From 24 hours after operation 5ml of aspirated fluid is injected down the fine tube into the distal

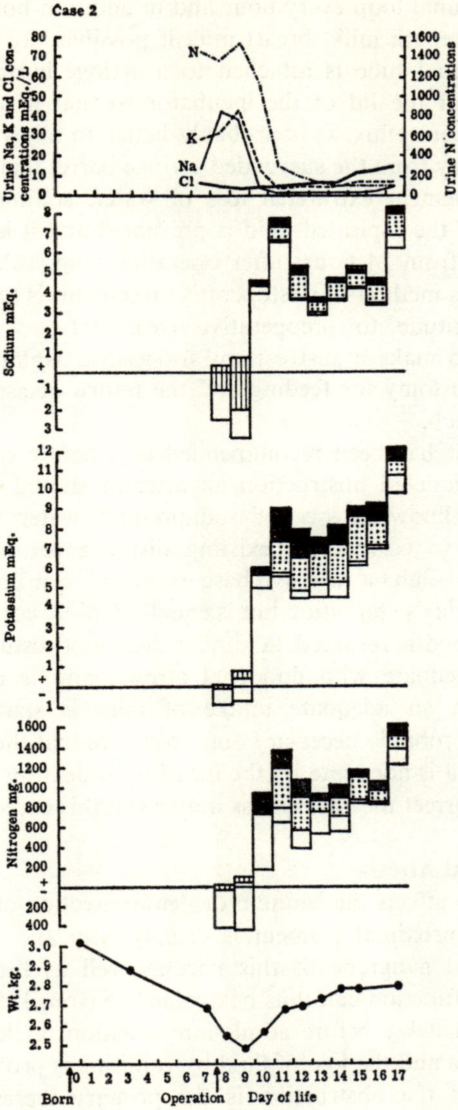

FIGURE. 15. Metabolic balance study, male, birth weight 3·1 kg, with duodenal obstruction due to volvulus of midgut with Ladd's bands. Small feeds of breast milk started 24 hours after relief of obstruction, uneventful recovery with large positive balances from third day after operation (Wilkinson *et al.*, 1965).

(Reproduced by kind permission of the Editor of the *British Journal of Surgery*.)

limb of the jejunal loop every hour and in addition hourly feeds of 5 ml of full-strength milk, breast milk if possible, are started. The end of the jejunal tube is attached to a syringe barrel suspended from the top of the lid of the incubator so that if necessary the injected fluid can reflux. It is probably better to allow the fluid to run in by gravity from the suspended syringe barrel than to inject it. By this arrangement extrarenal loss of water, sodium and other constituents of the aspirated fluid is prevented and it is possible to feed the baby from 24 hours after operation (Fig. 16). When it is known that this method of postoperative treatment is to be adopted a different attitude to preoperative treatment is justified. An alternative is to make a gastrostomy for gastric aspiration and an ordinary jejunostomy for feeding and the return of aspirated fluid from the stomach.

In the past it has been recommended that before operation on babies with duodenal obstruction an attempt should be made to replace the unknown losses of sodium and water which have occurred, and to correct the existing disturbances of acid base equilibrium. In adults a negative base excess of 15 mEq may result from only two day's starvation but is equally rapidly corrected when the intake of food is resumed. A similar degree of disturbance may occur in the neonate with duodenal atresia, and is also rapidly corrected when an adequate intake of milk is started. Before operation it is probably necessary only to ensure that the circulating volume of blood is adequate by the infusion of dextran in saline or blood and to correct the base excess only when this exceeds 15 mEq.

Jejunal and Ileal Atresia

When atresia affects the jejunum or ileum resection of the dilated hypertrophied proximal segment is usually easy and the risks of perforation and gangrene of this part as well as the prolonged disturbance of function can thus be avoided (Nixon, 1956). In these types of atresia delay before admission is seldom as long as with duodenal atresia and the loss of fluid by vomiting is probably not as great. Relief of the obstruction is the primary therapeutic consideration and should be deferred only to pass a soft tube to empty the stomach by aspiration, and if necessary to restore blood volume by the transfusion of dextran or blood. Although after resection of the dilated proximal blind segment most surgeons prefer to make a primary anastomis between the ends of the small intestine, when the atresia is high in the jejunum there is much to be said for the alternative of making an end-to-side enterostomy of the type described by Bishop and Koop (1957). The proximal stump of intestine is anastomosed to the antimesenteric border of the distal piece of bowel about 3 inches (7·5 cm) from its proximal end which is then brought out as a terminal enterostomy. Little fluid is lost from the enterostomy but gas escapes freely from it. Fluid sucked off the stomach and milk feeds can be injected into the enterostomy This method of anastomosis was originally devised for use in meconium obstruction when pancreatic extract is injected into the enterostomy as well as being given by mouth. The prevention of extrarenal losses by the instillation of fluid sucked from the stomach into the enterostomy has greatly reduced or avoided the need for parenteral fluid therapy.

Massive Intestinal Resection

The effects of resecting much of the small intestine depends first on how much of the small bowel remains, secondly on which part is left, and thirdly on the age of the patient. The mean length at birth of the normal jejunum and ileum is 253 cm (range 152 to 355 cm) in boys and 243 cm (range 149 to 338 cm) in girls (Scammon and Calkin, 1929; Ellis, 1951; Reiquam *et al.*, 1965). In adults the mean is 6·9 m (22 ft 6 in) in men and 7 m (23 ft 4 in) in women (range 4·7 m to 9·7 m (15 ft 6 in to 31 ft 10 in) (Treves, 1885). In the living subject the small intestine is shorter than in the dead. The length of the small intestine, in a full-term baby at birth may be much reduced by multiple atresias or by infarction of the midgut in a volvulus. It now seems likely that at least 20 cm is needed for independent survival in the neonate but the type of intestine which remains is almost as important as its length. Babies and young children need more small intestine than older subjects who have stopped growing. The ileocaecal valve should always be preserved if possible and ileum is of more value than an equal length of jejunum. Both in animals and in the human neonate the large bowel can be completely excised without much disturbance of nutrition (Wilkinson and McCance, 1973). Opinion is conflicting on whether the remaining bowel dilates or hypertrophies in the absence of distal obstruction, but the balance of the evidence suggests that it does not, nor does growth in length exceed that to be expected in a normal subject (McCance and Wilkinson, 1967). In infants and children the time taken for the transit of marked food or barium from the mouth to the anus is usually very short and may be as

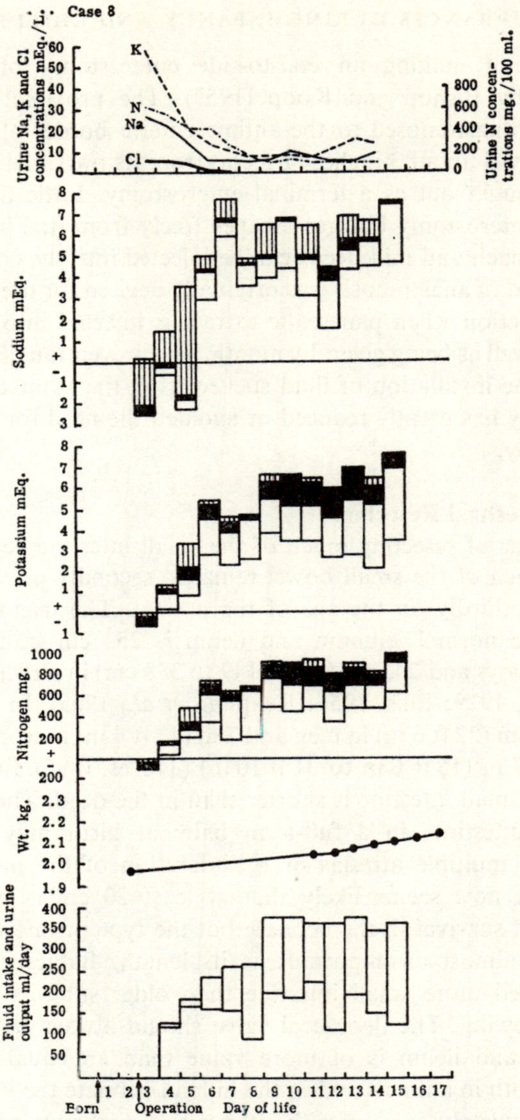

FIGURE 16 (*a*). Metabolic balance study, male, weight on admission 1·98 kg with duodenal atresia treated by duodeno-jejunostomy and gastrostomy with intubation of distal limb. Baby fed from 24 hours by jejunal tube. The vertical lines indicate the quantities in the aliquots of fluid, removed by gastric aspiration, which were kept for analysis, the rest of this aspirated fluid being injected through the jejunal tube. Positive nitrogen and potassium balances from second day after operation and of sodium from fourth day. The volume of urine was very small at first, and then as its volume rose the concentrations of its constituents fell to very low levels.

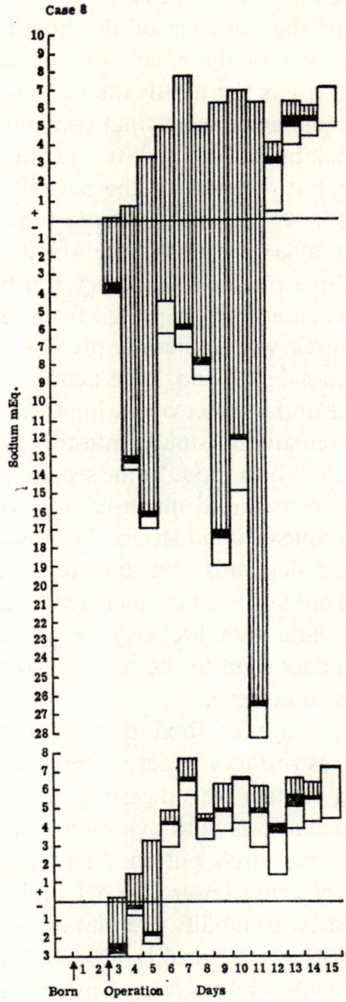

FIGURE 16 (*b*). In the lower graph the sodium balance is plotted as in (*a*) and in the upper graph is shown the sodium balance as it would have been if all the fluid sucked out of the stomach had been thrown away instead of being injected into the jejunostomy tube. During 9 days of aspiration 1887 ml of fluid containing 105 mEq sodium were sucked out of the stomach (Wilkinson *et al.*, 1965).

(Reproduced by kind permission of the Editor of the *British Journal of Surgery*.)

little as 15 minutes. It has been suggested that a short segment of the most distal remaining small intestine should be reversed so as to delay the passage of the contents of the bowel. There have been some favourable reports of the effects of this procedure in adults but not in children; it has the disadvantage that the more effective it is in delaying the passage of intestinal contents the more likely it is to cause also malabsorption and to encourage the growth of bacteria in the stagnant contents of the partially obstructed bowel (Hammer *et al.*, 1955, 1959; Venables *et al.*, 1967).

At any age after a large part of the small intestine has been resected there are three phases of recovery (Pullan, 1959). At first, after a day or two when nothing is passed from the bowel; but then for up to two or three weeks there is profuse diarrhoea with excoriation of the perianal skin and large quantities of intestinal secretions may be lost. For days after operation there may be dilation of the stomach and remaining small intestine with transient accumulation of secretions and food. In the second phase although the intake of food has been started much of it is lost unchanged and unabsorbed in the frequent liquid stools. This usually lasts for some weeks or months and demands constant attention and vigilance, if sudden severe losses are not to cause such acute and severe depletion of the extracellular fluid that life may be endangered. The third stage is that of full adaptation to the new situation which may take as long as two years to achieve.

The very rapid passage of food through the short remaining piece of intestine gives rise to a variety of problems. The short time for which food is in contact with digestive juices in the bowel and the mucous membrane affects both digestion and absorption. In the large bowel undigested starch putrefies and produces much gas, and unabsorbed fatty acids lower the pH and irritate the colon. The objective should be to modify the diet in such a way that it is predigested and fortified with readily absorbed materials, such as glucose and amino acids, and its rate of passage should be reduced by removing all irritant substances from it.

Animal fat should be excluded from the diet because it is so irritant. In the neonate this means that the feeds should be based on reconstituted dried skimmed milk, unless a carbohydrate intolerance also exists. The feed should be made with less than the usual amount of water, thickened with arrowroot and predigested with Benger's food (Wilkinson *et al.*, 1963). The caloric content may be increased by adding olive oil, or a medium chain triglyceride preparation should be substituted on an equicaloric basis for the excluded milk fat (Winawer *et al.*, 1966; Wilkinson, 1967). Dilute feeds should not be used and the oral consumption of fluid should be limited to prevent undue stimulation of intestinal secretion. The faeces should be collected and their volume measured and transit time regularly measured with a carmine marker.

If frequent liquid stools result in large losses of intestinal secretions the extracellular fluid volume must be restored promptly by the rapid intravenous infusion of sufficient 0·9 per cent saline, Darrow's solution and if necessary sodium bicarbonate; lactate should be avoided because of the adverse effects it has on the absorption of magnesium. When such losses are repeated and the intake of food is poor the liability to magnesium depletion must be remembered, especially if the replacement of potassium losses does not result in improvement. Although the ultimate objective is the oral consumption of sufficient food to provide for growth as well as the daily maintenance requirements it may often be necessary to control the loss of intestinal contents by stopping oral feeds. Parenteral feeding then has an important place for a limited time. By maintaining nutrition with the intravenous infusion of a hydrolysate of beef fibrin and concentrated glucose solution Dudrick *et al.* (1969) were able to keep alive a baby with only 3 cm of ileum for 22 months until thrombosis of all the available veins defeated them. Wilmore *et al.* (1971) found that after resection of 90 per cent of the small intestine from 10 week old beagle puppies growth and function of the remaining intestine was improved when adequate nutrition was maintained by intravenous feeding for 30 days. Subsequently body weight was much nearer normal but there was no greater increase in the length of the bowel than would normally have occurred but the mucosa was thicker and the calibre of the bowel was increased.

Success depends on constant watchfulness and regular repeated reviews of the whole situation at the bedside. Provided such babies can be carried through the early weeks until the bowel function becomes more stable, they can survive and grow though not as fast or as much as normal children.

Neonatal Volvulus

When *neonatal volvulus* is intermittent it is less likely to cause a severe circulatory disturbance than when a persisting tight twist leads to a closed loop obstruction and interference with the blood supply of a segment which may extend throughout the midgut.

Volvulus is less common in the neonatal period than atresia. The addition of blood loss into the vessels, lumen and wall of the twisted segments may cause circulatory failure and blood transfusion may be needed before operation can be started. Strangulation is usually indicated by the sudden and unexpected deterioration in the general condition of the baby and rapid transfusion of blood through the umbilical vein is the best form of resuscitation.

Acute Intususception

This is still probably the commonest acute abdominal emergency between the ages of two weeks and two years, although both the incidence and the mortality have recently fallen. Diagnosis is made early in about three-quarters of the cases, and with rare exceptions only in the remainder are blood loss into the bowel wall and lumen and fluid loss by vomiting likely to cause so severe a disturbance that blood transfusion is necessary. When resection is required it is usually also necessary to replace lost blood by transfusion When there is any doubt about the need for transfusion it is almost always better to give the blood.

Hirschsprung's Disease

Apart from oesophageal atresia and anomalies of the anus and rectum this is now the commonest single cause of intestinal obstruction in the first month after birth. When such obstruction is not relieved by colostomy or ileostomy, but is treated by rectal or colonic lavage, there may be recurrent abdominal crises marked by gross distension, vomiting and the passage of copious and often offensive loose faeces. There may then be rapid reduction in extracellular fluid volume with acute circulatory failure, which resembles that found in some other forms of severe diarrhoea, and requires to be corrected by the fast intravenous infusion of 0·9 per cent saline. Hirschsprung's disease may also be complicated by enterocolitis, which causes the rapid loss of fluid into the bowel which may be followed by acute peripheral circulatory faliure. This complication, which may also affect part or the whole of the small intestine and even the stomach, is almost certainly not due to infection but may be caused by some form of hypersensitivity reaction. As well as replacing the lost fluid by the very rapid intravenous infusion of sufficient 0·9 per cent saline, the bowel must be emptied by a rectal tube, and obstruction relieved by making a colostomy or ileostomy in normally innervated bowel. Enterocolitis varies in severity but may occur before any treatment has been started, after obstruction has been relieved and even after treatment by resection of the aganglionic bowel has been completed and the child has returned home and normal bowel function has been established and it may be recurrent. The risk of water intoxication due to washing out the bowel with hypotonic solutions instead of with 0·9 per cent, saline is now well recognised.

Inguinal Hernia

The diagnosis of acute intestinal obstruction due to incarceration of bowel in an inguinal hernia is seldom so long delayed that significant loss of fluid occurs either by vomiting or into the lumen of the bowel. Strangulation or its surgical relief may cause the loss of so much blood that transfusion is needed.

Peritonitis

This may be associated with a large change in blood volume in infants as in older children and adults. Blood transfusion is of most value before, during or immediately after operative treatment and should not be routinely followed by the infusion of solutions of glucose or glucose saline. Only when vomiting recurs or persistent ileus has led to prolonged gastric aspiration should a short rapid infusion of a carefully judged volume of saline be used.

Congenital Hypertrophic Pyloric Stenosis

This is now usually diagnosed so early and treated so promptly by operation that severe disturbance of the body fluids seldom occurs, but in a few patients for one reason or another repeated vomiting continues for several weeks. Such babies are shrunken, dry and quiet and may weigh less than at birth. It is important to recognise that while they have lost a large part of their extracellular fluid and that this can be acutely replaced by the rapid infusion of saline with marked improvement in their appearance and condition, a lot of fat and protein have also been destroyed during the period of vomiting and starvation, and this can be restored only by the feeding of milk and the reconstitution of the lost tissues. Moderate depletion of potassium can be readily corrected by starting milk feeds soon after operation, especially when potassium chloride is added to the feeds. In the rare baby who is sleepy, inactive and limp even after the infusion of an adequate volume of saline, up to 5 mEq potassium, as potassium chloride, and 3 mEq of magnesium, as magnesium chloride, per kilogram body weight may be infused during 24 hours provided the urinary output exceeds 120 ml per 24 hours. Very occasionally even this treatment is ineffective. It is then best to make a jejunostomy under local analgesia and to feed the baby through it with full strength milk containing supplementary potassium and magnesium chlorides for two or three weeks before operating on the pyloric tumour. Fluid which is sucked out of the stomach should be injected into the jejunum between the feeds.

PREOPERATIVE TREATMENT

Infants can be fed until four hours before deliberate operation, the last feed being of 5 per cent glucose solution. Older children should not drink for 4 to 6 hours before operation, but none should be purged. The complicated disturbances of body composition which result from prolonged illness and its treatment can be modified only to a very limited degree before operation, and in general a normal state is not restored for some weeks after a successful operation. Severe malnutrition can be corrected only by the consumption of a diet suitable to the age of the child and containing enough protein, calories, minerals and vitamins to enable lost tissue to be replaced in addition to the requirements for daily metabolism and growth.

Maintenance of Blood Volume

Newborn children tolerate thoracotomy and laparotomy very well, provided their blood volume is maintained. To do this it is necessary to keep a close watch on the rate and total quantity of blood loss, and this is most conveniently done by weighing the discarded blood-stained swabs and measuring the volume of the blood in the sucker bottle. No neonate should be subjected to a major operation unless blood is available for the prompt replacement of an excessive loss. During operation blood loss can be minimised by the use of the diathermy while opening the chest or abdomen; not more than 5 to 10 ml should be lost in thoracotomy or laparotomy and a loss of this size does not usually need to be replaced. In neonates blood may be transfused intermittently by the injection of small volumes (up to 10 ml) into the cannula of a scalp vein infusion, into a vein on the back of the hand, or into a cannula inserted into the umbilical vein (Wilkinson, 1963). The umbilical vein is divided in the transverse upper abdominal incision which is usually used for laparotomy in the newly born and a large Portex cannula (size 6D) can readily be tied into the upper stump of the vein; but because the cannula is removed when the wound is closed blood replacement must be completed during the operation. When the umbilical vein is used for transfusion the injected blood very rapidly reaches the inferior vena cava and the right side of the heart. The very rapid injection of cold or old blood may have very adverse effects in the neonate and cause cardiac arythmias or arrest. Blood should always be as fresh as possible and, even at the risk of being wasted, should be brought to the theatre and warmed before use.

POSTOPERATIVE TREATMENT

Unless the alimentary tract has been the site of operation, children should be allowed to drink suitably limited quantities of water, fruit juice or milk as soon as they ask for a drink. After operations under local or general analgesia for pyloric stenosis, feeding should be started within 4 hours of operation. Although after major abdominal operations there is a similar disturbance of gastric motility and absorption to that found in adults, it seldom lasts as long, nor is it usually necessary to stop drinking for more than 24 hours after operation. During this period older children should be allowed to relieve their thirst by sucking gauze moistened with cold water or small pieces of ice. After 24 hours small drinks should be allowed, starting with 5 ml every hour and so long as the child does not vomit the quantity can be gradually increased.

Routine parental administration of fluid has no place in paediatric surgical practice, and intravenous infusions should be reserved for the few patients who, as well as being unable to eat or drink, suffer large losses of body fluids. If replacement is then to be exact, it is essential that the fluid which is being lost from the body and the urine should be collected; the completeness with which this is achieved is directly related to the skill and adequacy of the nursing staff. The volume and the sodium and potassium content of the collected fluids are measured and used as a guide to treatment, and the replacements should seldom exceed the losses. If gastric aspiration is necessary either a fine soft Portex nasogastric tube can be used or a gastrostomy can be made. Whichever type of tube is used suction should be intermittent and if the amount of fluid obtained is small it is usually better to allow free drainage into a plastic pot at the same level as the stomach. Gastric aspiration should be stopped as soon as the aspirated fluid smells clean and is clear.

It is very important to remember that in the neonate and young child the requirements for growth as well as maintenance must be supplied or else they must be met as far as possible from the patients own body. We still do not know exactly how much of the various amino acids are needed for growth at different ages nor how these needs may be affected by disease or injury or by intravenous administration. It follows that every solution used clinically should have been previously shown at least to support normal growth in other species than man but this has seldom been done. It seems likely that the work of Adkins *et al.* (1966) and Jurgens and Dolif (1968) on the effect of proline on growth may lead to further improvements in amino acids solutions for intravenous use in man.

Munro (1972) reviewed the varying published reports on protein requirements and concluded that the mean requirements for infants were 1·6 of nitrogen per kg body weight of which 43 per cent must be 'essential' amino acids and for adults was 0·425 g per kg with 19 to 20 per cent 'essential' amino acids. These estimates should be followed in designing amino acid combinations for intravenous feedings until there is more evidence about variations in requirements for 'essential' amino acids in particular clinical circumstances, for example after severe injury, during infection, or in severely wasted and depleted patients.

Fomon and May (1958) found that when infants were growing well on a milk diet the intake of protein was 2·4 g per kg per 24 hours in the first month and 1·5 g per kg 24 hours during the fourth to sixth months.

Although reliable and nutritionally adequate amino acid solutions are now available for intravenous infusion many clinicians still prefer to use human plasma or reconstituted dried serum for this purpose. Williams *et al.* (1949) recommended that 1·0 g per lb body weight of plasma protein should be given daily to the post-operative patient. Such use of plasma protein or of an amino acid solution is theoretically sound only if the intake of calories apart from those derived from protein is high enough to satisfy the daily energy requirements. Thus an infant who weighs 7 lb (3·5 kg) ought to receive 7·0 g plasma protein in about 150 ml plasma or 7·0 g amino acids in 200 ml of solution. In addition the child should receive at least 200 non-protein calories per 24 hours so that the protein contributes about 12·5 per cent of the total calorie intake.

These additional calories can be provided by some combination such as 20 per cent fructose solution, a glucose, fructose, ethanol mixture or a fat emulsion. Strong solutions of fructose, and any solution containing glucose which has been autoclaved irritate the veins and soon cause thrombophlebitis. This is bad enough when a superficial peripheral vein is involved but is very serious indeed if the infusion is being given into a deep vein such as the superior or inferior vena cava. Infection of the needle puncture or incision for the insertion of a cannula is very common because of lack of care and attention to asepsis both when the infusion is first started and thereafter. Septicaemia due to such infection, often with antibiotic resistant organisms, is now so common that prolonged intravenous infusions should be maintained only when they are essential to survival and after most careful consideration. The achievement of Dudrick and his colleagues (1969) in maintaining a baby entirely by intravenous feeding for 22 months depended on their devotion to meticulous attention to aseptic practice and was terminated by the thrombosis of all the available veins.

It is uncertain how long daily infusions of fat emulsion can be safely used, since after some days they are liable to cause disturbances of blood coagulation with petechial haemorrhages in the skin and mucous membranes. The daily dose of fat should probably not exceed 3 g per kg body weight and a specimen of blood should be drawn daily six hours after the last injection of fat and examined to ensure that the injected fat is being cleared satisfactorily from the blood.

The daily transfusion of plasma has also been recommended to maintain the circulating plasma protein concentration which in children, as in adults, declines during the first week after operation. Since this decline is probably related in children as in adults to postoperative protein catabolism, the transfusion of plasma alone without an adequate accompaniment of calories does not do much good. A compound vitamin supplement should be administered either daily in the intravenous solution or weekly by intramuscular injection. Trace elements can be provided by giving 10 ml human plasma per kg body weight twice a week; commercial preparations are also available.

Deficiency of disaccharidases may be a feature of diseases like sprue and kwashiorkor but it is now recognised to be not uncommon in neonates after colostomy or ileostomy. Lactase deficiency lasts longest and special milks may have to be used for several months until the intestinal production of the enzyme returns to normal. True congenital deficiency of lactase seems to be very rare. One form of disaccharide intolerance is due to a deficiency of disaccharidase in the brush border. The disaccharide cannot be hydrolysed and absorbed and remains in the intestinal lumen and retains water there also. The volume of intestinal fluid stimulates peristalsis and the more rapid transit of intestinal contents leads to diarrhoea. These effects are enhanced if in addition disaccharide is converted to lactic acid in the distal ileum or colon.

Control of Treatment

Before treatment is begun it is essential to have a clear idea of the nature of the disturbance and of the kind of fluid loss which has caused it. A plan of treatment should then be made and reviewed and if necessary modified each time the state and progress of the infant are assessed, which in acute illness should be at intervals of 6 hours. Oral and parenteral intakes and the output in stools, urine, vomitus or aspirations should be recorded hourly by the nursing staff. It is essential that once every 24 hours all the data from preceding days of the illness are reconsidered. A suitable allowance for the insensible loss of water must be included in the daily total of loss from the body. This should be based on the basal caloric consumption of a normal baby of the same weight, rather than on surface area which involves too many doubtful assumptions. It is probably best to base decisions about the total quantity of water, sodium or potassium which should be given, as in adults, on the clinical history and the state of the patient and the response to treatment. Many clinicians calculate the deficits of sodium or potassium from the changes in serum concentration of these ions ignoring the associated changes in body water content. Darrow (1946) estimated that in severe depletion a third of the extracellular sodium and water might be lost, equivalent to about 80 ml per kg of 0·9 per cent saline in an infant, or 60 ml per kg in an older child or adult.

Methods of Administration of Fluid

Subcutaneous infusions should be used only for administration of small quantities of isotonic solutions and are not of much value when extracellular fluid volume is so far reduced as to cause obvious signs of reduction in blood volume. The addition of hyaluronidase increases the rate of absorption of subcutaneous infusions. *Rectal infusions* are unreliable, especially in surgical patients, in whom disorders of the gastrointestinal tract are the commonest cause of severe fluid loss. Because of the risk of infection with resistant organisms and osteomyelitis the *intramedullary* route should never be used. *Intraperitoneal* injection can be employed when the intra-abdominal organs are not involved, but its clinical applications are few.

INTRAVENOUS INFUSION is the most reliable method, since it allows a greater control of the rate of administration and of the volume used than any other, but its technique must be modified for use in small babies. The insertion of a fine needle into the superficial veins of an infant is usually difficult and demands considerable skill and practice. In the limbs the veins in the back of the hand are usually more easily seen than any others. In the scalp, however, the tributaries of the superficial temporal vein are usually readily seen even in small premature neonates, and with practice and a suitable needle, can be entered more easily than any others. When intravenous feeding is being maintained for a long time it is necessary to use the superficial veins on the trunk as well as those in the limbs and this is preferable to the use of the great veins with its much greater associated risks.

Umbilical vein. The umbilical vein is readily accessible as it runs from the umbilicus to the liver in the falciform ligament. It is divided in the transverse upper abdominal incision which affords the best access for laparotomy in the neonate, but it can also be exposed at the same point under local analgesia when rapid resuscitation is necessary in a collapsed baby. At laparotomy the vein should be secured and drawn up and divided between forceps before the peritoneum is opened. The butt end of a 6D Portex cannula is then passed under the towel at the upper edge of the wound to the anaesthetist who connects it to the infusion set and fills the cannula with fluid. The proximal stump of the vein is then cut across with scissors and the cannula is inserted and tied in. The umbilical vein remains patent for up to 15 days after birth. The large size of cannula allows the rapid injection of blood which should not be cold or so old that its serum potassium concentration is excessively high. When blood loss has been full replaced and the final dose of relaxant has been given the cannula is withdrawn and the vein is tied off as the wound is closed. The use of the umbilical vein avoids delay in finding and cannulating a small peripheral vein especially in premature babies in bad condition, and is of great value in acute emergency (Wilkinson, 1963).

TECHNIQUE OF SCALP VEIN INFUSION. The bottle and tubing should first be connected and filled with fluid. One half of the scalp is then shaved and cleaned with a 1 per cent solution of cetrimide. The baby is then laid across the cot in a good light and with the shaved side uppermost the head is held firmly in both hands by an assistant. The operator compresses the main stem of the superficial temporal vein just above the ear and chooses a suitable tributary. A fine needle (21 BWG) is now available with a double flap of plastic material at the butt and attached to a short length of plastic tubing with a butt for attachment to a syringe. The needle and tubing are filled with sterile 0·9 per cent saline and when the needle enters the vein blood can be seen in the plastic tubing which is then connected to the adaptor on the end of the infusion set tubing. When the veins are constricted it may be necessary to use a finer needle (25 BWG). The needle is fixed in position on the scalp by its plastic flaps with several strips of adhesive plaster.

During a prolonged intravenous infusion to ensure accurate control of the volume and rate of infusion a graduated cylinder should be included in the infusion system so that volumes of up to 30 ml can be measured and administered over a period of several hours; the longer and narrower the graduated cylinder is, the more accurate the measurements will be. Disposable infusion sets are now available which include a graduated cylinder. When several solutions are being repeatedly administered it is convenient to connect the bottles by tubing to the inlet side of a three-way tap; this is especially important when fat emulsions and protein hydrolysates are being used. The technique of cutting down on a vein in an infant is the same as that used in adults (p. 260); local analgesia should always be used because this helps to reduce spasm in the vein, but it is seldom easy to find and to enter the fine vein amidst the subcutaneous fat of a baby's limbs.

APPENDIX I

TABLE XXIII

The normal range of concentrations of blood constituents

	mg/100 ml	*mEq/litre*
Serum		
Sodium	316 to 340	137 to 148
Potassium	15 to 20	3·8 to 5·1
Magnesium	1·9 to 2·5	1·7 to 2·2
Calcium	9·6 to 11·0	4·8 to 5·4
Chloride	570 to 620 (as NaCl)	97 to 106
Whole blood		
Chloride	450 to 530 (as NaCl)	77 to 90
CO_2 combining power	52 to 72 (ml CO_2)	
Total bicarbonate		23 to 32
Non-protein nitrogen	25 to 40	
Urea nitrogen	9 to 16	
	g/100 ml	*mEq/litre*
Serum		
Total protein	5·5 to 7·6	13·4 to 18·5
Albumin	3·3 to 5·3	
Globulin	1·9 to 2·8	

TABLE XXIX

Atomic weights, valencies and equivalent weights

	Atomic weight	*Valency*	*Equivalent weight*
Sodium	23	1	23
Potassium	39	1	39
Magnesium	24	2	12
Calcium	40	2	20
Chlorine	35·5	1	35·5
Phosphorus	31	1·8	17·2
Sulphur	32	2	16

TABLE XXX

Milliequivalents per gram

1·0 g	Sodium	contains 43·5 mEq	Sodium
	Potassium	26·0	Potassium
	Magnesium	85·0	Magnesium
	Calcium	50·0	Calcium
	Chloride	29·0	Chloride
	Sodium chloride	17·0	Sodium
		17·0	Chloride
	Potassium chloride	13·4	Potassium
		13·4	Chloride
	Sodium lactate	9·0	Sodium
		9·0	Lactate
	Sodium acetate	12·0	Sodium
		12·0	Acetate
	Sodium bicarbonate	11·9	Sodium
		11·9	Bicarbonate
	Magnesium chloride	21·0	Magnesium
		21·0	Chloride
	Magnesium Sulphate	16·6	Magnesium
		16·6	Sulphate

APPENDIX II

Milliequivalents

The clinical convention that the concentrations of the constituents of body fluids should be expressed in milligrams per 100 ml describes the concentration of the individual constituents by weight but does not give any indication of their chemical activity. The biological activity of any element depends largely on its chemical 'equivalence' or value rather than on its gravimetric weight. The universal chemical convention is to express concentrations in terms of the equivalent weights of the constituents of a solution; by reference in this way to a common factor of equivalence, the hydrogen atom, it is possible to compare directly the chemical value or activity of different solutions and their constituents. The clinical importance of recognising alterations in the composition of body fluids is undisputed. Unless however the concentrations of the constituents of such fluids are expressed in terms of chemical equivalence, as milliequivalents per litre, the recognition and assessment of alterations in composition are made difficult and indirect.

The equivalent weight of an element is that quantity of it expressed in grams which is chemically equivalent to, or will displace or react with, one gram of hydrogen. The equivalent weight is also equal to the atomic weight of the element divided by the valency. A milliequivalent is the equivalent weight of an element expressed in milligrams. The elements which are of clinical importance together with their atomic weights, valencies and equivalent weights are shown in Table XXIX. Most of these elements are monovalent, and for these the equivalent weight in the same as the atomic weight. In the case of phosphorus, however, within the normal range of pH of extracellular fluid, 20 per cent of the phosphate is monovalent (BH_2PO_4) and 80 per cent is divalent (B_2HPO_4). The valency of phosphorus in this mixed phosphate is therefore $0.2+(0.8\times0.2)=$ 1·8. Because the pH may not be known, or has not been measured, most biochemists express the value of phosphate in milligrams per

100 ml of serum. Clinical convention has led to the expression of concentrations of bicarbonate ($BHCO_3$) and carbonic acid ($HHCO_3$) in terms of volumes of carbon dioxide per 100 ml; this figure can be converted to mEq litre by dividing by 2·22.

Milligrams can be converted to milliequivalents by dividing by the equivalent weight and vice versa. To convert a concentration expressed in milligrams per 100 ml to milliequivalents per litre the first step is to multiply by 10 to convert to milligrams per litre. Milligrams are then converted to milliequivalents by dividing by the equivalent weight; this is the same as dividing the valency by the atomic weight.

For example

$$\text{mg per 100 ml} \times 10 = \text{mg per litre}$$

$$\frac{\text{mg per litre}}{\text{equivalent weight}} = \text{mg per litre} \times \frac{\text{valency}}{\text{atomic weight}}$$

$$= \text{mEq per litre.}$$

For sodium

$$325 \text{ mg per 100 ml} \times 10 = 3250 \text{ mg per litre}$$

$$\frac{3250 \text{ mg per litre}}{\text{equivalent weight}} = 3250 \text{ mg per litre} \times \frac{\text{valency}}{\text{atomic weight}}$$

$$= \frac{3250 \times 1}{23}$$

$$= 141 \text{ mEq per litre.}$$

A *millimole* (mmol) is the molecular weight of a substance expressed in milligrams.

A *milliosmole* (mosmol) is the quantity in milligrams of a substance which, when dissolved in 22·4 litres of water at 0°C will exert an osmotic pressure of one thousandth of an atmosphere. Osmotic pressure depends on the number of particles in a solution rather than on the number of electrical charges, so the osmotic effect or 'osmolar weight' of a divalent ion is the same as its atomic weight and is independent of its valency.

The osmolality or osmotic activity of a soultion depends on the number of osmotically active particles which it contains, whatever their size, and whether they are ionised or not. Broadly speaking, osmolality is inversely proportional to the molecular weight of a substance; for example a large protein molecule has less osmotic effect than the much smaller sodium ion; urea and glucose or other non-electrolytes may, however, exert considerable osmotic pressure when they are present in high concentrations in the urine. Protein osmotic pressure is effective only when protein is confined by a cell membrane. The osmolality of the plasma can be estimated from the concentrations of sodium and potassium in mEq per litre. Since these cations are derived from salts and at neutral pH are balanced by equivalent numbers of anions the osmolality is approximately double the concentration in mEq per litre of potassium and sodium, plus some addition for un-ionised substances like urea and glucose. In most disease states there are other unknown and variably active substances in the plasma which are almost certainly of much more importance than sodium and potassium, but we know little or nothing about most of these substances.

In any solution the particles of solutes have marked effects on the properties of the solvent, which in the case of living bodies is water. At temperatures below 0°C water is frozen and cystalline and so has an orderly structure. Between 0° and 100°C it is a liquid and its structure varies with the temperature from the perfect order of the ice crystal to the molecular freedom of water vapour at 100°C and above. In solutions the concentrations of the solutes affect the vapour pressure, and depress the freezing point and raise the boiling point of water; both these latter effects can be used to measure the solute concentrations or osmolality of a solution, but the measurement of depression of the freezing point is the more convenient. An osmole, or 1000 milliosmoles, dissolved in 1000 g of water will lower the freezing point by 1·86°C.

The osmolality of the extracellular fluid is remarkably constant in spite of the many variations in its content of osmotically active substances, consequent on exercise, metabolic activity and the eating of food, and only body temperature is as finely regulated.

The normal range of osmolality of blood serum is 280 to 300 mosmol per kg of serum water, or about twice the serum concentration of sodium in mEq per litre. In normal adults the osmolality of the urine varies from 250 to 1300 mosmol per kg of urine water. The specific gravity of the urine is the weight of a volume of urine divided by the weight of an equivalent volume of distilled water. Thus osmolality expresses the number of osmotically active particles and specific gravity merely measures their weight, and number is of much more importance than size. While in many circumstances there is a close relationship between the osmolality and specific gravity of urine this is not true when the urine contains a lot of substances of high molecular weight but low osmotic activity, such as protein. These substances increase the specific gravity of the urine much more than its osmotic activity, which is related to the numbers of particles but not their size. Osmolality for this reason is often a better index than specific gravity of renal functional capacity and activity.

The osmolality of urine is usually about twice that of serum during the day and about three times as much in the urine first passed in the morning. Inability to vary the urine osmolality in this way is a good indication of poor renal capacity to concentrate or dilute the urine. In diabetes insipidus the osmolality of the urine may be as low as 50 mosmol per kg urine water and will remain lower than that of the plasma even when the water intake is curtailed or stopped, whereas in normal subjects it would rise to 1000 mosmol per kg urine water or more.

APPENDIX III

Method of Charting Metabolic Data

The method of charting metabolic balance data is shown in Figure 17. (*a*) Intake is plotted up from the baseline and (*b*) output is then plotted down from the top of the intake line. When output is less than intake the balance is said to be positive (*c*) and there is a clear space above the baseline. When output exceeds intake it will lie below the baseline and the balance is then negative (*d*).

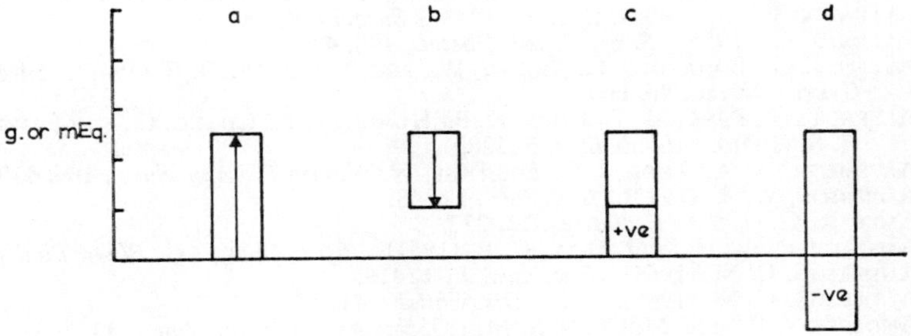

FIGURE 17.

In the charts faecal loss is shown in solid black, urine is shown by a clear area and material recovered from nappy washings and the soaking out of bedding is shown by dotted areas. Material removed in fluid aspirated from the stomach is shown by vertical lines. When the volume of fluid intake and urine are plotted, intake is again plotted up from the baseline and urine volume down from the top of the intake line.

References

Abbott, W. E., and Albertsen, K. (1963). *Nutr. et Dieta, Basel*, **5**, 339.

Abbott, W. E., Kreiger, H., Holden, W. D., Bradshaw, J., and Levey, S. (1957). *Metabolism*, **6**, 691.

Adolph, E. F. (1947). *The Physiology of Man in the Desert.* New York: Interscience Publishers Inc.

d'Agostino, A., Leadbetter, W. F., and Schwartz, W. B. (1953). *J. clin. Invest.*, **32**, 444.

Albright, F. (1943). *Harvey Lect.*, **38**, 123.

Alcock, N. W., MacIntyre, I., and Radde, I. (1960). *J. clin. Path.*, **13**, 506.

Alcock, N. W., MacIntyre, I., and Radde, I. (1965). *Nature*, **206**, 89.

Allen, A. W., and Welch, C. E. (1941). *Surgery*, **9**, 163.

Allen, J. G. (1955). *Surg. Gynec. Obstet.*, **100**, 495.

Allen, J. G., Bogardus, G., Egner, W., and Phemister, D. B. (1948). *Surg. Gynec. Obstet.*, **86**, 604.

Allen, T. H., Peng, M. T., Chen, K. P., Huang, T. F., Chang, C., and Fang, H. S. (1956). *Metabolism*, **5**, 328.

Altemeier, W. A., Todd, J. C., and Inge, W. W. (1967). *Ann. Surg.*, **166**, 530.

Amberson, W. R. (1937). *Biol. Rev.*, **12**, 48.

Ames, R. G. (1953). *Pediatrics*, **12**, 272.

Amspacher, W. H., and Artz, C. P. (1951). *Proc. Amer. Ass. Blood Banks.*

Anderson, C. M. (1965). *Brit. med. J.*, **1**, 419.

Anderson, C. M. (1966). *Arch. Dis. Childh.*, **41**, 571.

Andersson, B., and McCann, S. M. (1955). *Acta physiol. scand.*, **33**, 333.

Andersson, G., Brohult, J., and Sterner, G. (1969). *Acta pediatr. scand.*, **58**, 301.

Arden, F. (1934). *Aust. J. exp. Biol. med. Sci.*, **12**, 111, 121.

Arturson, G., Granath, K., Thoren, L., and Wallenius, G. (1964). *Acta chir. scand.*, **127**, 543.

Astrup, P., Jorgensen, K., Sigaard Andersen, O., and Engel, K. (1960). *Lancet*, **1**, 1035.

Atwater, W. O., and Benedict, F. G. (1902). *Mem. nat. Acad. Sci.*, **8**, 231.

Babior, B. M. (1966). *Amer. J. Med.*, **41**, 615.

Badoe, E. A. (1968). *Ghana med. J.*, **7**, 59.

Baker, D. R., Schrader, W. H., and Hitchcock, C. R. (1964). *J. Amer. med. Ass.*, **190**, 586.

Baldwin, D., Robinson, P. K., Zierler, K. L., and Lilienthal, J. L. (1952). *J. clin. Invest.*, **31**, 850.

Baldwin, E. (1949). *An Introduction to Comparative Biochemistry.* 3rd edn. Cambridge University Press.

Barcroft, H., Edholm, O.G., McMichael, J., and Sharpey-Schafer, E. P. (1944). *Lancet*, **1**, 489.

Barker, E. S., Elkinton, J. R., and Clark, J. R. (1959). *J. clin. Invest.*, **36**, 1733.

Bartter, F. C. (1956). *Metabolism*, **5**, 369.

Bayliss, L. E. C., Kerridge, P. M. T., and Russell, D. S. (1933). *J. Physiol.*, **77**, 386.

BAYLISS, W. M. (1916). *Proc. roy. Soc.*, **B, 89**, 380.
BAYLISS, W. M. (1919). Special Report Series, Medical Research Council, No. 26.
BEHNKE, A. R. (1942). *Harvey Lect.*, **37**, 198.
BENEDICT, F. G. (1915). *A Study of Prolonged Fasting.* Washington: Carnegie Institute of Washington.
BENEDICT, F. G., and ROOT, H. F. (1926). *Arch. intern. Med.*, **38**, 1.
BENEDICT, F. G., and TALBOT, F. B. (1915). *The Physiology of the Newborn Infant. Character and Amount of the Katabolism.* Carnegie Inst. Pub. No. 233. Washington.
BENEDICT, F. G., and TALBOT, F. B. (1921). *Metabolism and Growth from Birth to Puberty.* Carnegie Inst. Pub. No. 302. Washington.
BERGSTROM, B., DAHLQUIST, A., LUNDH, G., and SJOVALL, J. (1957). *J. clin. Invest.*, **26**, 1521.
BERGSTROM, J., FURST, P., JOSEPHSON, B., and NORÉE, L-O (1970). *Life Sci.*, **9**, 787.
BERGSTROM, W. H., and WALLACE, W. M. (1954). *J. clin. Invest.*, **33**, 867.
BERLINER, R. W., (1952). *Fed. Proc.*, **11**, 695.
BERLINER, R. W., KENNEDY, T. J., and HILTON, J. G. (1950). *Amer. J. Physiol.*, **162**, 348.
BERLYNE, G. M., JANABI, K., SHAW, A. B. and HOCKEN, A. G. (1966). *Lancet*, **1**, 169.
BERNARD, C. (1856). *Physiologie expérimentale, Paris*, **II**, 50.
BERNARD, C. (1877). *Leçons sur le Diabété et la Glycogenese animal*, p.210, Paris: Baillière.
BEST, C. H., and TAYLOR, N. B. (1955). *The Physiological Basis of Medical Practice*, 6th edn. London: Baillière, Tindall & Cox.
BISHOP, H. C., and KOOP, C. E. (1957). *Ann. Surg.*, **145**, 410.
BLACK, D. A. K. (1953). *Lancet*, **1**, 305.
BLALOCK, A. (1931). *Arch. Surg.*, **22**, 314, 598. 610.
BLIXENKRONE-MØLLER, N. (1949). *Acta chir. scand.*, **97**, 300.
BLOCKER, T. G., LEVIN, W. C., NORVINSKI, W. W., LEWIS, S. R. and BLOCKER. V. (1955). *Ann. Surg.*, **141**, 589.
BLOCKER, T. G., LEVIN, W. C., PERRY, S. R., LEWIS, S. R. and BLOCKER, V. (1957). *A.M.A. Arch Surg.*, **74**, 792.
BOLING, E. A. (1963). *Ann. N.Y. Acad. Sci.*, **110**, 246.
BOLLMAN, J. L. (1951). *Arch. Surg.*, **63**, 749.
BOOTH, C. C., BABOURIS, N., HANNA, S., and MACINTYRE, I. (1963). *Brit. med. J.*, **2**, 141.
BØRRESEN, H. C., CORAN, A. G., and KNUTRUD, O. (1970). *Ann. Surg.*, **172**, 291.
BORST, J. G. G. (1948). *Lancet*, **1**, 824.
BOYD, E. (1935). *Growth of Surface Area of Human Body.* Minneapolis: University of Minnesota Press.
BOYLE, R. (1663). *Some Considerations touching the Usefulness of Experimental Natural Philosophy*, etc. Oxford.
BRØNSTED, F. N. (1923). *Rec. Trav. chim. Pays-Bas*, **42**, 718.
BROWN, H. R., CLARK, W. F., JONES, N., WALTHER, J., and WARREN, S. L. (1943). *J. clin. Invest.*, **22**, 471.
BROŽEK, J., and KEYS, A. (1952). *Science*, **116**, 140.
BRÜCK, K. (1961). *Biologia Neonat.*, **3**, 65.
BRYANT, M. F., HOWARD, J. M., and DRAWHORN, C. W. (1957). *Surgery, Gynec. & Obstet.*, **105**, 417.
BULL, G. M., JOEKES, A. M., and LOWE, K. G. (1949). *Lancet*, **2**, 229.
BULL, G. M., JOEKES, A. M., and LOWE, K. G. (1950). *Clin. Sci.*, **9**, 379.
BULL, J. P., RICKETTS, C., SQUIRE, J. R., MAYCOCK, W. d'A., SPOONER, S. J. L., MOLLISON, P. L., and PATERSON, J. C. S. (1949). *Lancet*, **1**, 134.
BUTLER, A. M. (1950). *New Engl. J. Med.*, **243**, 648.
BUTLER, A. M., and TALBOT, N. B. (1944). *New Engl. J. Med.*, **231**, 585.
BUTLER, A. M., TALBOT, N. B., CRAWFORD, J. D., MACLACHLAN, E. A., and APPLETON, J. (1946). *Amer. J. Dis. Child.*, **72**, 481.

Bywaters, E. G. L. (1944). *J. Amer. med. Ass.*, **124**, 1103.
Bywaters, E. G. L., and Joekes, A. M. (1948). *Proc. R. Soc. Med.*, **41**, 420.
Cairnie, A. B., Campbell, R. M., Pullar, J. D., and Cuthbertson, D. P. (1957). *Brit. J. exp. Path.*, **38**, 504.
Calcagno, P. L., Rubin, M. I., and Singh, W. S. (1955). *Pediatrics*, **16**, 619.
Caldwell, F. T. (1962). *Ann. Surg.*, **155**, 119.
Calloway, D. H., and Margen, S. (1971). *J. Nutr.*, **101**, 204.
Camerer, W., Soldner, and Herzog (1902). *Z. Biol.*, **43**, i.
Cameron, G. R., Allen, J. W., Coles, R. F. G., and Rutland, J. P. (1945). *J. Path. Bact.*, **57**, 37.
Campbell, R. M., and Cuthbertson, D. P. (1967). *Quart. J. exp. Physiol.*, **52**, 114.
Campbell, R. M., Sharp, G., Boyne, A. W., and Cuthbertson, D. P. (1954). *Brit. J. exp. Path.*, **35**, 566.
Cannon, W. B. (1918). *J. Amer. med. Ass.*, **70**, 611.
Cason, J. S. (1966). In *Research in Burns*, Ed. A. B. Wallace and A. W. Wilkinson, p. 1. Edinburgh: Livingstone.
Chambers, R. (1948). *Nature, Lond.*, **162**, 835.
Chaplain, H., Mollison, P. L., and Vetter, H. (1953). *J. clin. Invest.*, **32**, 1309.
Clarke, A. M., Chirnside, A., Hill, G. L., Pope, G., and Stewart, M. K. (1967). *Lancet* **2** 740.
Clarke, R., Topley, E,. and Flear, C. T. G. (1955). *Lancet*, **1**, 629.
Cohen, B. D. (1962). *Ann. intern. Med.*, **57**, 204.
Coleman, W., and Dubois, E. F. (1914). *Arch. intern. Med.*, **13**, 786.
Colle, E., and Paulsen, E. P. (1959). *Pediatrics*, **23**, 1063.
Coller, F. G., Maddock, W. G. (1935). *Ann. Surg.*, **102**, 947.
Conn, J. W. (1949). *Arch. intern. Med.*, **83**, 416.
Conn, J. W. (1956). *Arch. intern. Med.*, **97**, 135.
Conway, E. J. (1956). *Mem. Soc. Endocrin.*, **5**, 3.
Cooke, R. E., Segar, W. E., Cheek, D. B., Coville, F. E., and Darrow, D. C. (1952). *J. clin. Invest.*, **31**, 798.
Cooper, C. E., and Nelson, D. H. (1962). *J. clin. Invest.*, **41**, 1599.
Cope, O., and Moore, F. D. (1944). *J. clin. Invest.*, **23**, 241.
Corsa, L., Olney, J. M., Steenburg, R. W., Ball, M. R., and Moore, F. D. (1950). *J. clin. Invest.*, **29**, 1280.
Costeff, H. (1966). *Arch. Dis. Childh.*, **41**, 681.
Counsell, P. B., and Goligher, J. C. (1952). *Lancet*, **2**, 1045.
Craig, A. B., and Waterhouse, C. (1955). *J. clin. Invest.*, **34**, 928.
Crockson, R. A., Payne, J. A., Ratcliff, A. P., and Soothill, J. F. (1966). *Clin. chim. Acta*, **14**, 435.
Cuthbertson, D. P. (1930). *Biochem. J.*, **24**, 1244.
Cuthbertson, D. P. (1932). *Quart. J. Med.*, **25**, 233.
Cuthbertson, D. P. (1936). *Brit. J. Surg.*, **23**, 505.
Cuthbertson, D. P. (1945). *Brit. med. Bull.*, **3**, 96.
Cuthbertson, D. P. (1957). *Z. Tierernähr*, **12**, 259.
Cuthbertson, D. P., Smith, C. M., and Tilstone, W. J. (1968). *Brit. J. Surg.*, **55**, 513.
Darrow, D. C. (1946). *J. Pediat.*, **28**, 515.
Darrow, D. C., and Pratt, E. L. (1950). *J. Amer, med. Ass.*, **143**, 365, 432.
Darrow, D. C., Pratt, E. L., Flett, J., Gamble, A. H., and Wiese, H. F. (1949). *Pediatrics*, **3**, 129.
Davies, J. W. L. (1964). *Clin Sci.*, **26**, 429.
Davies, J. W., and Topley, E. (1956). *Clin. Sci.*, **15**, 135.
Davies, J. W. L., Liljedahl, S. O., Birke, G. (1969). *Injury*, **1**, 43.
Dawkins, M. J. R., and Hull, D. (1963). *J. Physiol .*, **169**, 101 P.
Dawkins, M. J. R., and Hull, D. (1964). *J. Physiol .*, **172**, 216.
Dawson, A. M. (1965). *Recent Advances in Gastroenterology*. London: Churchill.
Day, R. (1943). *Amer. J. Dis. Child.*, **65**, 376.
Day, S., and Buckell, M. (1971). *Proc. Nutr. Soc.*, **30**, 184.

DEAN, R. B. (1941). *Biol. Symp.*, **3**, 331.
DEANE, N., and SMITH, H. W. (1952). *J. clin. Invest.*, **31**, 197.
DEMING, Q. B., and LUETSCHER, J. A. (1950). *Proc. Soc. exp. Biol., N.Y.*, **73**, 171.
DIEFENBACH, W. C. L., FISK, S. C., and GILSON, S. B. (1951). *New Engl. J. Med.*, 244, 326.
DILL, D. B., JONES, B. F., EDWARDS, H. T., and OBERG, S. A. (1933). *J. biol. Chem.*, **100**, 755.
DILLON, J., LYNCH, L. J., and MYERS, R. (1966). *Surg. Gynec. Obstet.*, **122**, 967.
DRAWHORN, C. W., and HOWARD, J. M. (1957). *Ann. Surg.*, **146**, 239.
DRUCKER, W. R., HOLDEN, W. D., KINGSBURY, B., and WOODWARD, H. (1962). *J. Trauma*, **2**, 567.
DUBOIS, E. F. (1936). *Basal Metabolism in Health and Disease.* 3rd edn. London: Baillière, Tindall & Cox.
DUBOIS. D., and DUBOIS, E. F. (1916). *Arch. intern. Med.*, **17**, 863.
DUCKWORTH, J., and GODDEN, W. (1943). *Biochem. J.*, **37**, 595.
DUCKWORTH, J., and WARNOCK, G. M. (1942). *Nutr. Abstr. Rev.*, **12**, 167.
DUDRICK, S. J., GROFF, D. B., and WILMORE, D. W. (1969). *Surgery, Gynec. & Obstet.* **129**, 805.
DUKE, J. H., JØRGENSEN, S. B., BROELL, J. R., LONG, C. L., and KINNEY, J. M. (1970). *Surgery*, **68**, 168.
EDELMAN, I. S., HALEY, H. B., SCHLOERB, P. R., SHELDON, D. B., FRIIS-HANSEN, B. J., STOLL, G., and MOORE, F. D. (1952). *Surg. Gynec. Obstet.*, **95**, 1.
EDELMAN, I. S., JAMES, A. H., BADEN, H., and MOORE, F. D. (1954). *J. clin. Invest.*, **33**, 122.
EGGLETON, M. G. (1940). *J. Physiol.*, **98**, 228, 239.
EHRENPREIS, T., and SANDBLOM, P. (1949). *Acta pediat., Stockh.*, **38**, 109.
EIK-NES, K., SANDBERG, A. A., MIGEON, C. J., TYLER, F. H., and SAMUELS, L. T. (1955). *J. clin. Endocrin.*, **15**, 13.
EISEMAN, B. (1954). *Arch. Surgery*, **68**, 167.
EISENSTEIN, A. B., WENNEKER, A. S., and LONDE, A. M. (1962). *Proc. Soc. exp. Biol. Med.*, **109**, 947.
ELEBUTE, E. A., (1969). *Brit. J. Surg.*, **56**, 213.
ELKINTON, J. R., and TARAIL, R. (1950). *Amer. J. Med.*, **9**, 200.
ELKINTON, J. R., WINKLER, A. W., and DANOWSKI, T. S. (1944). *Yale J. Biol. Med.*, **17**, 383.
ELPHICK, M. C., and WILKINSON, A. W. (1968). *Lancet*, **2**, 539.
ENGEL, F. L. (1951). *Recent Progr. Hormone Res.*, **6**, 277.
ESPINER, E. Q. (1966). *J. Endocr.*, **8**, 23.
EVANS, E. I., PURNELL, O. J., ROBINETT, P. W., BATCHELOR, A., and MARTIN, M. T. (1952). *Ann. Surg.*, **135**, 804.
FELLERS, F. X., BARNETT, H. L., HARE, K., and MCNAMARA, H. (1949). *Pediatrics*, **3**, 622.
FINE, J., and SELIGMAN, A. M. (1943). *J. clin. Invest.*, **22**, 285.
FINE, J., and SELIGMAN, A. M. (1944). *J. clin. Invest.*, **23**, 720.
FISCHER, A. (1947). *Biol. Rev.*, **22**, 178.
FLEXNER, L. B., WILDE, W. S., PROCTOR, N. K., COWIE, D. B., VOSBURGH, G. J., and HELLMAN, L. M. (1947). *J. Pediat.*, **30**, 413.
FLETCHER, R. F., HENLY, A. A., SAMMONS, H. G., and SQUIRE, J. R. (1960). *Lancet*, **1**, 522.
FLINK, E. B., STUTZMAN, F. L., ANDERSON, A. R., and KONIG, T. J. (1953). *J. clin. Invest.*, **32**, 568.
FOLIN, O. (1905). *Amer. J. Physiol.*, **13**, 66.
FOMON, S. J., DE MAEYER, E. M., and OWEN, G. M. (1965). *J. Nutr.*, **85**, 235.
FOMON, S. J., and MAY, C. D. (1968). *Pediatrics*, **22**, 1134.
FORBES, G. B., and PERLEY, A. (1951). *J. clin. Invest.*, **30**, 566.
FOURMAN, P. (1952). *Lancet*, **1**, 1042.
FOX, C. L. (1944). *J. Amer. med. Ass.*, **124**, 207.
FOX, C. L., and BAER, H. (1947). *Amer. J. Physiol.*, **151**, 155.
FOX, C. L., WINFIELD, J. M., SLOBODY, L. B., SWINDLER, C. M., and LATTIMER, J. K. (1952). *J. Amer. med. Ass.*, **148**, 827.
FRANKENTHAL, L. (1916). *Virchows Arch,.* **222**, 332.

FRIEDMAN, E., GRABLE, E., and FINE, J. (1966). *Lancet*, **2**, 609.
FRIIS-HANSEN, B. J., HOLIDAY, M., STAPLETON, T., and WALLACE, W. M. (1951). *Pediatrics*, **7**, 321.
FURMAN, R. A., HELLERSTEIN, H. K., and STARTZMAN, V. V. (1951). *J. Pediat.*, **38**, 45.
FÜRST, P., JOSEPHSON, B., MASCHIO, G., and VINNARS, E. (1969). *J. appl. Physiol.*, **26**, 13.
GAMBLE, J. L. (1947). *Harvey Lect.*, **42**, 247.
GAMBLE, J. L. (1954). *Chemical Anatomy, Physiology and Pathology of Extracellular Fluid.* 6th edn. London: Geoffrey Cumberlege.
GAMBLE, J. L., and ROSS, S. G. (1925). *J. clin. Invest.*, **1**, 403.
GANONG, W. T. (1963). *Advances in Endocrinology.* Urbana, Illinois: University of Illinois Press.
GARDNER, W. J., and STORER, J. (1966). *Surgery, Gynec. & Obstet.*, **123**, 792.
GARROW, J. S. (1965). *W. Indian med. J.*, **14**, 73.
GELIN, L. E. (1956). *Acta chir. scand.*, Suppl. 210.
GERBER, A., ROGERS, F. A., and SMITH, L. L. (1958). *Surg. Gynec. Obstet.*, **107**, 247.
GIBSON, J. G., and EVANS, W. A. (1937). *J. clin. Invest.*, **16**, 301.
GILMAN, A. (1937). *Amer. J. Physiol.*, **120**, 323.
GILMAN, A., and BRAZEAU, P. (1953). *Amer. J. Med.*, **15**, 765.
GIORDANO, C. (1963). *J. Lab. clin. Med.*, **62**, 231.
GOVAN, C. D., and DARROW, D. C. (1946). *J. Pediat.*, **28**, 541.
GRANT, R. T., and REEVE, E. B. (1941). *Brit. med. J.*, **2**, 293, 329.
GRINDON, A. J., HOLLAND, P. V., and SCHMIDT, P. J. (1967). *Amer. Heart J.*, **74**, 591.
GRÖNWALL, A., and INGELMAN, B. (1944). *Acta physiol. scand.*, **7**, 97.
GRÖNWALL, A., and INGELMAN, B. (1945). *Acta physiol. scand.*, **9**, 1.
GROSS, R. E. (1953). *The Surgery of Infancy and Childhood.* Philadelphia: W. B. Saunders.
GROTTE, G., KNUTSON, R. C., and BOLLMAN, J. L. (1951). *J. Lab. clin. Med.*, **38**, 577.
HADEN, R. L., and ORR, T. G. (1923). *J. exp. Med.*, **37**, 365.
HALLBERG, D. (1965). *Acta physiol. scand.*, **65**, Suppl. 254.
HALLBERG, D., HOLM, I., OBEL, A. L., SCHUBERTH, O., and WRETLIND, A. (1967). *Postgrad. med. J.*, **43**, 307.
HAMMARSTEN, J. F., HELLER, B. I., and EBERT, R. V. (1953). *J. clin. Invest.* **32**, 340.
HAMMER, J. M., SEAY, P. H., HILL, E. J., PRUST, F. H., and CAMPBELL, R. J. (1955). *Arch. Surg.*, **71**, 625.
HAMMER, J. M., SEAY, P. H., JOHNSON, R. L., HILL, E. J., PRUST, F. H., and CAMPBELL, R. J. (1959). *Arch. Surg.*, **79**, 537.
HANNA, S., HARRISON, M., MACINTYRE, I., and FRASER, R. (1960). *Lancet*, **2**, 172.
HANSEN, J. D. L., and SMITH, C. A. (1952). *Amer. J. Dis. Child.*, **84**, 477.
HANSEN, J. D. L., and SMITH, C. A. (1953). *Pediatrics*, **12**, 99.
HARDY, J. D., and DRABKIN, D. L. (1950). *Amer. J. med. Sci.*, **219**, 109.
HARDY, J. D., NEELY, W. A., WILSON, F. C., LOVELACE, J. R., and JABOUR, E. (1955). *Surg. Gynec. Obstet.*, **101**, 94.
HARRIS, I. M., and WILKINSON, A. W. (1971). *Lancet*, **2**, 735.
HARRISON, H. E., DARROW, D. C., and YANNET, H. (1936). *J. Biol. Chem.*, **113**, 515.
HARTMAN, F. W. (1951). *Arch. Surg.*, **63**, 728.
HARTMANN, A. F., and SMYTH, F. S. (1926). *Amer. J. Dis. Child.*, **32**, 1.
HASTINGS, A. B. (1941). *Harvey Lect.*, **36**, 91.
HATAI, S. (1902). *Anat. Anz.*, **21**, 369.
HAYNES, B. W. (1965). *J. Trauma*, **5**, 267.
HECHT, G., and WEESE, H. (1943). *Munch. med. Wschr.*, **90**, 11.
HENRIQUES, V., and ANDERSON, A. C. (1913). *Hoppe-Seyl. Z.*, **88**, 357.
HEY, E. N., and MOUNT, L. E. (1967). *Arch Dis. Childh.*, **42**, 75.
HEY, E. N., and O'CONNELL, B. (1970). *Arch. Dis. Childh.*, **45**, 335.

HILL, J. R. (1959). *J. Physiol.*, **149**, 346.
HILL, J. R., and RAHIMSULLA, K. A. (1965). *J. Physiol.*, **180**, 239.
HILLS, A. G., CHALMERS, T. M., WEBSTER, G. D., and ROSENTHAL, O. (1953). *J. clin. Invest.*, **32**, 1236.
HOLLIDAY, M. A., and SEGAR, W. E. (1957). *Pediatrics*, **19**, 823.
HOWARD, J. E., BIGHAM, R. S., EISENBERG, H., WAGNER, D., and BAILEY, E. (1946). *Johns Hopk. Hosp. Bull.*, **78**, 282.
HOWARD, J. M. (1955). *Surg. Gynec. Obstet.*, **100**, 69.
HOWARD, J. M., and SCOTT, R., (1954). *Surgery, Gynec. & Obstet.*, **99**, 703.
HOWARD, J. M., TENG, C. T., and LOEFFLER, R. K. (1956). *Ann. Surg.*, **143**, 369.
HUGHES, E. A., STEVENS, L. H., and WILKINSON, A. W. (1964). *Arch. Dis., Childh.*, **39**, 598.
HUGHES, E. A., STEVENS, L. H., TOMS, D. A., and WILKINSON, A. W. (1965)., *Brit. J. Surg.*, **52**, 403.
HUME, D. M., and EGDAHL, R. H. (1959). *Ann. Surg.*, **150**, 607.
IKKOS, D., LUFT, R., and SJÖGREN, B. (1954). *Metabolism*, **3**, 400.
INGLE, D. J. (1951). *Ann. intern. Med.*, **35**, 652.
INGLE, D. J. (1952). *J. Endocrin.*, **8**, xxiii.
INGLE, D. J., WARD E., and KUIZENGA, M. H. (1947). *Amer. J. Physiol.*, **149**, 510.
JACKSON, D. M., and CASON, J. S. (1965). *Arch. Dis. Childh.*, **39**, 598.
JACOBS, A., and STIRLING, W. B. (1952). *Brit. J. Urol.*, **24**, 259.
JOHNSON, J. B. (1941). *J. clin. Invest.*, **20**, 101.
JOHNSTON, I. D.A. (1964). *Ann. R. Coll. Surg. Engl.*, **35**, 270.
JURGENS, P., and DOLIF, D. (1968). *Klin. Wschr.*, **45**, 131.
KANAGHINIS, T., LUBRAN, M., and COGHILL, N. F. (1963). *Gut*, **4**, 322.
KENNEDY, A. C., LINTON, A. L., and EATON, J. C. (1962). *Lancet*, **1**, 410.
KERPEL-FRONIUS, Ö. (1935). *Z. Kinderheilk.*, **57**, 489.
KERPEL-FRONIUS, Ö. (1938). *Acta paediat., Stockh.*, **22**, 143.
KEYS, A., BROZEK, J., HENSCHEL, A., MICKELSEN, O., and TAYLOR, H. L. (1950). *The Biology of Human Starvation*, Vol. 1, p. 176. Minneapolis: University of Minnesota Press.
KINNEY, J. M., DUKE, J. H., LONG, C. L., and GUMP, F. E. (1970). *J. clin. Path.*, **23**, Suppl. 4 (Roy. Coll. Path.)
KINNEY, J. M. (1960). *Bull. N.Y. Acad. Med.*, **36**, 617.
KOJ, A. (1970). In *Energy Metabolism after Injury*, p. 79. Ciba Foundation Symposium. London: Churchill.
KUMAR, R., HILL, C. M., MCGEOWN, M. G. (1973). *Lancet*, **1**, 90.
LADELL, W. S. S. (1945). *Brit. med. Bull.*, **3**, 175.
LADELL, W. S. S. (1947). *Brit. med. Bull.*, **5**, 9.
LADELL, W. S. S. (1955). *J. Physiol.*, **127**, 11.
LADELL, W. S. S. (1957). *Trans. R. Soc. trop. Med. Hyg.*, **51**, 189.
LASCH, W. (1923). *Z. Kinderheilk.*, **36**, 42.
LAWSON, L. J., BLAINEY, J. D., DAWSON EDWARDS, P., and TONGUE, S. M. (1962). *Brit. med. J.*, **2**, 293.
LEONSINS, A. J. (1951). *S. Afr. med. J.*, **25**, 127.
LEQUESNE, L. P., and LEWIS, A. A. G. (1953). *Lancet*, **1**, 153.
LESCHKE, E. (1918). *Arch. Psychiat. Nervenkr.*, **59**, 773.
LEVEY, S., ABBOTT, W. E., KREIGER, H., and DAVIS, J. H. (1956). *J. Lab. clin. Med.*, **47**, 437.
LEVINE, S. Z., and MARPLES, E. (1930). *Amer. J. Dis. Child.*, **40**, 269.
LEVISON, L. M. (1972). *Archs. intern. Med.*, **130**, 225.
LEWIS, T. (1927). *The Blood Vessels of the Human Skin and their Responses.* London: Shaw & Son.
LIPSITZ, P. J., and ENGLISH, I. C. (1967), *Pediatrics*, **40**, 856.
LOWE, K. G. (1953). *Clin. Sci.*, **12**, 57.
LOWERY, B. D., CLOUTIER, C. G., and CAREY, L. C. (1971). *Surgery, Gynec. & Obstet.*, **133**, 273.
LOWRY, T. M. (1923). *Chem. Ind., Lond.*, **42**, 43.
LUCKÉ, B. (1946). *Milit. Surg.*, **99**, 371.

Luke, R. C., Dinwoodie, A. J., Linton, A. L. and Kennedy, A. C. (1964). *J. Lab. clin. Med.*, **64**, 731.
Lynch, J. B., Bray, J. P., Lewis, S. R., and Blocker, T. G. (1964). *J. surg. Res.*, **4**, 226.
Macbeth, R. A. L., and Mabbott, J. D. (1964). *Surg. Gynec. Obstet.*, **118**, 748.
McCallister, R., Prasad, A. S., Doe, R. P., and Flink, E. B. (1958). *J. Lab. clin. Med.*, **52**, 928.
McCance, R. A. (1936). *Proc. roy. Soc.*, **B**, **119**, 245.
McCance, R. A. (1950). *Amer. J. Med.*, **9**, 229.
McCance, R. A., Naylor, N. J. B., and Widdowson, E. M. (1954). *Arch. Dis. Child.*, **29**, 104.
McCance, R. A., and Widdowson, E. M. (1939). *Biochem. J.*, **33**, 523.
McCance, R. A., and Widdowson, E. M. (1951). *Proc. roy. Soc.*, **B**, **138**, 115.
McCance, R. A., and Wilkinson, A. W. (1967). *Brit. J. Nutr.*, **21**, 731.
McCance, R. A., and Young, W. F. (1941). *J. Physiol.*, **99**, 265.
Macintyre, I. (1963). In *Scientific Basis of Medicine*. London: The Athlone Press.
Maclaurin, J. C. (1966). *Arch. Dis. Childh.*, **41**, 286.
MacLean, L. D., Mulligan, W. G., MacLean, A. P. H., and Duff, J. H. (1962). *Ann. Surg.*, **166**, 543.
McMichael, J., Sharpey-Schafer, E. P., Mollison, P. L., and Vaughan, J. M. (1943). *Lancet*, **1**, 637.
McMurrey, J. D., Davis, J. M., Boling, E. A, and Moore, F. D. (1955), *Surg. Forum*, **6**, 14.
Mahler, R. F., and Stanbury, S. W. (1956). *Quart. J. Med.*, **49**, 21.
Maizels, M. (1949). *J. Physiol.*, **108**, 247.
Markley, K., Bocanegra, M., Bazan, A., Temple, R., Chiappori, M., and Morales, G. (1956). *J. Amer. med. Ass.*, **161**, 1465.
Markley, K., Bocanegra, M., Ego-Aguirre, E., Chappori, M., and Morales, G. (1950). *Surgery*, **47**, 489.
Marriott, H. L. (1947). *Brit. med. J.*, **1**, 245, 285, 328.
Marshall, M. E., and Deutsch, H. F. (1950). *Amer. J. Physiol.*, **163**, 461.
Marston, N. A. (1954). *Lancet*, **2**, 688.
Martensen-Larsen, O. (1954). *Brit. med. J.*, **2**, 464.
Martin, H. E., Mehl, J., and Wertman, M. (1952). *Med. Clin. N. Amer.*, **36**, 1157.
Martin, H. E., Reynolds, T. B., Snyder, E. N., Berne, C. J., Homann, R. E., Edmondson, H. A., Blatherwick, N., Felds, I., Wertman, M., and Westover, L (1951). *J. Amer. med. Ass.*, **147**, 24.
Mellanby, E. (1919). *Med. Res.Coun., Spec. Rep. Ser.*, No. 31.
Mellemgaard, K., and Astrup, P. (1960). *Scand. J. clin. Lab. Invest.*, **12**, 187.
Melrose, D. G., and Shackman, R. (1951). *Lancet*, **1**, 1144.
Metcalf, W., Rousselot, L. M., and Gilbertson, F. E. (1954). *Surg. Forum*, **5**, 520.
Meyer, H W. (1962). *Surgery*, **51**, 755.
Miksche, L. W., and Caldwell, F. T. (1967). *Surgery*, **62**, 66.
Miller, J. F. (1944). *Amer. J. Dis. Child.*, **67**, 117.
Milne, M. D., Muehrcke R. C., and Aird, I. (1957). *Quart. J. Med.*, **26**, 317.
Mitchell, A. D., and Valk, W. L. (1953). *J. Urol.*, **69**, 82.
Moore, D. C., and Karp, M. (1945). *Surg. Gynec. Obstet.*, **80**, 523.
Moore, F. D. (1954). *Ann. Surg.*, **139**, 253.
Moore, F. D., and Ball, M. R. (1952). *The Metabolic Response to Surgery*. Springfield, Ill.: C. C. Thomas.
Moore, F. D., Edelman, I.S., Olney, J. M., James, A. H., Brooks, L., and Wilson, G. M. (1954). *Metabolism*, **3**, 334.
Moore, R. E., and Underwood, M. C. (1960). *Lancet*, **1**, 1277.
Moyer, C. A., Coller, F. A., Iob, V., Vaughan, H. H., and Marty, D. (1944). *Ann. Surg.*, **120**, 367.

MOYER, C. A., LEVIN, M., and KLINGE, F. W. (1947). *Sth. med. J., Nashville*, **40**, 479.
MUELLER, S. (1939). *Surg. Clin. N. Amer.*, **19**, 401.
MUNRO, H. N. (1972). In *Parenteral Nutrition*, p. 34. Ed. Wilkinson, A. W. Edinburgh: Churchill Livingstone.
NADAL, J. W., PEDERSON, S., and MADDOCK, W. G. (1941). *J. clin. Invest.*, **20**, 691.
NADE, S. M. L., and DICKSON, J. A. S. (1970). *Brit. J. Surg.*, **57**, 540.
NADLER, C. S., BELLET, S., and LANNING, M. (1948). *Amer. J. Med.*, **5**, 838.
NEEDHAM, A. E. (1955). *J. Embryol. exp. Morphol.*, **3**, 189.
NEEDHAM, A. E. (1958). *J. exp. Zool.*, **138**, 369.
NEWBURGH, L. H., JOHNSTON, M. W., LASHMET, F. H., and SHEILDON, J. M., (1937). *J. Nutr.*, **13**, 203.
NIXON, H. H. (1956). *Great Ormond St. J.*, No. 11, p. 1.
NORTHFIELD, T. C., SMITH, T. (1970). *Lancet*, **2**, 584.
OLIVER, J., MACDOWELL, M., and TRACY, A. (1951). *J. clin. Invest.*, **30**, 1307.
OLIVER, T. K., and KARLBERG, P. (1963). *Amer. J. Dis. Childh.*, **105**, 427.
OLIVER, W. J., GRAHAM, B. D., and WILSON, J. L. (1958). *J. Amer. med. Ass.*, **167**, 1211.
PACE, N., and RATHBUN, E. N. (1945). *J. biol. Chem.*, **158**, 685.
PAPPENHEIMER, J. R. (1952). *Ann. N.Y. Acad. Sci.*, **55**, 465.
PARSONS, F. M., PYRAH, L. N., POWELL, F. J. N., REED, G. W., and SPIERS, F. W. (1952). *Brit. J. Urol.*, **24**, 317.
PAWAN, G. L. S. (1972). *Proc. Nutr. Soc.*, **31**, 82.
PETERS, J. P. (1948). *Surgery*, **24**, 568.
PETERS, J. P., and VAN SLYKE, D. D. (1931). *Quantitative Clinical Chemistry*. Vol. 1, p. 358. London: Baillière, Tindall & Cox.
PHLLIPS, R. A., VAN SLYKE, D. D., HAMILTON, P. B., DOLE, V. P., EMERSON, K., ARCHIBALD, R. M., and STANLEY, E. G. (1950). *J. Biol. Chem.*, **183**, 305.
PITTS, R. F. (1950). *Amer. J. Med.*, **9**, 356.
PITTS, R. F., and ALEXANDER, R. S. (1945). *Amer. J. Physiol.*, **144**, 239.
PRADERA, E. S., FERNANDEZ, E., and CALERIN, O. (1942). *Amer. J. Dis. Childh.* **64**, 977.
PRENTICE, T. C., SIRI, W., and JORNIER, E. E. (1952). *Amer. J. Med.*, **13**, 668.,
PRENTICE, T. C., SIRI, W., BERLIN, N. I., HYDE, G. M., PARSONS, R. J., JOINER, E. E., and LAWRENCE, J. H. (1952). *J. clin. Invest.*, **31**, 412.
PRUNTY, F. T. G., MCSWINEY, R. R., and MILLS, I. H. (1955). *Proc. R. Soc. Med.*, **48**, 629.
PULLAN, J. M. (1959). *Proc. R. Soc. Med.*, **52**, 31.
RAJASURIYA, K., HAMZOO, M. H. M. (1954). *Ceylon med. J.*, **2**, 251.
RATHBUN, E. N., and PACE, N. (1945). *J. biol. Chem.*, **158**, 667.
REIQUAM, C. W., ALLEN, R. P., and AKERS, D. R. (1965). *Amer. J. Dis. Childh.*, **109**, 447.
RELMAN, A. S. (1966). *Ann. N.Y. Acad. Sci.*, **133**, 160.
RHOADS, J. E., WOLFF, W. A., and LEE, W. E. (1941). *Ann. Surg.*, **113**, 955.
RICCA, R. A., FINK, K., STEADMAN, L. T., and WARREN, S. L. (1945). *J. clin. Invest.*, **24**, 140.
RICE, C. O., STRICKLER, J. H., and ERWIN, P. D. (1952). *Arch. Surg.*, **64**, 20.
ROBERTS, K. E., RANDALL, H. T., PHILBIN, P., and LIPTON, R. (1954). *Surgery*, **36**, 599.
ROBERTS, S. (1953). *J. biol. Chem.*, **200**, 77.
ROBERTSON, J. D. (1964). In *Cellular Membranes in Development*. Ed. M. Locke. New York: Academic Press.
ROBINSON, J. R. (1950). *Proc. roy. Soc.*, **B, 137**, 378.
ROBINSON, J. R. (1953). *Biol. Rev.*, **28**, 158.
ROBINSON, R. A. (1951). Conference on Metabolic Interrelation. *Transactions of the Third Conference, New York, N.Y.*, p. 271. New York: Josiah Macy, Jr., Foundation.
ROBSON, J. S., DUDLEY, H. A., HORN, D. B., and STEWART, C. P. (1956). *Clin. chim. Acta*, **1**, 533.

ROE, C. F., and KINNEY, J. M. (1965). *Ann. Surg.*, **161**, 140.
ROSE, W. C. (1949). *Fed. Proc.*, **8**, 546.
ROSENQUIST, H., and THORSÉN, H. G. R. (1951). *Arch. Surg.*, **62**, 524.
ROSENTHAL, S. M., and TABOR, H. (1945). *Arch. Surg.*, **51**, 244.
ROSS, B., WATSON, B. W., and KAY, A. W. (1963). *Gut*, **4**, 77.
RUBNER, M. (1931). *S.B. preuss. Akad. Wiss., phys.-math. Kl.*, Nos. 16-18, p. 272.
SANDBERG, A. A., EIK-NES, K., SAMUELS, L. T., and TYLER, F. H. (1954). *J. clin. Invest.*, **33**, 1509.
SCATCHARD, G. (1952). *Ann. N.Y. Acad. Sci.*, **55**, 455.
SCHACHTER, D., FREINKEL, N., and SCHWARTZ, I. L. (1950). *Amer. J. Physiol.*, **160**, 512.
SCHACHTER, D., and ROSEN, S. M. (1959). *Amer. J. Physiol.*, **196**, 357.
SCHLOERB, P. R., FRIIS-HANSEN, B. J. EDELMAN, I. S., SOLOMON, A. K., and MOORE, F. D. (1950). *J. Clin. Invest.*, **29**, 1296.
SCHOENHEIMER, R. (1942). *The Dynamic State of Body Constituents.* Cambridge, Mass.: Harvard University Press.
SCHOLER, J. F., and CODE, C. F. (1954). *Gastroenterology*, **27**, 565.
SCHRADER, G. A., PRICKETT, C. O., and SALMON, W. D. (1937). *J. Nutr.*, **14**, 85.
SCHROEDER, H. A. (1949). *J. Amer. med. Ass.*, **141**, 117.
SCHUBERTH, O. (1964). *Acta chir. scand.*, Suppl. 325, 43.
SCHULTZE, M. O. (1956). *J. Nutr.*, **60**, 35.
SCHWARTZ, W. B., and RELMAN, A. S. (1967). *New Engl. J. med.*, **276**, 383, 452.
SCHWARTZ, I. L., and THAYSEN, J. H. (1956). *J. clin. Invest.*, **35**, 114.
SCHWARTZ, W. B. (1949). *New Engl. J. Med.*, **240**, 173.
SCHWARTZ, W. B., and RELMAN, A. S. (1953). *J. clin. Invest.*, **32**, 258.
SCOPES, J. W. (1966). *Brit. med. Bull.*, **22**, 88.
SELYE, H. (1950). *The Physiology and Pathology of Exposure to Stress; a Treatise based on the Concepts of the General-Adaptation-Syndrome and the Diseases of Adaptation.* Montreal: Acta Inc.
SHAFFER, P. A., and COLEMAN, W. (1909). *Arch. intern. Med.*, **4**, 538.
SHARPEY-SCHAFER, E. P. (1944). *Clin. Sci.*, **5**, 125.
SHEARBURN, E. W. (1942). *Proc. Soc. exp. Biol., N.Y.*, **50**, 140.
SHIBOLET, S., COLL, R., GILAT, T., and SOHAR, E. (1967). *Quart. J. Med.*, **36**, 525.
SHIELDS, R. (1965). *Brit. J. Surg.*, **52**, 774.
SHIRES, T., WILLIAMS, J., and BROWN, F. (1961). *Ann. Surg.*, **154**, 803.
SIGAARD ANDERSEN, O., and ENGEL, K. (1960). *Scand. J. clin. Lab. Invest.*, **12**, 177.
SIGAARD ANDERSEN, O., ENGEL, K., JØRGENSEN, K., and ASTRUP, P. (1960). *Scand. J. clin. Lab. Invest.*, **12**, 172.
SILVERMAN, W. A., and BLANC, W. A. (1957). *Pediatrics*, **20**, 477.
SIMPSON, S. A., TAIT, J. F., WETTSTEIN, A., NEHER, R., VON EUW, J., SCHINDLER, O., and REICHSTEIN, T. (1954). *Helv. chim. Acta*, **37**, 1163.
SINCLAIR, I. S. R. (1956). *Brit. J. Surg.*, **44**, 250.
SMALLEY, R. L., and DRYER, R. L. (1963). *Science, N.Y.*, **140**, 1333.
SMITH, C. A. (1951). *The Physiology of the Newborn Infant.* 2nd edn. Oxford: Blackwell Scientific Publications.
SOBERMAN, R., BRODIE, B. B., LEVY, B. B., AXELROD, J., HOLLANDER, V., and STEELE, J. M. (1949). *J. biol. Chem.*, **179**, 31.
STANBURY, S. W., and THOMSON, A. E. (1951). *Clin. Sci.*, **10**, 267.
STEENBURG, R. W., LENNIHAN, R., and MOORE, F. D. (1956). *Ann. Surg.*, **143**, 180.
STEMMER, E. A., HEAD, L. R., and ALLEN, J. G. (1955). *Surg. Forum*, **6**, 38.
STEPHENS, R. V., BURY, K. D., DE LUCA, F. G., and RANDALL, H. T. (1972). *Amer. J. Surg.*, **123**, 374.
STERLING, K., LIPSKY, S. R., and FREEDMAN, L. J. (1955). *Metabolism*, **4**, 343.
STEVENS, L. H., HUGHES, E. A., and WILKINSON, A. W. (1962). *Arch. Dis. Childh.*, **37**, 485.
STEWART, J. D., and ROURKE, G. M. (1942). *J. clin. Invest.*, **21**, 197.
STONE, H. H. (1971). *Surgery, Gynec. & Obstet.*, **134**, 669.

STRØMME, J. H., NESBAKKEN, R., NORMAN, T., SKJØRTEN, F., SKYBERG, D., and JOHANNSEN, B. (1969). *Acta pediat. scand.*, **58**, 433.

SWAN, R. C., and MERRILL, J. P. (1953). *Medicine, Baltimore*, **32**, 215.

TAKAORI, M., and SAFAR, P. (1967). *J. Amer. med. Ass.*, **199**, 297.

DE TAKATS, G. (1931). *Amer. J. Surg.*, **11**, 39.

TARAIL, R., and ELKINTON, J. R. (1949). *J. clin. Invest.*, **28**, 99.

TAYLOR, H. L., ERICKSON, L., HENSCHEL, A., and KEYS, A. (1945). *Amer. J. Physiol.*, **144**, 227.

TAYLOR, W. H. (1957). *Lancet*, **2**, 703.

TERNER, C., EGGLESTON, L. V., and KREB, H. A. (1950). *Biochem. J.*, 47, 139.

TESCHAN, P. E., POST, R. S., SMITH, L. H., ABERNATHY, R. S., DAVIS, J. H., GRAY, D. M., HOWARD, J. M., JOHNSON, K. E., KLOPP, E., MUNDY, R. L., O'MEARA, M. P., and RUSH, B. F. (1955). *Amer. J. Med.*, **18**, 172.

THERON, P. H., and WILSON, W. C. (1949). *Lancet*, **1**, 172.

THOMPSON, G. N. (1956). *Alcoholism.* Springfield, Illinois: C. C. Thomas.

THOMSON, J. (1944). *Arch. Dis. Childh.*, **19**, 169.

THOREN, L. (1963). *Acta chir. scand.*, Suppl. 306.

THORSEN, G., and HINT, H. (1950). *Acta chir. scand.*, Suppl. 154.

TINCKLER, L. F. (1966). *Brit. med. J.*, **1**, 1263.

TSINGOGLOU, S., and WILKINSON, A. W. (1971). *Arch. Dis. Childh.*, **46**, 452.

TSINGOGLOU, S., PHILLIPS, H., and WILKINSON, A. W. (1972). *Arch. Dis. Childh.*, **47**, 941.

UPJOHN, H. L., CREDITOR, M. C., and LEVENSON, S. M. (1957). *Metabolism*, **6**, 607.

USSING, H. H. (1952). *Advanc. Enzymol.*, **13**, 21.

VAN ITALLIE, T. B., WADDELL, W. R., GEYER, R. P., and STARE, F. J. (1952). *Arch. intern. Med.*, **89**, 353.

VAN SLYKE, K. K., and EVANS, E. I. (1947). *Ann. Surg.*, **126**, 545.

VENABLES, C. W., ELLIS, H., and SMITH, A. D. M. (1966). *Lancet*, **2**, 1390.

VERNEY, E. B. (1947). *Proc. roy. Soc.*, **B**, **135**, 25.

VERNEY, E. B. (1954). *Irish J. med. Sci.*, p. 377.

WACKER, W. E. C., IIDA, C., and FUWA, K. (1965). *Nature*, **209**, 90.

WADSTROM, L. B. (1958). *Acta chir. scand.*, **116**, 395.

WALL, A. J., and KIRSNER, J. B. (1971). *Modern Treatment*, **8**, 944.

WARREN, R., and MCKITTRICK, L. S. (1951). *Surg. Gynec. Obstet.*, **93**, 555.

WATCHORN, E., and MCCANCE, R. A. (1937). *Biochem. J.*, **31**, 1379.

WEBSTER, D. R., HENRIKSON, H. W., and CURRIE, D. J. (1950). *Trans. Amer. surg. Ass.*, **68**, 458.

WECKESSER, E. C., CHINN, A. B., SCOTT, M. W., and PRICE, J. W. (1949). *Amer. J. Surg.*, **78**, 706.

WEECH, A. A. (1938). *Harvey Lectures*, p. 57. Baltimore: The Williams and Wilkins Coy.

WEECH, A. A., WOLLSTEIN, M., and GOETTSCH, E. (1937). *J. clin. Invest.*, **16**, 719.

WEINSTEIN, J. J., and ROE, J. H. (1952). *J. Lab. clin. Med.*, **40**, 39.

WELLS, C., RAWLINSON, K., TRINCKLER, L., JONES, M., and SAUNDERS, J. (1964). *Lancet*, **1**, 4.

WELT, L. G., HOLLANDER, W., and BLYTHE, W. R. (1960). *J. chron. Dis.*, **11**, 213.

WIDDOWSON, E. M. (1960). In *Transactions of 4th Conference on Physiology of Prematurity, p.* 97. Ed. Lanman, J. T., New York: Josiah Macy Foundation.

WIDDOWSON, E. M., MCCANCE, R. A., and SPRAY, C. M. (1951). *Clin. Sci.*, **10**, 113.

WIDDOWSON, E. M., and SPRAY, C. M. (1951). *Arch Dis. Childh.*, **26**, 205.

WILKINSON, A. W. (1954). *Post Grad. med. J.*, **30**, 405.

WILKINSON, A. W. (1955). *Proc. Nutr. Soc.*, **14**, 124.

WILKINSON, A. W. (1956 a). *Lancet*. **1**, 184.

WILKINSON, A. W. (1956 b). *Lancet*, **2**, 428.

WILKINSON, A. W. (1956 c). *Lancet*, **2**, 604.

WILKINSON, A. W. (1958). *Brit. J. plast. Surg.*, **10**, 275.

WILKINSON, A. W. (1963). *Lancet*, **1**, 86.
WILKINSON, A. W. (1965). In *The Adaptation of the Newborn Infant to Extra Uterine Life*. Ed. Jonxis, J. H. P., Visser, H. K. A., and Troelstra, J. A. Leiden: H. E. Stenfert Kroese N.V.
WILKINSON, A. W. (1966). In *Wound Healing*. Ed. Sir Charles Illingworth. London: J. & A. Churchill.
WILKINSON, A. W. (1967). *Symposium on Malabsorption, Zurich*. Basel: Karger.
WILKINSON, A. W. (1972). In *Parenteral Nutrition*, p. 242. Ed. Wilkinson, A. W. Edinburgh: Churchill Livingstone.
WILKINSON, A. W., BILLING, B. H., NAGY, G., and STEWART, C. P. (1949). *Lancet*, **1**, 640.
WILKINSON, A. W., BILLING, B. H., NAGY, G., and STEWART, C. P. (1950a), *Lancet*, **1**, 533.
WILKINSON, A. W., BILLING, B. H., NAGY, G., and STEWART, C. P. (1950b). *Lancet*, **2**, 135.
WILKINSON, A. W., HUGHES, E. A., and STEVENS, L. H. (1965). *Brit. J. Surg.*, **52**, 410.
WILKINSON, A. W., HUGHES, E. A., and TOMS, D. A. (1963). *Brit. J. Surg.*, **50**, 715.
WILKINSON, A. W., and MCCANCE, R. A. (1973). *Arch. Dis. Childh.*, **48**, 121.
WILKINSON, A. W., STEVENS, L. H., and HUGHES, E. A. (1962). *Lancet*, **1**, 983.
WILKINSON, A. W., and STOREY, I. D. E. (1953). *Lancet*, **2**, 956.
WILKINSON, A. W., and STOREY, I. D. E. (1954). *Lancet*, **1**, 1269.
WILLIAMS, J. A., and FINE, J. (1961). *New Engl. J. Med.*, **264**, 842.
WILLIAMS, Y. J., BISHOP, E. A., and YOUNG, W. F. (1949). *Arch. Dis. Childh.*, **24**, 159.
WILMORE, D. W., DUDRICK, S. J., DALY, J. M., and VARS, H. M. (1971). *Surgery, Gynec. & Obstet.*, **132**, 673.
WILMORE, D. W., GROFT, D. B., BISHOP, H. C., and DUDRICK, S. J. (1969). *J. paed. Surg.*, **4**, 181.
WILSON, G. M. (1963). *Brit. med. J.*, **1**, 285.
WILSON, G. M., EDELMAN, I. S., BROOKS, L., MYRDEN, J. A., HARKEN, D. E., and MOORE, F. D. (1954). *Circulation*, **9**, 199.
WILSON, R. F., SARVER, E., and BIRKS, R. (1971). *Surgery, Gynec. & Obstet.*, **132**, 631.
WILSON, W. C., MACGREGOR, A. R., and STEWART, C. P. (1938). *Brit. J. Surg.*, **25**, 826.
WINAWER, S. J., BROITMAN, S. A., WOLOCHOW, D. A., OSBORNE, M. P., and ZAROCHEK, N. (1966). *New Engl. J. Med.*, **274**, 72.
WINITZ, M., SEEDMAN, D. A., and GRAFF, J. (1970). *Amer. J. clin. Nutr.*, **23**, 525.
WOLF, A. V. (1950). *Amer. J. Physiol.*, **161**, 75.
YLPPO, A. (1919). *Z. Kinderheilk.*, **20**, 212.
YOUNG, V. R., and SCRIMSHAW, N. S. (1968). *Brit. J. Nutr.*, **22**, 9.
ZIMMERMANN, B., and WANGENSTEEN, O. H. (1952). *Surgery*, **31**, 654.
ZUIDEMA, G. D., GAISFORD, W. D., KOWALCZK, R. S., WOLFMAN, E. F., and KIRSH, M. M. (1964). *Surg. Gynec. Obstet.*, **119**, 790.
ZWEYMULLER, E. (1970). *Arch. Dis. Childh.*, **45**, 815.

Index

Printed by A. Brown & Sons Ltd.